TRANSCRANIAL MAGNETIC STIMULATION IN CLINICAL PSYCHIATRY

TRANSCRANIAL MAGNETIC STIMULATION IN CLINICAL PSYCHIATRY

Edited by

Mark S. George, M.D.

Robert H. Belmaker, M.D.

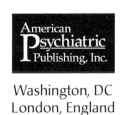

Washington, DC
London, England

Note: The authors have worked to ensure that all information in this book is accurate at the time of publication and consistent with general psychiatric and medical standards, and that information concerning drug dosages, schedules, and routes of administration is accurate at the time of publication and consistent with standards set by the U.S. Food and Drug Administration and the general medical community. As medical research and practice continue to advance, however, therapeutic standards may change. Moreover, specific situations may require a specific therapeutic response not included in this book. For these reasons and because human and mechanical errors sometimes occur, we recommend that readers follow the advice of physicians directly involved in their care or the care of a member of their family.

Books published by American Psychiatric Publishing, Inc., represent the views and opinions of the individual authors and do not necessarily represent the policies and opinions of APPI or the American Psychiatric Association.

To buy 25 –99 copies of this or any other APPI title at a 20% discount, please contact APPI Customer Service at appi@psych.org or 800-368-5777. For 100 or more copies of the same title, please e-mail bulksales@psych.org for a price quote.

Copyright © 2007 American Psychiatric Publishing, Inc.
ALL RIGHTS RESERVED

Manufactured in the United States of America on acid-free paper
10   09   08   07   06   5   4   3   2   1
First Edition

Typeset in Adobe's AGaramond and CastleT.

American Psychiatric Publishing, Inc.
1000 Wilson Boulevard
Arlington, VA 22209-3901
www.appi.org

Library of Congress Cataloging-in-Publication Data
Transcranial magnetic stimulation in clinical psychiatry / edited by
    Mark S. George, Robert H. Belmaker. — 1st ed.
        p. ; cm.
    Includes bibliographical references and index.
    ISBN 1-58562-197-8 (pbk. : alk. paper)
    1. Magnetic brain stimulation. 2. Psychiatry. I. George, M. S. (Mark S.),
1958– . II. Belmaker, Robert H.
    [DNLM: 1. Nervous System Diseases—therapy. 2. Transcranial Magnetic
Stimulation. 3. Brain—physiology. 4. Mental Disorders—therapy.
    WL 140 T772 2007]
    RC386.6.M32T732 2007
    616.89--dc22
                                                                2006023466

British Library Cataloguing in Publication Data
A CIP record is available from the British Library.

TABLE OF CONTENTS

CONTRIBUTORS

Berry Anderson, B.S.N., R.N.
Clinical Research Manager, Central Study Coordinator for OPT-TMS, Brain Stimulation Laboratory, Medical University of South Carolina, Charleston, South Carolina

Julia Applebaum, M.D.
Senior Psychiatrist, Women's Inpatient Psychiatry Service, and Lecturer in Psychiatry, Ben Gurion University of the Negev, Beersheva, Israel

R.H. Belmaker, M.D.
Hoffer-Vickar Professor of Psychiatry, Ben Gurion University of the Negev, Beersheva, Israel

Daryl E. Bohning, Ph.D., D.A.B.R.
Professor, Department of Radiology, Medical University of South Carolina, Charleston, South Carolina

Jeffrey Borckardt, Ph.D.
Assistant Professor, Brain Stimulation Laboratory and Departments of Psychiatry and Behavioral Sciences and Anesthesiology and Perioperative Medicine, Medical University of South Carolina, Charleston, South Carolina

Bella Chudakov, M.D.
Senior Psychiatrist and Lecturer in Psychiatry, Emergency Psychiatry Services, Ben Gurion University of the Negev, Beersheva, Israel

Stewart Denslow, Ph.D.
Assistant Professor, Radiology Department, Medical University of South Carolina, Charleston, South Carolina

Paulien M. De Vries, M.S.
MD/PhD student, Neurology, University Medical Center Groningen, University of Groningen, Groningen, the Netherlands

Charles M. Epstein, M.D.
Professor, Department of Neurology, Emory University School of Medicine, Rehabilitation Research and Development Center, Atlanta VA Medical Center, Atlanta, Georgia

Mark S. George, M.D.
Distinguished University Professor of Psychiatry, Radiology and Neuroscience; Director, Brain Stimulation Laboratory and Center for Advanced Imaging Research, Medical University of South Carolina, Charleston, South Carolina

Benjamin D. Greenberg, M.D., Ph.D.
Professor, Brown Medical School, Department of Psychiatry and Human Behavior, Butler Hospital, Providence, Rhode Island

Nimrod Grisaru, M.D.
Director of Emergency Psychiatry and Senior Lecturer in Psychiatry, Ben Gurion University of the Negev, Beersheva, Israel

Mark Hallett, M.D.
Human Motor Control Section, National Institute of Neurological Disorders and Stroke, National Institutes of Health, Bethesda, Maryland

Ralph E. Hoffman, M.D.
Professor of Psychiatry, Yale University School of Medicine, New Haven, Connecticut

Richard Holt, M.D.
Chief Resident, Psychiatry, Brain Stimulation Laboratory, Medical University of South Carolina, Charleston, South Carolina

Kevin A. Johnson, B.E.
Ph.D. program, Department of Neurosciences and Brain Stimulation Laboratory, Medical University of South Carolina, Charleston, South Carolina

Alex Kaptsan, M.D.
Director, Dual Diagnosis Unit, and Lecturer in Psychiatry, Ben Gurion University of the Negev, Beersheva, Israel

Jejo Koola, B.S.
M.D. program, Brain Stimulation Laboratory, Medical University of South Carolina, Charleston, South Carolina

Samet Kose, M.D.
Brain Stimulation Laboratory, Medical University of South Carolina, Charleston, South Carolina

F. Andrew Kozel, M.D., M.S.C.R.
Assistant Professor, Department of Psychiatry, University of Texas Southwestern Medical Center, Dallas, Texas; Adjunct Assistant Professor, Brain Stimulation Laboratory and CAIR, Medical University of South Carolina, Charleston, South Carolina

Xingbao Li, M.D.
Instructor, Brain Stimulation Laboratory, Medical University of South Carolina, Charleston, South Carolina

Sarah H. Lisanby, M.D.
Associate Professor of Clinical Psychology, Brain Stimulation and Neuromodulation Division, New York State Psychiatric Institute, Columbia University, New York, New York

Jeffrey P. Lorberbaum, M.D.
Assistant Professor, Anxiety, Stress, and Trauma Research, Psychiatry Department, Pennsylvania State College of Medicine, Hershey, Pennsylvania

Antonio Mantovani, M.D.
Postdoctoral Research Fellow, Columbia University, Ph.D. student, Siena University, Siena, Italy

Christine Molnar, Ph.D.
Clinical Research Psychologist, Behavior Therapy Laboratory, Pennsylvania State College of Medicine, Hershey, Pennsylvania

Ziad Nahas, M.D., M.S.C.R.
Associate Professor; Director, Mood Disorders Program; and Medical Director, Brain Stimulation Laboratory, Medical University of South Carolina, Charleston, South Carolina

Robert M. Post, M.D.
Professor of Psychiatry, Pennsylvania State School of Medicine, Hershey, Pennsylvania. Work emanated from the Intramural Program of the National Institute of Mental Health, Bethesda, Maryland

David Ramsey, M.S.
Vice President–Research Services, South Carolina Research Authority, BioMedical Applications Research Institute, Communications and Computing Infrastructure Technology, North Charleston, South Carolina

Komal Rastogi
Brain Stimulation Laboratory, Medical University of South Carolina, Charleston, South Carolina

Raffaella Ricci, Ph.D.
Assistant Professor, Brain Stimulation Laboratory, Medical University of South Carolina, Charleston, South Carolina, and Department of Psychology, University of Turin, Turin, Italy

Alona Shaldubina, Ph.D.
Scientist, Psychopharmacology Unit, Division of Psychiatry, Ben Gurion University of the Negev, Beersheva, Israel

Andrew M. Speer, M.D.
Clinical Fellow, National Institute of Mental Health, National Institutes of Health, U.S. Department of Health and Human Services, Bethesda, Maryland

Ulf Ziemann, M.D.
Professor, Department of Neurology, Johann Wolfgang Goethe-University of Frankfurt, Frankfurt, Germany

The following contributors to this book have indicated a financial interest in or other affiliation with a commercial supporter, a manufacturer of a commercial product, a provider of a commercial service, a nongovernmental organization, and/or a government agency, as listed below:

Jeffrey J. Borckardt, Ph.D. *Research Grant Support:* National Institute of Neurological Disorders and Stroke (National Institutes of Health [NIH]); Cyberonics, Inc.; Neurosciences Institute of Medical University of South Carolina (MUSC). *Other:* MUSC has filed two patents or invention disclosures in Dr. Borckardt's name regarding brain stimulation techniques and/or technologies.

Charles M. Epstein, M.D. *Research Grant Support/Honoraria:* UCB Pharma. The clinical use of UCB Pharma products is not discussed in Chapter 4. *Consultation:* Neuronetics, Inc. Neither Neuronetics nor its branded products are named in Chapter 4.

Mark S. George, M.D. *Pharmaceutical Companies:* Current—Argolyn Pharmaceuticals, consultant; Aventis Pharmaceuticals Inc., consultant; DarPharma, Inc., imaging research grant; GlaxoSmithKline Inc., imaging research grant/speaker's bureau; Jazz Pharmaceuticals, consultant; Parke-Davis (Pfizer Inc.), speaker's bureau. Past (≥3 years ago)—Cortex Pharmaceuticals, Inc., clinical trial research grant; Eli Lilly and Company, imaging research grant/speaker's bureau; Janssen, imaging research grant/ speaker's bureau; Parke-Davis, imaging research grant; Solvay Duphar, imaging research grant. *Imaging and Stimulation Device Companies:* Current—Cephos Corporation, advisory board and research grant; Cyberonics, Inc., clinical research grants/ imaging grant/speaker's bureau/depression advisory board/mechanisms of action advisory board; Dantec (Medtronic, Inc.), formal research collaborations (TMS, DBS); Neuronetics, Inc., clinical research grants, consultant; NeuroPace, Inc., advisory board. Past—DuPont Pharma, Inc., imaging research grant; Mediphysics/Amersham, imaging research grant/speaker's bureau; Neotonus, Inc. (now Neuronetics), clinical research grants, consultant; Picker International (now Philips), formal research collaboration (MRI)/speaker's bureau. *Other:* No equity ownership in any device or pharmaceutical company. Total industry-related compensation is <10% of university salary. MUSC has filed six patents or invention disclosures in Dr. George's name regarding brain imaging and stimulation.

Benjamin D. Greenberg, M.D., Ph.D. *Pharmaceutical Companies:* Past (≥3 years ago)— Forest Laboratories, Inc.; Pfizer Inc., speaker's bureau. *Medical Device Companies:* Aspect Neuroscience (scientific advisory board and formal research collaboration); Medtronic, Inc. (research support; formal research collaboration; unpaid consultation). *Other:* No equity ownership in any device or pharmaceutical company. No industry-related compensation in past 2 years; No patents, inventions, or intellectual property claims.

Ralph E. Hoffman, M.D. *Research Grant Support:* The studies described in Chapter 8 were supported by two Independent Investigator Awards from the National Alliance for Research on Schizophrenia and Depression (NARSAD); two grants from the National Institute of Mental Health (NIMH); grants from the Dana Foundation and the Donaghue Medical Foundation to Dr. Hoffman; and a grant from the NIH/National Center for Research Resources/General Clinical Research Centers (NCRR/GCRC).

Frank Andrew Kozel, M.D., M.S.C.R. *Research Grant Support:* Current—Cephos Corporation; Department of Defense Polygraph Institute; NIMH K23 (candidate); Stanley Foundation Center subgrant (no salary support). Past (1–3 years ago)—Cyberonics, Inc.; GlaxoSmithKline Inc.; NIMH; Veterans Affairs special fellowship in psychiatric research/neurosciences. *Other:* Cephos Corporation, scientific advisory board (no compensation); 2004 monthly case discussion group sponsored by AstraZeneca; educational materials and continuing medical education meals from multiple companies. No equity ownership in any device or pharmaceutical company, except possibly through mutual funds. MUSC has filed patents or invention disclosures in Dr. Kozel's name regarding brain imaging and stimulation.

Sarah H. Lisanby, M.D. *Research Grant Support:* Current—American Foundation for Aging Research; Cyberonics, Inc.; Dana Foundation; Defense Advanced Research Projects Agency (DARPA); John F. Kennedy Institute of Denmark; NARSAD; Neuronetics, Inc.; NIH; Stanley Foundation; institutional grants from Columbia University and the Research Foundation for Mental Hygiene. Past (> 1 year ago)—Cortex Pharmaceuticals, Inc., consultation; Cyberonics, Inc., speaker's bureau, travel, and honoraria; Magstim Company, research grant, consultation; Neuronetics, Inc., travel and consultation; Novartis, consultation; Pfizer Inc., co-investigator on research grant (no compensation). *Other:* Defense Sciences Study Group, member (unrelated to brain stimulation devices); Janssen translation neuroscience fellowship to a postdoctoral mentee (no compensation); Magstim Company, travel support, unpaid beta testing, unpaid collaboration on development of technology for magnetic seizure therapy (no patents, investments, or royalties); Naval Services International, board of directors (unrelated to brain stimulation devices); NIH Study Section Review Group, honoraria; consultation to investment firms on health care issues. No equity ownership in any device or pharmaceutical company. Columbia University has filed an invention disclosure for a novel stimulation device developed in Dr. Lisanby's laboratory, where the principal investigator on the disclosure is a postdoctoral fellow.

Ziad Nahas, M.D. *Research Grant Support:* Cyberonics, Inc.; Eli Lilly Company; Integra LifeSciences; Medtronic, Inc.; Neuronetics, Inc.; NeuroPace, Inc.; NIMH. *Consultant:* Avanir Pharmaceutical; Aventis Pharmaceuticals Inc.; Cyberonics, Inc.; Neuronetics, Inc.; NeuroPace, Inc. *Speaker's Bureau:* Cyberonics, Inc.

Robert M. Post, M.D. *Consultation:* Current—Eli Lilly and Company; GlaxoSmithKline Inc.; Memory Pharmaceuticals; Shire Pharmaceuticals Group; UCB Pharma. Past—Abbott; AstraZeneca; Bristol-Myers Squibb; Janssen; Novartis. *Speaker's Bureau/Honoraria:* Abbott; AstraZeneca; Bristol-Myers Squibb; GlaxoSmithKline Inc.; Novartis.

Ulf Ziemann, M.D. *Pharmaceutical Company Support (investigator-initiated trial grants):* Current—Teva Pharmaceuticals. Past—Biogen Idec; Schering.

1

Overview of Transcranial Magnetic Stimulation

History, Mechanisms, Physics, and Safety

Mark S. George, M.D.
Daryl E. Bohning, Ph.D., D.A.B.R.
Jeffrey P. Lorberbaum, M.D.
Ziad Nahas, M.D., M.S.C.R.
Berry Anderson, B.S.N., R.N.
Jeffrey J. Borckardt, Ph.D.
Christine Molnar, Ph.D.
Samet Kose, M.D.
Raffaella Ricci, Ph.D.
Komal Rastogi

HISTORY OF TRANSCRANIAL MAGNETIC STIMULATION

Transcranial magnetic stimulation (TMS) allows scientists to stimulate the brain noninvasively in awake, alert adults and simultaneously to observe changes in behavior. Clinicians are now using TMS as a potential treatment for many neuropsychiatric disorders. In the history of ideas, TMS is a tool that builds on an intellectual progression of the idea of localizing function within the brain.

1

Localization of Function in the Brain

Most modern neuroscientists are so firmly embedded in the idea that functions are organized into discrete brain regions that it strikes many as odd that this was not always the prevailing paradigm. Perhaps the first evidence of behavior-brain links came from the work of preliterate shamans who practiced *trepanning*, that is, hollowing out a hole in the skull in a living patient. Remarkably, some of these patients survived the trepanning, which was performed without anesthetics or antibiotics. Skulls have been found with bone growth around the edges of trepanned holes, indicating that the patient lived for some time after the operation. It seems clear that these prehistoric humans theorized about some link between specific brain regions and behavior, although one can only speculate about the underlying notions of mind and brain and exactly why these operations were performed.

The concept of the brain as the supreme organizer of behavior is a relatively new phenomenon in the Western tradition. For many centuries, the writings of Hippocrates and then later Galen attributed movements, wishes, thoughts, and emotions not to brain activity but rather to the fluids or "humors" that interacted in the body (McHenry 1969, p. 23). All diseases were the result of an imbalance of the mixture of the four humors, and "therapy" (i.e., bloodletting, purgatives, cathartics) was aimed at restoring the balance. Up until the 1800s, in general, the cerebral hemispheres were thought to have no specific function other than being the seat of the *sensorum commune,* and there was no specific functional localization. It is somewhat surprising that this idea persisted despite the ancient knowledge that injury to one side of the brain causes damage to the limbs on the opposite side.

The seventeenth century saw a renewal in theories of localization of brain function. Several writers, including Sir Thomas Willis, rejected Galenic thinking and wrote of the brain and behavior. Willis was one of the first to equate mental disease with altered brain function. Almost as soon as electrical current (galvanic) was introduced as an experimental tool, a host of researchers performed direct electrical studies in animals, through which they began to build the case for cerebral localization of function.

It was the pioneering work of Franz Joseph Gall and other "localizationists" in the early 1800s that formed the basis of modern neuroscience's ideas of brain localization of function. Ironically, although these investigators laid the basis for localization, they also contributed to a delay in adopting these ideas by overextrapolating localization in the "science" of phrenology (Critchley 1965). Later in that century, Pierre Paul Broca described his celebrated patient "Tan," who lost speech function as an adult (except to say "tan" for everything) and then developed weakness in the right leg and arm. Broca argued that motor speech was located in the left hemisphere and that the dysfunction in this patient had started in the "speech" area and then spread. His autopsy confirmed a lesion in the left frontal lobe. In 1861 Broca described eight cases of patients with loss of speech, all of whom had lesions in the third left frontal convolution (Broca 1865, 1878, 1879).

Broca's work in humans was paralleled by work in animals by Sir David Ferrier and others. Ferrier, working at the West Riding Lunatic Asylum in York, England, under the protection of Sir James Crichton-Browne, performed pioneering studies with direct electrical stimulation of animals. These meticulous studies confirmed that discrete brain regions controlled and coordinated specific behaviors. Sherrington and others extended this work in more modern times.

Working in a clinical setting, John Hughlings Jackson struck an intermediate line between supreme localization and more systemic views of brain function (Hughlings-Jackson 1879; Jackson 1873, 1874; Jackson and Stewart 1899). Working primarily with patients with epilepsy, Jackson made several important distinctions that might have importance in the modern use of TMS as a brain-mapping tool. Jackson argued that while it may be possible to localize a lesion, it is much more difficult to localize a function. He also pioneered the concept of negative (ablative) versus positive (irritative) aspects of lesions and brain function. A lesion in the same part of the brain might produce different symptoms depending on whether it destroyed tissue or instead irritated neurons and caused them to carry out their normal functions in a pathological way. Many TMS researchers would do well to remember these two ideas from Jackson: that lesions can be localized more easily than functions, and that lesions (or TMS) might have different effects depending on whether normal function is interrupted or augmented.

The pendulum of thought about brain localization swung too far with the growing influence of the phrenologists, who argued, along with the localizationalists, that each complex behavior was localized to a specific region. However, the phrenologists went further and also theorized that different aptitudes of behavior in an individual could be discerned by examination of skull shapes and morphologies. Modern researchers using TMS, with the study of behavioral changes with discrete stimulation, might do well to remember the lessons of the phrenologists and not over-interpret the specificity of location of effects.[1]

In the modern area, after the phrenologists had been curbed, the pioneering work of Wilder Penfield again rekindled the interest in brain stimulation and localization of function (Penfield 1975; Penfield and Erickson 1941; Penfield and Evans 1935; Penfield and Jasper 1954; Penfield and Perot 1963; Penfield et al.

---

[1]For example, consider the effects of a single TMS pulse into superficial cortex. The adult human brain is massively interconnected and has 25 billion cells, of which at least 10% are neurons (thus, at least 2.5 billion neurons). If one assumes that each neuron has at least two synapses (and some have many, many more) in an adult, there are at least 5 billion synapses in the brain. If one assumes that there are 2.5 million neurons in 1 cc of tissue, and a TMS pulse causes depolarization of 1 cc of cortex, then a TMS pulse will have secondary effects at as many as 5 million neurons—many of them remote from the TMS site!

1939). Penfield, working at McGill University in Montreal, Canada, performed a series of studies in epileptic patients undergoing surgery for intractable seizures. He clearly outlined the motor and sensory homunculus and also reported fascinating evocation of smells, musical passages, and even complex memories (which were all part of the seizure aura) when stimulating over the temporal lobes of these patients. The entire field of brain surgery for psychiatric disorders then followed on these ideas of brain localization. The significance of the work in this era was overemphasized, leading to overapplication of a modality that was not understood (for reviews: Ballantine et al. 1986; Lisanby and Sackeim 2000).

In related work, Robert Heath at Tulane University in New Orleans, Louisiana, recorded electrical activity from deep brain regions in awake patients with schizophrenia and demonstrated behavior-specific activity in these regions. He even experimented with low-level direct current stimulation of the cerebellum in schizophrenia patients, with claims of pronounced improvement (Heath and Mickle 1960). Unfortunately, the invasiveness of this procedure, and the lack of a sham condition, made this work unattractive, and it has not been repeated.

With the advent of modern neuroimaging tools, the entire localization debate has reemerged, with a great deal more sophistication and clarity. Ever more elaborate neuropsychological paradigms for brain activation have been coupled with positron emission tomography (PET), single-photon emission computed tomography (SPECT), and now magnetic resonance imaging (MRI) scanners to help advance knowledge of brain localization. The advance in knowledge has been remarkably rapid in some areas of neuroscience (e.g., vision, movement), modestly so in others (e.g., memory), and slower in other areas of the brain (e.g., basis of mood dysregulation, psychotic thinking). However, even tools like PET and SPECT scanning suffer from the epistemological problem of determining the causal relationship between activation in a given brain region and the behavior under study (for further discussion, see Chapter 9, "Transcranial Magnetic Stimulation and Brain Imaging," in this volume). TMS offers a unique tool for effecting advances in this area.

TMS as a Treatment Modality: Comparison With ECT

The preceding discussion has revolved around the development of TMS as a neuroscience investigational tool. The area that is capturing the most popular press attention at the moment, however, is TMS as a therapeutic tool, particularly for the treatment of depression (for further discussion, see Chapter 5, "Transcranial Magnetic Stimulation in Major Depression," in this volume).

TMS resembles electroconvulsive therapy (ECT), since both are somatic interventions that alter neuronal activity and change mood. However, the history of the development of ECT is different from the more recent history of the use of TMS as an antidepressant (for reviews of the history of ECT, see Impastato 1960; Lisanby and

Sackeim 2000). ECT was first considered as a potential therapeutic treatment following the probably faulty observation that patients with schizophrenia had no seizures or that epileptic patients were not psychotic (subsequent work has shown that both of these statements are likely false). Thus, generalized seizures were given to patients with psychosis, some of whom improved (probably those with psychotic depression). Years of ECT use then allowed the clinical winnowing of applications to its current use profile in treating patients with mood disorders and occasionally patients with catatonia or Parkinson's disease. In fact, the history of ECT can be seen as the over-application of a powerful brain intervention to many conditions, with clinical use narrowing both the clinical applications for which it is effective and the methods of application that affect efficacy. Thus, physicians used ECT for 30 years before it was determined that prefrontal application of the electrodes, and not parietal, was necessary for therapeutic effect, regardless of whether a generalized seizure occurred (Sackeim et al. 1993).

In the context of this history, TMS may be starting off better than did ECT. In the chapters that follow, current clinical researchers describe how they now have elaborate "roadmaps" of the brain regions putatively involved in the disorders of interest, with focal TMS as their method of first testing the roadmaps in challenge studies and then modifying the maps, if possible, for therapeutic effects.

Development of Modern TMS

TMS depends on the principle of *electromagnetic induction*—the process by which electrical energy is converted into magnetic fields, and vice versa—discovered by Faraday in 1831 (Faraday 1831/1965). Magnetic fields were then applied by many investigators to the human central nervous system (CNS), but in most cases the magnetic field was not of the strengths commonly used today (for a detailed review, see Geddes 1991). D'Arsonval, in 1896, was perhaps the first to apply something that resembles modern TMS to the nervous system. He reported that placing one's head inside a powerful magnetic coil (110 V, 30 A, 42 Hz) could produce phosphenes, vertigo, and even syncope (d'Arsonval 1896). In 1902, Berthold Beer reported that phosphenes could be produced by applying a magnetic field to the head (Beer 1902). Perhaps the first written idea of applying a modality like TMS for a neuropsychiatric condition was a patent filed that same year by Adrian Pollacsek and Berthold Beer of Vienna, Austria, to use an electromagnetic coil, placed over the skull, to pass vibrations into the skull and treat "depression and neuroses" (Figure 1–1). It is unclear whether the researcher wished for TMS to work its effects by inducing electrical current in the brain or rather by causing changes in fluid flow through vibration.

Several researchers in 1910 and 1911 constructed different magnetic stimulators to research the area of phosphene production (Dunlap 1911; Magnusson and Stevens 1911; Thompson 1910) (Figure 1–2). However, as can be seen in Figure 1–2, the capacitors of the day did not permit either high-intensity or rapid-

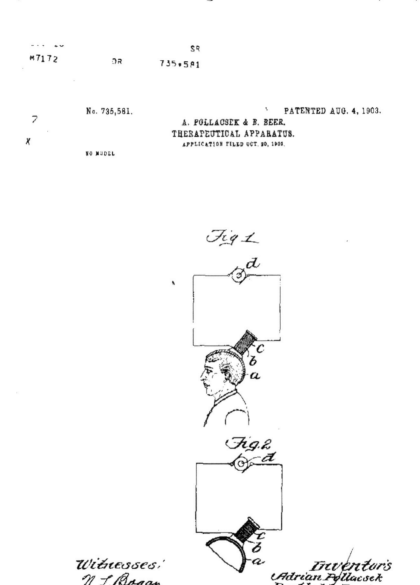

Figure 1–1. 1903 patent from Adrian Pollacsek and Berthold Beer for an electromagnetic device to be used in treatment of depression and neuroses.

Source.   Library of Mark S. George, M.D.

frequency use. It is unclear whether phosphenes were produced in these studies by occipital cortex stimulation or, more likely, through direct stimulation of the retina. In 1959 Kolin and colleagues were the first to demonstrate that a magnetic field could stimulate a peripheral frog muscle preparation (Kolin et al. 1959).

The modern age of TMS began in 1985 when A. T. Barker and colleagues in Sheffield, England, developed the first modern TMS device (Barker et al. 1985, 1987) (Figure 1–3). This laboratory has continued with new developments until the present day. The initial TMS devices were slow to recharge, and the coils would overheat with constant use. Currently there are at least three known commercial manufacturers of TMS devices, which have provided the hardware for an explosion of TMS-related research.

It is ironic that as TMS has arrived as a neuroscience tool, there is also a resurgence of interest in magnets in general as potential "alternative" therapies. In general, TMS involves the production of magnetic fields in the range of 1 tesla (T)—a strength powerful enough to cause neuronal depolarization. It is unclear how and whether TMS relates to use of constant low-level magnetic fields as therapies; the latter area has been less well studied, and many claims have not been investigated with the same scientific rigor as in the field of TMS. Thus, claims of the utility of low-intensity magnetic fields affecting the brain are not covered in this book. Similarly, it is not clear how TMS relates to claims of therapeutic effects by chronic low-level electrical stimulation (termed *transcranial direct current stimulation,* or tDCS), much of the work on which was done initially by Russian scientists (Klawansky et al. 1995). Recently, Paulus and colleagues in Germany have revived interest in this method, with exciting early findings (Antal et al. 2004a, 2004b, 2004c; Lang et al. 2004a, 2004b; Liebetanz et al. 2003; Nitsche et al. 2004; Rogalewski et al. 2004). This technique, as well as other types of brain stimulation techniques (e.g., deep brain stimulation, or DBS; vagus nerve stimulation, or VNS), are not covered in this book (George 2003; George et al. 2003).

THE PHYSICS BEHIND TMS

Physical Principles

TMS involves several relevant physics principles, from the current pulse through the TMS coil to the charge density involved in depolarizing neurons (Wagner et al. 2004). By applying these in a simplified, but hopefully consistent, approximation to a simple circular current loop model, we wish to convey a reasonably complete picture of TMS physics and the relative magnitude of the values of the important quantities involved. The reader is referred to the references cited in this section for in-depth discussions of this topic that more realistically take into account the actual conditions of stimulation in the human brain.

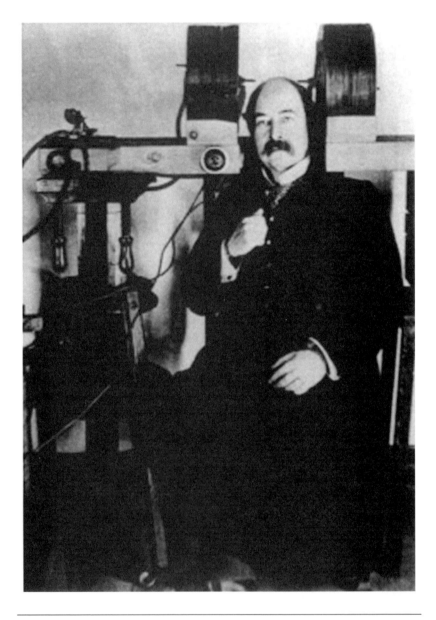

Figure 1–2.   Sylvanus P. Thompson and his apparatus to produce phosphenes via magnetic stimulation.

Source.   Thompson SP: "A Physiological Effect of an Alternating Magnetic Field." *Proceedings of the Royal Society of London* B82:396–399, 1910.

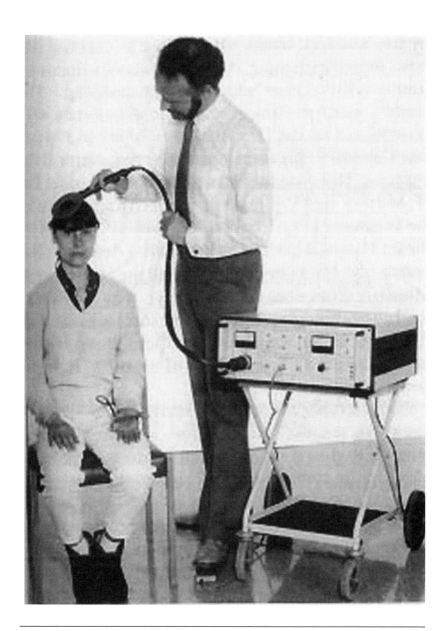

Figure 1–3. A.T. Barker with his transcranial magnetic stimulation (TMS) machine (in 1985), which set the stage for the modern work with TMS.

Source. Reprinted from Barker AT, Jalinous R, Freeston IL: "Non-invasive Magnetic Stimulation of the Human Motor Cortex," *The Lancet* 1:1106–1107, 1985, copyright 1985, with permission from Elsevier.

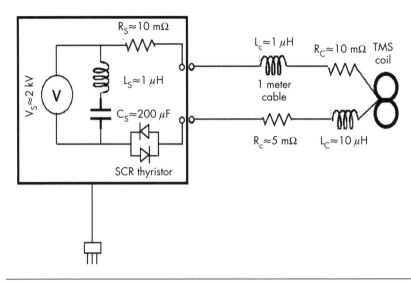

Figure 1–4. A typical transcranial magnetic stimulation (TMS) circuit diagram.

SCR = silicon controlled rectifier.

Source.   Courtesy of Daryl E. Bohning, Ph.D.

The TMS Stimulator Power Supply and Control Unit

The TMS apparatus is relatively simple, consisting of a power supply to charge a bank of large capacitors, which are then rapidly discharged through the TMS coil to create the magnetic field pulse. The circuit schematized in Figure 1–4 shows the basic configuration. Ancillary circuits include those for temperature monitoring and for setting the intensity and frequency of pulsing. A button is sometimes built into the handle of the coil so the operator can pulse the coil while still holding it in position with both hands. In addition, most units include a means of remotely triggering the system via TTL (transistor-transistor logic) pulse, and some even include programming capability so that a pattern of pulses and interpulse delays can be stored and then later recalled for execution.

Typical peak voltages are on the order of 2,000 V, and currents are around 10,000 A. The high-voltage electronic switch (thyristor) is crucial for creating the very short pulse (approximately 250 microseconds, or 1/4,000 of a second) needed for effective stimulation (Roth et al. 1991), and heavy copper cables are required to connect the TMS coil to the stimulator to carry the high currents involved.

Though the first generation of stimulators was designed to generate pulses that mimicked those found most effective for electrical stimulation, bipolar pulses are now the norm. Essentially a single cycle of a sine wave, such an oscillatory waveform achieves stimulation at lower levels of peak magnetic field than a monophasic one, allowing it to operate with less storage energy. At the end of the stimulating pulse, approximately 40% of the original energy stored in the capacitor has returned to it—a feature that is highly desirable for repetitive TMS.

Figure 1–5(1) shows a plot of a bipolar pulse of current through a TMS coil, the corresponding magnetic field, and the electric field that the magnetic field induces. The exact parameters of the oscillation are determined by the relative values of the storage capacitor, the inductance of the TMS coil, and the circuit resistance. Because the current has its maximum rate of change at the instant it is switched on, the induced electric field is also at its maximum at that point. As the current approaches its maximum value, its rate of increase slows, and the induced electric field drops, until at its maximum value its rate of change and the induced electric field are both zero. The current then starts to decrease, ever more rapidly, and then, as it passes through zero and reverses direction, decreases at its maximum rate, creating another peak, though of opposite sign, in the electric field induced. As the fall in current slows, the electric field induced begins to increase, passing through zero as the current reaches its minimum value. At the end of the cycle, as the current increases to zero, its rate of change also increases, creating another positive pulse in the induced electric field. In effect, there are two electric field pulses, the first approximately 100 μsec long, and the second about 50% longer and 30% less intense.

The TMS Coil

Two main coil types are used: circular coils and the figure-eight (or "butterfly") coil. They are designed to achieve a peak magnetic field of 1.5–2.5 T at the face of the coil. For comparison, this field is similar in strength to the constant field in an MR scanner and about 30,000–50,000 times greater than the earth's magnetic field.

Circular coils are usually about 8 cm in diameter and consist of one or more turns of pure, low-resistance copper wound in a flattened doughnut configuration. For a circular coil, there is no real focus. The field is strongest adjacent to the windings and the same all around the circumference, falling rapidly with distance. The field is fairly uniform in the center of the coil but about 30% less intense than close to the windings. For a coil with radius R, the magnetic field along a line perpendicular to the coil and through its center is proportional to

$$B \propto \frac{R^2}{2 \cdot (R^2 + z^2)^{3/2}}$$

where z is the distance from the coil along the central axis. Because the magnetic field of a simple circular coil is doughnut shaped, rapidly decreasing with distance from the loop, the sites where stimulation occurs are not in the center of the loop but at places around the loop where nerves pass across and close to the windings. This means that stimulation can occur at several different positions around the periphery of the coil unless the coil is placed on edge.

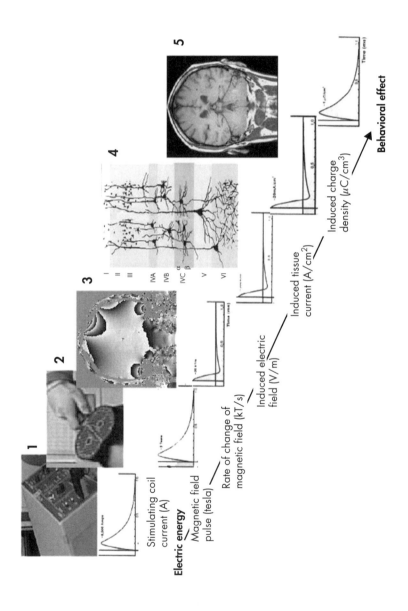

Stimulating coil current (A)

Electric energy

Magnetic field pulse (tesla)

Rate of change of magnetic field (kT/s)

Induced electric field (V/m)

Induced tissue current (A/cm²)

Induced charge density (μC/cm³)

Behavioral effect

Figure 1–5. Steps involved in transcranial magnetic stimulation (TMS).

TMS begins with the production of electrical current in the coil, the generation of a magnetic field around the coil, and the induction of electrical current in materials or tissues near the TMS coil, such as the brain. This process then produces an action potential or other changes in nervous tissue under the scalp. (1) TMS stimulator, (2) figure-eight TMS coil, (3) in vivo magnetic resonance phase map of magnetic field created by coil, (4) nerves in section of cerebral cortex and (5) functional magnetic resonance image of TMS induced activation.

Source. Reprinted from George MS, Nahas Z, Bohning DE, et al.: "Transcranial Magnetic Stimulation and Neuroimaging," in *Transcranial Magnetic Stimulation in Neuropsychiatry.* Edited by George MS, Belmaker RH. Washington, DC, American Psychiatric Press, 2000, pp. 253–268. Copyright 2000, American Psychiatric Press. Used with permission.

Since magnetic fields can be summed—that is, the magnetic field at each point near two separate current loops is the vector sum of the magnetic field vectors from the two separate loops—multiple loop configurations have been tried in attempts to improve on the penetration and focality of the circular coil. However, only the figure-eight configuration has gained wide acceptance. This is because the superposition of the magnetic fields of two adjacent current loops tends to make the field more uniform rather than focusing it, except where coils can be made to overlap with currents flowing in the same direction, as in a figure-eight configuration.

Figure-eight coils consist of two circular or D-shaped coils mounted adjacent to each other in the same plane and wired so that their currents circulate in opposite directions. This configuration has the effect of causing the fields of the two loops to add at their intersection, creating a cone-shaped volume of concentrated magnetic field, narrowing and decreasing in strength toward the apex. The panel at lower right in Figure 1–7 shows the pattern of the magnetic field intensity (magnitude) in a plane above a simple figure-eight coil. The other three panels of Figure 1–7 show the corresponding x, y, and z components of the magnetic field vector. Figure 1–6A shows a magnetic resonance (MR) image of the brain on which the magnetic field contours of a figure-eight coil have been superimposed. In Figure 1–6B, the plot of the field along the white line drawn on the image shows how the field intensity falls with distance, d, from the face of the coil. The decaying exponential (solid curve) gives a very good fit to the data.

An interesting issue is whether different coil designs can focus better or deeper in the brain. Though the field of a figure-eight coil is stronger and more focal than that of a circular coil (Cohen et al. 1990), there is still no remote focus in the sense of an isolated spot with high intensity surrounded by areas of lower intensity. According to Heller and Van Helsteyn (1992), at the frequencies used for extracranial stimulation of the brain, it is not possible to produce a three-dimensional local maximum of the electrical field strength inside the brain by using a superposition of simultaneous external current sources. In addition, even if the magnetic field were well localized, since the electric current density is induced around the magnetic flux lines, the greater the encircled flux, the greater the current density— which tends to "defocus" the electric current density.

There are also practical problems with having an array of coils for "focusing" TMS. In induction of neuron-depolarizing electric currents in tissue, very large and very short current pulses must be sent through the TMS coils. This necessitates low resistance, to prevent power loss and heating, and low inductance, to be able to minimize back electromotive force so that the short (approximately 250-μsec) pulses required can be created. In addition, there will be interactions between the electromagnetic fields of the two coils, changing the electromagnetic field of each and creating mechanical forces on them. However, several researchers are pursuing work in this area (Roth et al. 2005; B. Schneider, personal communication, February 2004).

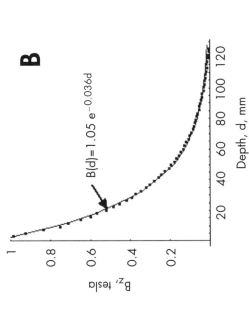

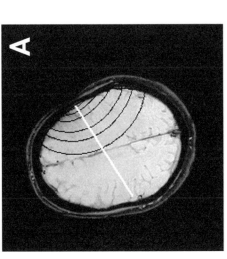

Figure 1–6. Magnetic resonance images of the actual magnetic fields induced by a transcranial magnetic stimulation (TMS) pulse.

(A) Transverse image of the brain with the TMS coil located over motor cortex. The black lines represent areas of consistent magnetic field strength, much as a contour map of the ground depicts altitude above sea level. (B) Actual field strength along the white line in Panel A is shown. Note how the field strength drops off rapidly with distance away from the coil.

Source. From Bohning DE, Pecheny AP, Epstein CM, et al.: "Mapping Transcranial Magnetic Stimulation (TMS) Fields in *Vivo* With MRI." *NeuroReport* 8:2535–2538, 1997. Copyright 1997, Lippincott Williams & Wilkins. Used with permission.

Because of its superior localization, the figure eight tends to be favored for TMS research studies of the brain, whereas circular coils are often used for peripheral nerve stimulation. For peripheral nerves, it is difficult to find an orientation in which the figure-eight coil effectively couples with tissue. Although the magnetic field itself does not require a coupling with the body part, being able to pass through air, the electric field induced does depend on the shape of the body part because the induced charge density depends on tissue shape and interfaces (Davey et al. 2004). That is, if there is no tissue, there are no current loops. Though stimulation can still be induced by the ends of a figure-eight coil, it is less likely to occur, because the field there is half as strong as at the center (approximately 2.0 T), and thus usually below threshold, and because the ends are usually poorly coupled with tissue.

Faraday's Law of Induction for Time-Varying Currents

The first quantitative observations relating time-varying electric and magnetic fields were made by Faraday in 1831. He observed that a transient current is induced in a circuit if 1) a steady current flowing in an adjacent circuit is turned on or off, 2) the adjacent circuit with a steady current flowing is moved relative to the first circuit, or 3) a permanent magnet is thrust into or out of the circuit (Faraday 1831/1965). Faraday attributed the transient current flow to a changing magnetic flux linked by the circuit. The changing flux induces an electric field around the circuit, the line integral of which he called the *electromotive force*. The electromotive force, in turn, in accordance with Ohm's law, causes a current flow.

Faraday's observations are summed up in a mathematical law known as *Faraday's law of electromagnetic induction.* The induced electromotive force around the circuit is proportional to the time rate of change of magnetic flux linking the circuit. It is worth noting that Faraday's law of induction can be derived from Maxwell's equations.

In TMS, Faraday's law of induction describes how the pulse of magnetic field that accompanies the pulse of current through the TMS coil and passes into the body induces an electric field (voltage differences between different points) in the tissue. Because body tissue is electrically conductive, this causes ionic currents to flow, with nerve depolarization as a consequence. Thus, by using the magnetic field as a "vector," TMS achieves "electrodeless" electrical stimulation.

Maxwell's classic paper published in 1864 provided a set of equations governing the relationships between electric and magnetic fields, including the observations of Faraday that figure so prominently in the theory of TMS (Maxwell 1864).

Electric Field Induced by Time-Varying Magnetic Field

Consider a path forming a circuit like C in Figure 1–4, which is closed over by the surface S. The induced electric field around C is proportional to the rate of change of the total magnetic flux normal to S. For a circular coil, the magnetic field forms a doughnut shape around the coil, being very intense near the windings and decreasing in intensity rapidly with distance from it. It turns out that the induced electric field in a plane below the coil is strongest in a ring the size of the coil. This is because a surface over such a circuit encloses the most magnetic flux. The flux through a small circuit near the windings would be more intense, but as it wraps around the winding, it would thread back through the loop canceling itself. A loop about the size of the coil surrounds the most flux in one direction—that is, before it starts to curve around the windings and begins canceling itself.

For a figure-eight coil, the magnetic flux is most intense under the intersection of the coils as shown in Figure 1–7, forming a cone-shaped volume of concentrated magnetic flux. The lower righthand panel (IBI) in Figure 1–7 shows a contour plot of the magnitude of the magnetic field in a plane below and parallel to the coil, and a region in the center where it is most intense. This pattern can also be seen in the magnetic field x-component contour plot in the upper lefthand panel of Figure 1–7, which shows that the x component dominates this "focus" in magnetic flux. Although there is clearly a "focus" directly under the coil, it is also apparent from the spreading contours that the field decreases rapidly, as is quantitatively shown in Figure 1–6(B), where the field as a function of distance from the coil is nicely fit with a decaying exponential. The electric current induced by a figure eight is essentially a superposition of the separate rings of current formed underneath the two circular coils that make up the figure eight, adding where the coils overlap, and partially canceling elsewhere.

A sense of the strength of the electric field induced can be gained by estimating the rate of change of magnetic flux through a small loop in the stimulated area. At the frequencies involved in TMS (<10 kilohertz), almost all of the electric field inside the head is induced by magnetic induction rather than by direct penetration of the electric field component of the electromagnetic field created by the coil; that is, radiative effects can be neglected (Polk and Postow 1986). Another way of looking at this is that the wavelength of the TMS pulse electromagnetic waves is on the order of kilometers, much greater than the size of the head.

Possible Mechanism of Action of TMS

Step 1: Creation of a Transmembrane Potential

The resting membrane potential (RMP) of a neuron, about −70 millivolts (intracellular minus extracellular), is determined by the relative intra- and extracellular concentrations of sodium (Na^+), potassium (K^+) and chloride (Cl^-) ions maintained by the sodium-potassium ion pump and passive diffusion. If the membrane of the neuron is depolarized from −70 mV to about −40 mV, the normally restrictive Na^+ channels open, and the cell responds with a brief, impulsive flow of ionic current that shifts the membrane potential to +20 mV and then back to −75 mV. This response

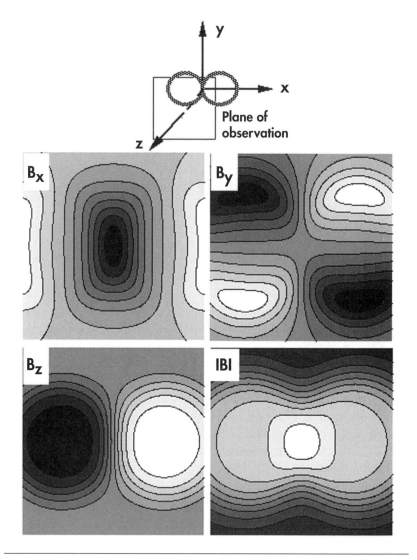

Figure 1–7.   Magnetic field components produced with the typical figure-eight transcranial magnetic stimulation (TMS) coil and their summation.

The figure shows how the summation of the different components produces the overall region where the TMS coil might produce focal changes.

Source.   From Bohning DE, He L, George MS, et al.: "Deconvolution of Transcranial Magnetic Stimulation (TMS) Maps." *Journal of Neural Transmission* 108:35–52, 2001. Copyright 2001, Springer-Verlag. Used with permission.

is known as the *action potential,* and the propagation of this impulse of current along the axon membrane is the mechanism by which neurons carry information.

Thus, although magnetic stimulation does not involve the direct passage of electric currents through the body like electrical stimulation, at the cellular level, the mechanisms of stimulation are the same, namely, an "electrodeless" electrical stimulation. Either directly, in the case of electrical stimulation, or indirectly, in the case of magnetic stimulation, charge is moved across an excitable cellular membrane, creating a transmembrane potential, or nerve depolarization voltage. If sufficient, this voltage can cause membrane depolarization and initiate an action potential, which then propagates along a nerve like any other action potential. Whether TMS has neurobiological effects in ways other than creating action potentials is unknown, though some animal studies have hinted at this possibility (Ji et al. 1998).

Step 2: Spatial Derivative of the Electric Field Along the Nerve

The general consensus has been that for a straight nerve in a relatively homogeneous conductive volume, excitation occurs where the negative-going first spatial derivative of the induced electric field parallel to the long axis of the nerve peaks (Cracco et al. 1987). Theoretical studies have also reached the conclusion that for a long axon, stimulation occurs not where the electric field is largest, but instead where its spatial derivative along the axon is largest. As explained by Barker and colleagues (1989), if the electric field is uniform and parallel to the nerve axon, it will cause current to flow both inside and outside but not across its membrane. However, by continuity, if the current within the axon changes along its length, a current equivalent to the change must pass through the membrane and can cause stimulation. The mathematical description of this change of electric field along the axon is the spatial derivative of the electric field along it. In the case of a bent nerve, even a spatially uniform electric field can cause stimulation. This stimulation occurs because at the place where the axon bends across the field, although the magnitude of the spatial derivative of the electric field does not change, its spatial derivative along the nerve will.

Step 3: Electric Field Distribution and Transmembrane Potential

It is not known what prediction is valid for stimulation of a short fiber, cell body, or dendritic tree. It is clear that the relative orientation of the nerve and the electric field is important (Amassian et al. 1990). Evidence also exists that the polarity of the current in the coil influences stimulation threshold (Sommer and Paulus 2003).

Observable Effects of TMS

Magnetic Field of TMS Coil

Since the magnetic field penetrates tissue with negligible distortion, the magnetic field of a TMS coil can be measured in the laboratory, or calculated if the current configuration of the coil is known. Hence, if the position of the TMS coil during the stimulations relative to a set of structural MR images is known, it would be possible to determine, through use of computer graphical methods, the strength of the field relative to the anatomy of the brain. However, it would be impractical to measure the three components of the magnetic field vector at the number of points necessary to give a high-resolution map of the field over a volume. For example, to map the 10 cm × 20 cm × 10 cm active volume of a typical figure-eight coil 10 cm deep at 1 mm resolution, it would take an astounding 6,000,000 measurements to obtain all three components of the magnetic field. Computer simulations are also possible, but exact current distribution in the coil is usually not known exactly.

Fortunately, if the coil is nonferromagnetic, it is a relatively straightforward procedure to obtain a three-dimensional map of the z component of the magnetic field in vivo in a magnetic resonance scanner (Bohning et al. 1997a). The z-component map (an example of which is shown in Figure 1–6A) can then be used as input to a difference method based on Maxwell's equations to obtain the complete three-dimensional vector magnetic field of the TMS coil in vivo (Bohning et al. 1998). The contours superimposed on the MR image show how the magnetic field of the TMS coil actually impinges on the brain. In Figure 1–6B, the plot of the field along the white line drawn on the image shows how the field intensity falls with distance from the coil.

Electric Field Induced by TMS Coil

At this time, we have no way of directly imaging the electric fields induced by the TMS coil, so determinations of the actual neuron depolarizing currents still depend on computer models. However, developing the ability to obtain high-resolution in vivo maps of the magnetic field of the TMS coil in relation to cerebral anatomy is a necessary first step toward the ultimate goal of imaging the induced current. Some have already begun using MRI techniques to determine tissue conductivity (Le Bihan et al. 2001).

Local Response to TMS Stimulation

By using one of the functional neuroimaging techniques (either PET, SPECT, electroencephalography, or MRI), it is now possible to observe the local response to TMS. This capability brings us a step closer to studying the in vivo neurophysiology of the brain—namely, observing the local response to electric fields induced in specific clusters of sensory nerve fibers. This capability would make it possible to directly study in vivo what could, in the past, only be inferred from measurements made in simplified model systems.

SAFETY OF TMS

After reviewing the history of the development of TMS and understanding how it works from a physics perspective, it is now important to ask whether TMS is safe.

TMS is generally regarded as safe and without lasting side effects. There have been no significant cognitive (Little et al. 2000; Triggs et al. 1999), neurological (Nahas et al. 2000), or cardiovascular sequelae reported as a result of repetitive TMS (rTMS). Single-pulse TMS has been in use for nearly 15 years. It is generally regarded as safe and virtually without lasting side effects. rTMS, on the other hand, can produce a range of lasting effects on cerebral function, some of which are desirable from the clinical point of view, such as the possible improvement of mood in depression, or from the experimental point of view, such as momentary disruption of cognitive function. It can also induce epileptic seizures predictably if it is not applied with limits on the stimulation parameters.

Single-Pulse Versus Repetitive TMS

In single-pulse TMS, single or paired pulses are delivered nonrhythmically and not more than once every few seconds (Wassermann 1998). This form of stimulation is usually used for physiological research or diagnostic purposes. With extensive experience and encouraging results in human safety studies (Bridgers 1991; Bridgers and Delaney 1989), a general consensus has arisen that single-pulse TMS can be performed safely in most individuals.

Precautionary measures for single-pulse TMS studies vary widely. Generally, all that is required from the point of view of safety is to obtain a brief screening history to rule out the presence of metal in the head or eyes, implanted electronic devices, and intracardiac lines. Guidelines for using single-pulse TMS are given in a publication of the International Federation of Clinical Neurophysiology (Rossini et al. 1994). Although seizures have occurred with single-pulse TMS in patients with cortical lesions such as infarcts, other investigators have had considerable difficulty producing seizures with stimulation delivered directly to epileptic foci (Hufnagel et al. 1990, 1995). To our knowledge, seizures have not occurred in healthy individuals undergoing single-pulse TMS, and reported adverse effects other than seizures have been limited to local discomfort and headache.

Since seizure thresholds may vary widely in the normal population, it is probably not sufficient to dose rTMS based on the absolute intensity of the stimulating pulse (Amiaz et al. 2001; Pridmore et al. 1998). Rather, a measure of the individual's sensitivity is required. The *evoked muscle twitch* or *motor evoked potential* (MEP) to stimulation of the primary motor area is the only TMS effect that can be quantified online, and the threshold intensity for producing the MEP is the best available index of an individual's sensitivity. While the MEP threshold (or motor threshold) varies widely across the normal population, the MEP threshold remains quite consistent over time within normal individuals (Wassermann 2002). Traditionally, MEPs have been recorded with surface electrodes and displayed online. However, the visible muscle twitch threshold may be as reliable (Pridmore et al. 1998). Because the MEP threshold is generally lowest in the hand

Table 1–1. Current safety guidelines for repetitive transcranial magnetic stimulation (rTMS): maximum safe duration (seconds) for single trains of rTMS

Frequency (Hz)	Intensity (% of MEP threshold)												
	100	110	120	130	140	150	160	170	180	190	200	210	220
1	>1800.00	>1800.00	360.00	>50.00	>50.00	>50.00	>50.00	27.00	11.00	11.00	8.00	7.00	6.00
5	>10.0	>10.00	>10.00	>10.00	7.60	5.20	3.60	2.60	2.40	1.60	1.40	1.60	1.20
10	>5.0	>5.00	4.20	2.90	1.30	0.80	0.90	0.80	0.50	0.60	0.40	0.30	0.30
20	2.05	1.60	1.00	0.55	0.35	0.25	0.25	0.15	0.20	0.25	0.20	0.10	0.10
25	1.28	0.84	0.40	0.24	0.20	0.24	0.20	0.12	0.08	0.12	0.12	0.08	0.08

Note. MEP=motor evoked potential.

Source. Wassermann EM: "Risk and Safety of Repetitive Transcranial Magnetic Stimulation: Report and Suggested Guidelines from the International Workshop in the Safety of Repetitive Transcranial Magnetic Stimulation, June 5–7, 1996." *Electroencephalography and Clinical Neurophysiology* 108:1–16, 1998.

Table 1–2. Current repetitive transcranial magnetic stimulation (rTMS): safe intertrain intervals (seconds)

Frequency (Hz)	rTMS intensity (% MT)	
	≤110% MT	>110% MT
≤20	5 seconds[a]	60 seconds[b]
>20	60 seconds[b]	60 seconds[b]

Note. MT = motor threshold.
[a]Perhaps less, but has not been worked out; definitely >1 second.
[b]Probably less, but has not been worked out.
Source. Adapted from Chen et al. 1997.

muscles, it is generally determined by using a low-threshold hand muscle such as the abductor pollicis brevis of the thumb. The recommended limits on rTMS parameters for preventing seizures (Chen et al. 1997; Wassermann 1998; see Tables 1–1 and 1–2) were determined with respect to a given individual's MEP threshold, the stimulation frequency, the train length, and the intertrain interval (when repeated trains are administered). They were based on the observation of motor phenomena during stimulation of the motor cortex (i.e., persistent electromyographic activity after the end of a pulse train; the apparent spread of activity to increasingly distant muscles; and, of course, seizures).

Adverse Events

Seizures: Experience With rTMS

Currently, the risk of causing a seizure is the primary safety concern with TMS. In contrast to single-pulse TMS, in which seizures have not been reported in healthy individuals, at least eight seizures have been caused by rTMS (Table 1–3). These seizures have occurred in an unknown sample size, but likely over several thousand rTMS sessions. Most of them have occurred with stimulation of the primary motor area; however, at least two occurred with prefrontal stimulation. Most have occurred in healthy volunteers who were subjects in early physiological experiments. However, one occurred in a patient with epilepsy when the stimulation site was in the hemisphere contralateral to the known seizure focus (Dhuna et al. 1990), and one was in a depressed patient who reportedly had recently been prescribed tricyclic and neuroleptic medications, which could have lowered the seizure threshold. Most of the seizures occurred with combinations of stimulation parameter settings that were outside of the published guidelines (Table 1–1) for motor cortex stimulation or in the presence of medications that might have lowered the seizure threshold (e.g.,the depressed patient described above), but two seizures were pro-

Table 1–3. Summary of seizures induced by repetitive transcranial magnetic stimulation (rTMS)

Subject condition	Seizure type	rTMS train Intensity (5 threshold)	Source
Temporal lobe epilepsy[b]	2° generalized	100	Dhuna et al. 1990
Normal	2° generalized	200	Pascual-Leone et al. 1992
Normal	2° generalized	250	Pascual-Leone et al. 1993
Normal[a]	2° generalized	105	Wassermann et al. 1996
Normal		110	
Normal	2° generalized	120	NINDS, unpublished data, 1997
Normal	Partial motor	130	B. Mercuri, unpublished data, 1996
Depression (subject taking medication)	2° generalized	90	A. Pascual-Leone, unpublished data, 1997
Depression	Pseudoabsence	110	Conca et al. 2000

Note. 2° = secondary; NINDS = National Institute of Neurological Disorders and Stroke.
[a]The intertrain interval did not appear to be a factor in seizure induction.
[b]The hemisphere contralateral to the side of seizure focus was stimulated.
Source. Modified from Wassermann 1998.

voked by trains delivered to the motor cortex—in the first case, by a 7-second train of 3-Hz stimulation at 130% of MEP threshold, and in the second, by a 2.5-second train of 15-Hz stimulation at 120% of MEP threshold (Wassermann 1998). These events make it clear that repetitive stimulation of the motor cortex, the most epileptogenic region of the neocortex, must always be performed with a high degree of caution. While Table 1–1 provides limits on combinations of intensity, train duration, and frequency, another critical parameter is the interval between stimulation trains. This was made clear when closely spaced trains that individually fell within the "safe" limits caused two seizures. Based on these events and some additional motor cortex experiments, guidelines have been provided for the safe interval between trains (Table 1–2).

To our knowledge there have been two publications since 1997 describing events during TMS that might be considered seizures. Conca and colleagues

(2000) reported on a patient who experienced a "pseudoabsence seizure"; it is unclear if this was a true seizure. Bernabeu and colleagues (2004) reported on a patient who had a seizure during rTMS. In this case, there was a brief interstimulus interval. None of the subjects who have experienced rTMS-induced seizures have suffered lasting physical sequelae. In most of them, electroencephalograms (EEGs) obtained immediately after the seizure showed the expected slowing but were normal within 1–2 days. Two subjects had neuropsychological testing before and after the seizures (Pascual-Leone et al. 1993; Wassermann et al. 1996). Both individuals had mild recall deficits, which disappeared within 24 hours.

Immediately following a routine therapeutic TMS session, subjects have been tested and do not show significant neurocognitive side effects. They are thus free to return to work or drive themselves home.

Hearing Loss

One report found evidence of short-term hearing loss in subjects who had been exposed to rTMS (Pascual-Leone et al. 1993). A study of single-pulse TMS in humans did not find any hearing loss (Pascual-Leone et al. 1992). To our knowledge, there has been only one study of TMS effects on hearing in rats (Counter et al. 1990). Further animal research is needed. Loo and colleagues (2001) found changes in auditory threshold in two depressed patients following a 2- to 4-week treatment regimen; although the changes were mild and transient, further safety testing appears warranted. The recently completed Neuronetics-sponsored trial of rTMS in depression (Aaronson et al., in press). performed auditory threshold measurement in more than 300 patients before and after 4 weeks of prefrontal rTMS and found no changes. All patients however wore ear plugs during treatment. However, in general, subjects in TMS studies wear earplugs to minimize potential ear damage.

Headache

Several studies have reported mild, transient tension-type headaches on the day of stimulation (Gershon et al. 2003; Nahas et al. 2004). At the Medical University of South Carolina, we studied 60 healthy young men in a sleep deprivation study (parietal cortex, 110% of MT [motor threshold], frequency range+1–20 Hz) (Anderson et al. 2006). They received large doses of TMS or sham TMS on three different days within a week. Of the 153 active TMS treatments delivered in the study, 19% were associated with reports of headache. Of the 29 sham treatments delivered, 17% were associated with headache. These differences were not significant. Rates of the occurrence and severity of headaches for this study are summarized in Tables 1–4 and 1–5, respectively.

In this study of healthy young men, active TMS was not associated with a significant increase in reported headaches compared to sham TMS. It should be noted, however, that sham TMS is not completely inert. Of course, only active

Table 1–4. Headache occurrence rates and standard errors associated with active and sham transcranial magnetic stimulation (TMS)

	Valid n	Headache occurrence	SE
All active TMS sessions	153	0.19	0.03
Active TMS (session 1)	62	0.13	0.04
Active TMS (session 2)	61	0.21	0.05
Active TMS (session 3)	30	0.23	0.08
Sham TMS sessions	29	0.17	0.07

Table 1–5. Headache severity counts and percentages associated with active and sham transcranial magnetic stimulation (TMS)

	Severe, n (%)	Moderate, n (%)	Mild, n (%)
Active TMS (session 1)	0 (0)	4 (6.5)	4 (6.5)
Active TMS (session 2)	1 (1.6)	4 (6.6)	8 (13.1)
Active TMS (session 3)	0 (0)	1 (3.3)	6 (20.0)
Sham TMS	0 (0)	1 (3.4)	4 (13.8)

TMS actually results in cortical stimulation; however, both active and sham TMS produce loud (~80 dB) clicks (i.e., pressure waves), and both active and sham TMS procedures require subjects to sit still with their chins in a mechanical head holder. Although subjects wear ear protection and efforts are made to ensure they are reasonably comfortable in the TMS chair, the effects of the noise and prolonged immobility may result in increased muscle tension, fatigue, and headache in some subjects, even if no cortical stimulation is occurring.

There is very little long-term (more than several weeks following treatment) safety data on subjects who have undergone TMS studies.

Dosing

There is also very little information on the maximum total daily or weekly exposure to TMS. The study described above again provides important safety information. In this study we administered up to 12,960 pulses within a day, and 38,880 pulses within a week, without adverse effects. The upper limit of TMS exposure in humans has not been determined.

The following classes of individuals should be excluded from rTMS studies, unless the benefits clearly outweigh the risks:

1. Individuals with focal or generalized encephalopathies (i.e., tumor, stroke, meningitis, encephalitis, epilepsy) or severe head trauma, which might be epileptogenic. Abnormalities on neurological examination suggesting cerebral dysfunction should be investigated with imaging prior to rTMS.
2. Individuals having first-degree relatives with idiopathic epilepsy. These individuals may be at increased risk of seizure and should be considered for exclusion.
3. Individuals with heavy consumption of alcohol or ongoing abuse of epileptogenic drugs such as cocaine. Individuals who consume large amounts of alcohol may be at increased risk of seizure if they stop consuming alcohol. Others suspected of ongoing abuse of epileptogenic drugs such as cocaine should be excluded unless abstinence can be guaranteed.
4. Individuals with significant heart disease or increased intracranial pressure who are at increased risk from seizure sequelae.

Precautionary Measures and Monitoring Procedures Specific to rTMS

General Precautionary and Monitoring Issues

For rTMS studies, a history that includes questions regarding the exclusion criteria above should be taken and a neurological examination should be performed. It is currently recommended that rTMS be performed in a room equipped with oxygen and with an emergency cart nearby (Belmaker et al. 2003). Before the initial rTMS session, the MEP motor threshold should be determined and treatment should then be performed with respect to this threshold and the safety parameters noted in Table 1–1. In rTMS studies that include multiple sessions, some suggest that the motor threshold also be checked prior to each treatment, or at least weekly. As well, before each rTMS session, some investigators routinely question subjects about events that might change the risk of seizures such as hours of sleep the night before, changes in medications (including over-the-counter medications), or drug or alcohol use (Keel et al. 2001) (see Appendix 1 in Chapter 2, "Methods of Administering Transcranial Magnetic Stimulation," this volume).

While electroencephalography is theoretically the most sensitive means of monitoring for epileptic activity and can be recorded from the site of stimulation, the electrical artifact produced by the stimulating pulse can be overwhelming, unless specialized artifact suppression circuits are used. To date, electroencephalography is not in routine use for monitoring during rTMS.

Management of Seizures in the TMS Laboratory

It is of particular importance that any laboratory using rTMS have a plan in place for the management of seizures. Until the safety of any specific stimulation regimen is firmly established, the plan should include the presence of medical personnel and the maintenance of emergency equipment and medication nearby. See Chapter 2, this volume, for a discussion of the management of TMS-induced seizures.

Effects of TMS on Paramagnetic or Conductive Objects in and on the Head

Like MR scanning, TMS may cause paramagnetic objects to move. Therefore, essentially the same precautions should be taken with TMS subjects regarding the presence of paramagnetic metal objects in the head or eye. Further, subjects with nonparamagnetic implanted metal hardware (i.e., aneurysm clips) should not receive rTMS because of the possibility of heating by the induced eddy currents. This phenomenon has been reported in conventional EEG electrodes fixed to the scalp near the stimulating coil during rTMS and can be prevented by radial notching, which interrupts the current path (Roth et al. 1992). Conductive objects, including electrodes, implanted in or on the brain pose another potential problem for single-pulse TMS as well because of their theoretical ability to provide a low-resistance pathway for induced current and locally high-charge densities that could cause tissue damage. However, single-pulse TMS has been carried out in patients with subdural and thalamic electrodes.

Exposure During Pregnancy

The potential effects of TMS on a gestating fetus when the stimulation is administered to the mother's head are not known. Therefore, pregnant women should not be exposed to TMS or other sources of powerful electromagnetic fields except when it is judged that the potential clinical benefit outweighs the risk. In the only reported therapeutic use of rTMS during pregnancy, Nahas and colleagues (1999) treated a woman with severe depression during the second trimester. She went on to deliver a healthy baby. Women of childbearing age should be questioned about the possibility of pregnancy before participating in rTMS studies and excluded unless the criterion of clinical benefit is met.

Exposure of Children

TMS has diagnostic applications in children as in adults, and some studies have used TMS to study the developing motor system by comparing the effects of motor stimulation on children in different age groups (Muller et al. 1997; Nezu et al. 1997). However repeated stimulation with rTMS could have particular effects on the developing brain. In studies of rats, electrical brain stimulation appears to be more effective in inducing ultrastructural changes associated with long-term synaptic potentiation in young than in aged animals (Geinisman et al. 1994), which suggests that children might be more vulnerable to such changes if such changes can be induced with rTMS. Therefore, rTMS should be used with caution in children and only when a clear clinical benefit is envisioned.

Effects of Stimulation on Neural Tissue

With one exception (Matsumiya et al. 1989, 1992), histological studies in animals (Counter 1994; Counter et al. 1991; Nishikiori 1996; Ravnborg et al. 1990; Sgro et al. 1991) and a single human biopsy specimen (Gates et al. 1992) after TMS exposure have failed to show pathological changes. In the single exceptional study (Matsumiya et al. 1992), microvacuolar changes were found in the cortex of rats exposed to more than 100 pulses at 2.8 T, which was approximately three times the rats' reported motor threshold. This stimulation intensity, while high, is not far beyond the range to which humans have been routinely exposed. However, this finding has not been reproduced. Rabbits exposed to 100–200 pulses per day for more than 30–42 days for a total of 5,000 pulses at 2.4 T showed no such changes (Nishikiori 1996), nor did rabbits exposed to 1,000 pulses at 2.0 T over a period of months (Counter et al. 1990). Some have questioned whether the findings in the exceptional case may have been caused by fixation artifact.

Structural MRIs obtained in depressed patients before and after ten 20-minute rTMS sessions showed no change (Nahas et al. 1998). Studies combining regional cerebral blood flow imaging with either TMS or transcranial electrical stimulation have shown that stimulation over the motor cortex does not increase cerebral blood flow more than does voluntary movement (Bohning et al 2003a, 2003b; Denslow et al. 2004, 2005a, 2005b). Although this subject needs further study, these imaging results suggest that short trains of rTMS at motor threshold and 1 Hz do not cause increases in blood flow that are much different from those produced in behavioral activation paradigms. One can directly measure water flow within axons within the brain using MRI diffusion (Le Bihan et al. 2001). An initial TMS study using diffusion failed to find any significant TMS-induced changes (Li et al. 1993), while a later, less rigorously controlled study did find differences (Mottaghy et al. 2003).

Theoretically, noxious effects on tissue are possible whenever the brain is stimulated with electrical currents, such as histotoxicity via mass hyperexcitation of neurons (excitotoxicity) or tissue heating. However, based on the extensive literature on the effect of electrical brain stimulation in animals (Agnew et al. 1983), the consensus among experts is that the danger of tissue damage from current TMS devices is negligible (Wassermann 1998). In the one comparable study performed on humans (Gordon et al. 1990), two patients with epilepsy received 50-Hz subdural electrical stimulation of the anterior temporal lobe for fairly brief periods with a maximum charge per phase of 4.5 μC and a charge density of 57 μC/cm^2 before resection of the temporal lobe. Light microscopy showed no evidence of histological damage to the stimulated tissue. It should be noted that this combination of parameters yields a combination of charge density and charge per phase that would have been unsafe according to McCreery and colleagues (1990). Manufacturers' estimates of the maximal charge density of currently available TMS devices are on the order of 2–3 μC/cm^2, and continuous 50-Hz stimulation is beyond the effective operating range of most magnetic stimulators. Therefore, the chance of producing excitotoxicity with rTMS seems to be remote. The only other known potential source of tissue injury from rTMS is heating of tissue by induced currents. Although theoretically such heating is possible in poorly perfused volumes, such as infarctions and cysts, it is not considered to be a significant hazard of rTMS.

Health Effects of Exposure to Magnetic Fields

The National Research Council concluded in 1996 that there are no proven health risks of prolonged exposure to low-intensity magnetic fields, such as those produced by power lines and household sources. Furthermore, the incidence of cancer does not appear to be increased in people such as MRI technicians, who have prolonged exposure to high-intensity magnetic fields that are similar in strength to the magnetic field produced by TMS (Baker and DeVos 1996). While these data are reassuring, TMS delivered focally and repeatedly to the same body site could have different risks. Also, the exposure of individuals habitually administering TMS may be more significant than that of subjects who are stimulated only occasionally.

Effects on Magnetic Media and Electronic Devices

Pagers, watches, credit cards, and magnetic data storage media may be adversely affected by magnetic fields. Therefore, these should be kept away from the discharging coil. Control devices for pacemakers and medication pumps are of particular concern, since a malfunction could be serious. However, Kofler and Leis (1998) have performed single-pulse TMS safely in patients with implanted electronic devices without causing any malfunctions.

Cardiovascular Effects

Foerster and colleagues (1997) continuously monitored blood pressure, pulse, and electrocardiograms while delivering rTMS serially to five scalp sites. In all subjects, there was a clear autonomic response with heart rate increases and blood pressure decreases. This autonomic response was significantly greater after real stimulation than after sham cortical stimulation. Nonetheless, Foerster et al. reported that no significant cardiovascular side effects occurred with stimulation. Because the autonomic response was not specific to a scalp site and correlated well with subjects' rating of stimulus discomfort, the authors concluded that the autonomic response was due not to direct cortical stimulation but rather to nonspecific arousal. This result is consistent with that of Niehaus and colleagues (1998), who also found a nonspecific arousal reaction when measuring the sympathetic skin response during rTMS over several scalp sites. Three other studies—one with single-pulse TMS (Chokroverty et al. 1995) and two with rTMS (Jahanshahi et al. 1998; Pascual-Leone et al. 1993)—assessed blood pressure and pulse changes but did not find any significant changes in blood pressure or heart rate.

CONCLUSION

TMS as a neuroscience probe fits within a historical current of attempting to localize functions within the human brain. As a potential therapy, TMS follows on the heels of ECT, although since its very beginning there have been important differences between these two techniques. TMS is emerging at a time of renewed popular interest in magnets and healing. TMS, at high fields and with intermittent stimulation, is unlike the low-level constant magnetic exposure of many of the more popular fad uses of magnets, which have not been subjected to serious and critical study. There are also other new attempts at modifying brain activity through somatic interventions (e.g., vagus nerve stimulation for epilepsy and perhaps depression, deep brain stimulation for Parkinson's disease).

The pulsed magnetic field, associated with the pulse of current through the TMS coil, penetrates tissue essentially unperturbed and, by Faraday's Law, induces neuron depolarizing electric currents in the brain under the coil. The magnetic field's distribution can be computed, and even measured in vivo, but the electric currents induced depend on the exact electrical characteristics of the specific tissue involved, which are not known. Hence, the distribution of the induced electric currents that actually depolarize the neurons is inferred from theoretical models and studies in phantoms and animals, which indicate that the currents are primarily parallel to the skull and fall rapidly with depth.

Animal studies indicate that the crucial quantity with respect to neuronal depolarization is the spatial derivative of the electric field along the nerve axon. This finding is consistent with the observation that excitation often originates at bends in fibers, where the spatial derivative of the electric field is large even in a uniform electric field. However, the extrapolation of these observations to humans is still widely debated, and recent studies have demonstrated nerve depolarization with electric fields perpendicular to the nerve fiber.

The most obvious and dangerous side effect of rTMS is the induction of epileptic seizures, and experience shows that currently available equipment is powerful enough to produce them readily. Present knowledge, however, suggests that if seizures are avoided, short-term exposure to rTMS at moderate intensities has no clear lasting adverse effects. In the one known case (Flitman et al. 1998) in which clear adverse effects on cognition were observed below the seizure threshold, the subjects were exposed to prolonged stimulation at high frequency and intensity and a seizure was caused in one subject. Therefore, the thresholds for cognitive deficits and overt seizure may be similar. Animal studies suggest that even with prolonged exposure to high intensities of stimulation, there is little likelihood of structural brain damage. However, in the clinical setting, where potentially therapeutic effects may involve neural reorganization and chronic rTMS exposure may be required, there is the possibility of lasting side effects at moderate combinations of parameter settings. Unfortunately, the potential for such effects and what form they might take are unknown, nor will reliable information be available until large and systematic studies are undertaken.

REFERENCES

Aaronson S, Avery D, Canterbury R, et al: Transcranial magnetic stimulation: effectiveness and safety in a randomized, controlled, multisite clinical trial and an open-label extension study (abstract). Neuropsychopharmacology (in press)

Agnew W, Yuen T, McCreery D: Morphologic change after prolonged electrical stimulation of the cat's cortex at defined charge densities. Exp Neuro 79:397–411, 1983

Amassian VE, Quirk GJ, Stewart M: A comparison of corticospinal activation by magnetic coil and electrical stimulation of monkey motor cortex. Electroencephalogr Clin Neurophysiol 77:390–401, 1990

Amiaz R, Stein O, Schreiber S, et al: Magnetic and seizure thresholds before and after six electroconvulsive treatments. J ECT 17:195–197, 2001

Anderson B, Mishory A, Nahas Z, et al: Tolerability and safety of high daily doses of repetitive transcranial magnetic stimulation in healthy young men. J ECT 22:49–53, 2006

Antal A, Nitsche MA, Kruse W, et al: Direct current stimulation over V5 enhances visuomotor coordination by improving motion perception in humans. J Cogn Neurosci 16:521–527, 2004a

Antal A, Varga ET, Kincses TZ, et al: Oscillatory brain activity and transcranial direct current stimulation in humans. Neuroreport 15:1307–1310, 2004b

Antal A, Varga ET, Nitsche MA, et al: Direct current stimulation over MT+/V5 modulates motion aftereffect in humans. Neuroreport 15:2491–2494, 2004c

Baker KA, DeVos D: Safety considerations with high field MRI. Radiol Technol 67:251–252, 1996

Barker AT, Jalinous R, Freeston IL: Non-invasive magnetic stimulation of the human motor cortex. Lancet 1:1106–1107, 1985

Barker AT, Freeston IL, Jalinous R, et al: Magnetic stimulation of the human brain and peripheral nervous system: an introduction and the results of an initial clinical evaluation. Neurosurgery 20:100–109, 1987

Barker AT, Freeston IL, Jarratt JA, et al: Magnetic stimulation of the human nervous system: an introduction and basic principles, in Magnetic Stimulation in Clinical Neurophysiology. Edited by Chokroverty S. Boston, MA, Butterworths, 1989, pp 55–72

Beer B: Über das Auftreten einer objektiven Lichtempfindung in magnetischen Felde. Klinische Wochenzeitschrift 15:108–109, 1902

Belmaker B, Fitzgerald P, George MS, et al: Managing the risks of repetitive transcranial stimulation. CNS Spectr 8:489, 2003

Bernabeu M, Orient F, Tormos JM, et al: Seizure induced by fast repetitive transcranial magnetic stimulation. Clin Neurophysiol 115:1714–1715, 2004

Bohning DE, Pecheny AP, Epstein CM, et al: In-vivo three dimensional transcranial magnetic stimulation (TMS) field mapping with MRI. Neuroimage 5(suppl):S522, 1997a

Bohning DE, Pecheny AP, Epstein CM, et al: Mapping transcranial magnetic stimulation (TMS) fields in vivo with MRI. Neuroreport 8:2535–2538, 1997b

Bohning DE, Shastri A, Nahas Z, et al: Echoplanar bold fMRI of brain activation induced by concurrent transcranial magnetic stimulation. Invest Radiol 33:336–340, 1998

Bohning DE, He L, George MS, et al: Deconvolution of transcranial magnetic stimulation (TMS) maps. J Neural Transm 108:35–52, 2001

Bohning DE, Denslow S, Bohning PA, et al: Interleaving fMRI and rTMS. Suppl Clin Neurophysiol 56:42–54, 2003a

Bohning DE, Denslow S, Bohning PA, et al: A TMS coil positioning/holding system for MR image–guided TMS interleaved with fMRI. Clin Neurophysiol 114:2210–2219, 2003b

Bridgers SL: The safety of transcranial magnetic stimulation reconsidered: evidence regarding cognitive and other cerebral effects. Electroencephalogr Clin Neurophysiol 43:170–179, 1991

Bridgers SL, Delaney RC: Transcranial magnetic stimulation: an assessment of cognitive and other cerebral effects. Neurology 39:417–419, 1989

Broca P: Sur le siége de la facult du language articulé. Bulletin d'Anthropologie 6:377, 1865

Broca P: Anatomie comparee des circonvolutions cerebrales. Le grand lobe limbique et la scissure limbique dans la serie des mammiferes. Revue d'Anthropologie 1:456–498, 1878

Broca P: Localisations cerebrales: recherches sur les centres olfactifs. Revue d'Anthropologie 2:382–455, 1879

Chen R, Gerloff C, Classen J, et al: Safety of different inter-train intervals for repetitive transcranial magnetic stimulation and recommendations for safe ranges of stimulation parameters. Neurology 48:1398–1403, 1997

Chokroverty S, Shah S, Chokroverty M, et al: Magnetic brain stimulation: safety studies. Electroencephalogr Clin Neurophysiol 97:36–42, 1995

Cohen LG, Roth BJ, Nilsson J, et al: Effects of coil design on delivery of focal magnetic stimulation: technical considerations. Electroencephalogr Clin Neurophysiol 75:350–357, 1990

Conca A, Konig P, Hausmann A: Transcranial magnetic stimulation induces "pseudoabsence seizure." Acta Psychiatr Scand 101:246–248, 2000

Counter SA: Auditory brainstem and cortical responses following extensive transcranial magnetic stimulation. J Neurol Sci 124:163–170, 1994

Counter SA, Borg E, Lofqvist L, et al: Hearing loss from the acoustic artifact of the coil used in extracranial magnetic stimulation. Neurology 40:1159–1162, 1990

Counter SA, Borg E, Lofqvist L: Acoustic trauma in extracranial magnetic brain stimulation. Electroencephalogr Clin Neurophysiol 78:173–184, 1991

Cracco RQ, Amassian VE, Maccabee PJ: Physiological basis of the motor effects of cortical stimulation, I: transcranial electrical stimulation. J Clin Neurophysiol 4:221–222, 1987

Critchley M: Neurology's debt to F. J. Gall (1758–1828). Br Med J 5465:775–781, 1965>

d'Arsonval A: Dispositifs pour la mesure des courants alternatifs de toutes fréquences. CR Societé Biologique (Paris), May 2, 1896, pp 450–451

Davey KR, Epstein CM, George MS, et al: Modeling the effects of electrical conductivity of the head on the induced electrical field in the brain during magnetic stimulation. Clin Neurophysiol 114:2204–2209, 2004

Denslow S, Lomarev M, Bohning DE, et al: A high resolution assessment of the repeatability of relative location and intensity of transcranial magnetic stimulation–induced and volitionally induced blood oxygen level–dependent response in the motor cortex. Cogn Behav Neurol 17:163–173, 2004

Denslow S, Bohning DE, Bohning PA, et al: An increased precision comparison of TMS-induced motor cortex BOLD fMRI response for image-guided versus function-guided coil placement. Cogn Behav Neurol 18:119–127, 2005a

Denslow S, Lomarev M, George MS, et al: Cortical and subcortical brain effects of transcranial magnetic stimulation (TMS)–induced movement: an interleaved TMS/functional magnetic resonance imaging study. Biol Psychiatry 57:752–760, 2005b

Dhuna A, Gates JR, Pascual-Leone A: Induction of seizures but lack of activation of epileptic foci in epileptic patients with rapid transcranial magnetic stimulation (abstract). Ann Neurol 28(suppl):264, 1990

Dunlap K: Visual sensations from the alternating magnetic field. Science 33:68–71, 1911

Faraday M: Effects on the production of electricity from magnetism (1831), in Michael Faraday. Edited by Williams LP. New York, Basic Books, 1965, p 531

Flitman SS, Grafman J, Wassermann EM, et al: Linguistic processing during repetitive transcranial magnetic stimulation. Neurology 50:175–181, 1998

Foerster A, Schmitz JM, Nouri S, et al: Safety of rapid-rate transcranial magnetic stimulation: heart rate and blood pressure changes. Electroencephalogr Clin Neurophysiol 104:207–212, 1997

Gates JR, Dhuna A, Pascual-Leone A: Lack of pathologic changes in human temporal lobes after transcranial magnetic stimulation. Epilepsia 33:504–508, 1992

Geddes LA: History of magnetic stimulation of the nervous system. J Clin Neurophysiol 8:3–9, 1991

Geinisman Y, deToledo ML, Morrell F: Comparison of structural synaptic modifications induced by long-term potentiation in the hippocampal gyrus of young adult and aged rats. Ann NY Acad Sci 747:452–466, 1994

George MS: Stimulating the brain: the emerging new science of electrical brain stimulation. Sci Am 289(3):66–73, 2003

George MS, Nahas Z, Bohning DE, et al: Transcranial magnetic stimulation and neuroimaging, in Transcranial Magnetic Stimulation in Neuropsychiatry. Edited by George MS, Belmaker RH. Washington, DC, American Psychiatric Press, 2000, pp 253–268

George MS, Rush AJ, Sackeim HA, et al: Vagus nerve stimulation (VNS): utility in neuropsychiatric disorders. Int J Neuropsychopharmacol 6:73–83, 2003

Gershon AA, Dannon PN, Grunhaus L: Transcranial magnetic stimulation in the treatment of depression. Am J Psychiatry 160:835–845, 2003

Gordon B, Lesser RP, Rance NE, et al: Parameters for direct cortical electrical stimulation in the human: histopathologic confirmation. Electroencephalogr Clin Neurophysiol 75:371–377, 1990

Heath RG, Mickle WA: Evaluation of seven years experience with depth electrode studies in human patients, in Electrical Studies of the Unanesthetized Brain. Edited by Ramey ER, O'Doherty D. New York, Paul B Hoeber, 1960, pp 214–247D

Heller L, Van Helsteyn DB: Brain stimulation using electromagnetic sources: theoretical aspects. Biophys J 63:129–138, 1992

Hufnagel A, Elger CE, Durwen HF, et al: Activation of the epileptic focus by transcranial magnetic stimulation of the human brain. Ann Neurol 27:49–60, 1990

Hufnagel A, Elger CE, Klingmuller D, et al: Activation of epileptic foci by transcranial magnetic stimulation: effects on secretion of prolactin and luteinizing hormone. J Neurol 237:242–246, 1995

Hughlings-Jackson J: On affections of speech from disease of the brain. Brain 2:202, 1879

Impastato DJ: The story of electroshock treatment. Am J Psychiatry 116:1113–1114, 1960

Jackson JH: Observations on the localisation of movements in the cerebral hemispheres. West Riding Lunatic Asylum Medical Reports 3:175–190, 1873

Jackson JH: On temporary mental disorders after epileptic paroxysms. West Riding Lunatic Asylum Medical Reports 5:103–129, 1874

Jackson JH, Stewart P: Epileptic attacks with a warning of a crude sensation of smell and with the intellectual aura (dreamy state) in a patient who had symptoms pointing to gross organic disease of the right temporo-sphenoidal lobe. Brain 22:534–549, 1899

Jahanshahi M, Profice P, Brown RG, et al: The effects of transcranial magnetic stimulation over the dorsolateral prefrontal cortex on suppression of habitual counting during random number generation. Brain 121:1533–1544, 1998

Ji RR, Schlaepfer TE, Aizenman CD, et al: Repetitive magnetic stimulation activates specific regions in rat brain. Proc Natl Acad Sci USA 95:15635–15640, 1998

Keel JC, Smith MJ, Wassermann EM: A safety screening questionnaire for transcranial magnetic stimulation (letter). Clin Neurophysiol 112:720, 2001

Klawansky S, Yeung A, Berkey C, et al: Meta-analysis of randomized controlled trials of cranial electrostimulation: efficacy in treating selected psychological and physiological conditions. J Nerv Ment Dis 183:478–484, 1995

Kofler M, Leis AA: Safety of transcranial magnetic stimulation in patients with implanted electronic equipment. Electroencephalogr Clin Neurophysiol 107:223–225, 1998

Kolin A, Brill NQ, Broberg PJ: Stimulation of irritable tissues by means of an alternating magnetic field. Proc Soc Exp Biol Med 102:251–253, 1959

Lang N, Nitsche MA, Paulus W, et al: Effects of transcranial direct current stimulation over the human motor cortex on corticospinal and transcallosal excitability. Exp Brain Res 156:439–443, 2004a

Lang N, Siebner HR, Ernst D, et al: Preconditioning with transcranial direct current stimulation sensitizes the motor cortex to rapid-rate transcranial magnetic stimulation and controls the direction of after-effects. Biol Psychiatry 56:634–639, 2004b

Le Bihan D, Mangin JF, Poupon C, et al: Diffusion tensor imaging: concepts and applications. J Magn Reson Imaging 13:534–546, 2001

Li X, Nahas Z, Lomarev M, et al: Prefrontal cortex transcranial magnetic stimulation does not change local diffusion: a magnetic resonance imaging study in patients with depression. Cogn Behav Neurol 16:128–135, 2003

Liebetanz D, Fauser S, Michaelis T, et al: Safety aspects of chronic low-frequency transcranial magnetic stimulation based on localized proton magnetic resonance spectroscopy and histology of the rat brain. J Psychiatr Res 37:277–286, 2003

Lisanby SH, Sackeim HA: Therapeutic brain interventions and the nature of emotion, in The Neuropsychology of Emotion. Edited by Borod J. New York, Oxford University Press, 2000, pp 456–492

Little JT, Kimbrell TA, Wassermann EM, et al: Cognitive effects of 1- and 20-hertz repetitive transcranial magnetic stimulation in depression: preliminary report. Neuropsychiatry Neuropsychol Behav Neurol 13:119–124, 2000

Loo C, Sachdev P, Elsayed H, et al: Effects of a 2- to 4 week course of repetitive transcranial magnetic stimulation on neuropsychological functioning, electroencephalogram, and auditory threshold in depressed patients. Biol Psychiatry 49:615–623, 2001

Magnusson CE, Stevens HC: Visual sensations induced by the changes in the strength of a magnetic field. Am J Physiol 29:124–136, 1911

Matsumiya Y, Yamamoto T, Miyauchi S, et al: Effect of pulsed magnetic stimulation of the head, II: neuropathological changes in the rat (abstract). J Clin Neurophysiol 6:354, 1989

Matsumiya Y, Yamamoto T, Yarita M, et al: Physical and physiological specification of magnetic pulse stimuli that produced cortical damage in rats (abstract). J Clin Neurophysiol 9:287, 1992

Maxwell JC: A dynamical theory of the electromagnetic field. Proc R Soc London 13:531–536, 1863–1864

McCreery DB, Agnew WF, Yuen TGH, et al: Charge density and charge per phase as cofactors in neural injury induced by electrical stimulation. IEEE Trans Biomed Eng 37:996–1001, 1990

McHenry LC: Garrison's History of Neurology. Springfiel, IL, Charles C Thomas, 1969

Mottaghy FM, Gangitano M, Horkan C, et al: Repetitive TMS temporarily alters brain diffusion (see comment). Neurology 60:1539–1541, 2003

Muller K, Kass-Iliyya F, Reitz M: Ontogeny of ipsilateral corticospinal projections: a developmental study with transcranial magnetic stimulation. Ann Neurol 42:705–711, 1997

Nahas Z, Speer AM, Lorberbaum JP, et al: Safety of rTMS: MRI scans before and after 2 weeks of daily left prefrontal rTMS for depression (abstract). Biol Psychiatry 43:95s-#316, 1998

Nahas Z, Bohning DE, Molloy M, et al: Safety and feasibility of repetitive transcranial magnetic stimulation in the treatment of anxious depression in pregnancy. J Clin Psychiatry 60:50–52, 1999

Nahas Z, DeBrux C, Chandler V, et al: Lack of significant changes on magnetic resonance scans before and after 2 weeks of daily left prefrontal repetitive transcranial magnetic stimulation for depression. J ECT 16:380–390, 2000

Nahas Z, Li X, Kozel FA, et al: Safety and benefits of distance-adjusted prefrontal transcranial magnetic stimulation in depressed patients 55–75 years of age: a pilot study. Depress Anxiety 19:249–256, 2004

Nezu A, Kimura S, Uehara S, et al: Magnetic stimulation of motor cortex in children: maturity of corticospinal pathway and problem of clinical application. Brain Dev 19:176–180, 1997

Niehaus L, Meyer BU, Roricht S: Magnetic stimulation over different brain regions: no differential effects on the elicited sympathetic skin responses. Electroencephalogr Clin Neurophysiol 109:94–99, 1998

Nishikiori O: Studies on transcranial magnetic stimulation, Part 2: pathological findings of rabbit brain after long-term stimulation based on characteristics of intracerebral induced voltage. Nippon Ganka Gakkai Zasshi 100:489–495, 1996

Nitsche MA, Niehaus L, Hoffmann KT, et al: MRI study of human brain exposed to weak direct current stimulation of the frontal cortex. Clin Neurophysiol 115:2419–2423, 2004

Pascual-Leone A, Cohen LG, Shotland LI, et al: No evidence of hearing loss in humans due to transcranial magnetic stimulation. Neurology 42:647–651, 1992

Pascual-Leone A, Houser CM, Reese K, et al: Safety of rapid-rate transcranial magnetic stimulation in normal volunteers. Electroencephalogr Clin Neurophysiol 89:120–130, 1993

Penfield W: The Mystery of the Mind: A Critical Study of Consciousness and the Human Brain. Princeton, NJ, Princeton University Press, 1975

Penfield W, Erickson T: Epilepsy and Cerebral Localization. Springfield, IL, Charles C Thomas, 1941

Penfield W, Evans J: The frontal lobe in man: a clinical study of maximum removals. Brain 58:115–133, 1935

Penfield W, Jasper H: Epilepsy and the Functional Anatomy of the Human Brain, 8th Edition. Boston, MA, Little, Brown, 1954

Penfield W, Perot P: The brain's record of auditory and visual experience: a final summary and discussion. Brain 86:595–696, 1963

Penfield W, VonSantha K, Cipriani A: Cerebral blood flow during induced epileptiform seizures in animals and man. J Neurophysiol 2:257–267, 1939

Polk C, Postow E: CRC Handbook of Biological Effects of Electromagnetic Fields. Boca Raton, FL, CRC Press, 1986

Pridmore S, Filho JAF, Nahas Z, et al: Motor threshold in transcranial magnetic stimulation: a comparison of a neurophysiological and a visualization of movement method. J ECT 14:25–27, 1998

Ravnborg M, Knudsen GM, Blinkenberg M: No effect of pulsed magnetic stimulation on the blood-brain barrier in rats. Neuroscience 38:277–280, 1990

Rogalewski A, Breitenstein C, Nitsche MA, et al: Transcranial direct current stimulation disrupts tactile perception. Eur J Neurosci 20:313–316, 2004

Rossini PM, Barker AT, Berardelli A, et al: Non-invasive electrical and magnetic stimulation of the brain, spinal cord and roots: basic principles and procedures for routine clinical application: report of an IFCN committee. Electroencephalogr Clin Neurophysiol 91:79–92, 1994

Roth BJ, Cohen LG, Hallett M: The electric field induced during magnetic stimulation, in Magnetic Motor Stimulation: Basic Principles and Clinical Experience (EEG Suppl 43). Edited by Lecy WJ, Cracco RQ, Barker AT, et al: Amsterdam, Elsevier Science, 1991, pp 268–278

Roth BJ, Pascual-Leone A, Cohen LG, et al: The heating of metal electrodes during rapid-rate magnetic stimulation: a possible safety hazard. Electroencephalogr Clin Neurophysiol 85:116–123, 1992

Roth Y, Zangen A, Voller B, et al: Transcranial magnetic stimulation of deep brain regions: evidence for efficacy of the H-coil. Clin Neurophysiol 116:775–779, 2005

Sackeim HA, Prudic J, Devanand DP, et al: Effects of stimulus intensity and electrode placement on the efficacy and cognitive effects of electroconvulsive therapy. N Engl J Med 328:839–846, 1993

Sgro JA, Ghatak NR, Stanton PC, et al: Repetitive high magnetic field stimulation: the effect upon rat brain. Electroencephalogr Clin Neurophysiol Suppl 43:180–185, 1991

Sommer M, Paulus W: Pulse configuration and rTMS efficacy: a review of clinical studies. Electroencephalogr Clin Neurophysiol Suppl 56:33–41, 2003

Thompson SP: A physiological effect of an alternating magnetic field. Proceedings of the Royal Society of London Series B 82(557):396–399, 1910

Triggs WJ, McCoy KJ, Greer R, et al: Effects of left frontal transcranial magnetic stimulation on depressed mood, cognition, and corticomotor threshold. Biol Psychiatry 45:1440–1446, 1999

Wagner TA, Zahn M, Grodzinsky AJ, et al: Three-dimensional head model simulation of TMS. IEEE Transactions on Biomedical Engineering 51:1586–1597, 2004

Wassermann EM: Risk and safety of repetitive transcranial magnetic stimulation: report and suggested guidelines from the International Workshop in the Safety of Repetitive Transcranial Magnetic Stimulation, June 5–7, 1996. Electroencephalogr Clin Neurophysiol 108:1–16, 1998

Wassermann EM: Variation in the response to transcranial magnetic brain stimulation in the general population. Clin Neurophysiol 113:1165–1171, 2002

Wassermann EM, Grafman J, Berry C, et al: Use and safety of a new repetitive transcranial magnetic stimulator. Electroencephalogr Clin Neurophysiol 101:412–417, 1996

2

METHODS OF ADMINISTERING TRANSCRANIAL MAGNETIC STIMULATION

Ziad Nahas, M.D., M.S.C.R.
F. Andrew Kozel, M.D., M.S.C.R.
Christine Molnar, Ph.D.
David Ramsey, M.S.
Richard Holt, M.D.
Raffaella Ricci, Ph.D.
Kevin A. Johnson, B.E.
Jejo Koola, B.S.
Mark S. George, M.D.

In light of the growing interest in using transcranial magnetic stimulation (TMS) in a variety of experimental and therapeutic settings, the International Society of Transcranial Stimulation (ISTS) recognized the need to formulate a consensus statement to assist the field in developing guidelines for its safe application. Repetitive TMS (rTMS) may provoke a seizure (see Chapter 1, "Overview of Transcranial Magnetic Stimulation," in this volume, for more details). The risk of a seizure is in part related to certain central nervous system pathologies and/or concomitant psychotropic drugs (Wassermann 1998). Use of treatment parameters that exceed the dose parameter guidelines summarized in the published 1998 National Institute of Neurological Disorders and Stroke workshop report (discussed in Chapter 1), may also increase the potential risk of seizure.

In the summer of 2002, the ISTS issued a consensus statement on managing the risks of rTMS (Belmaker et al. 2003; available online at http://www.ists.unibe.ch/consensus.html). It is recommended that rTMS should only be administered in a medical setting where a procedure for seizure management and basic life support can be instituted. In addition, rTMS administration should also be done with the direct involvement and supervision of a licensed physician knowledgeable in the technology and fully trained in neurology, psychiatry, or another appropriate specialty. rTMS administrators should be skilled in assessing the risk factors for the procedure and be trained in recognizing and carrying out first-line management of an epileptic seizure. Finally, the use of rTMS should comply with regulations put forward by local regulatory bodies, medical professional organizations, and medical licensing boards.

TMS is particularly attractive to probe various aspects of brain function, as it has minimal side effects. Research studies should be approved by local ethics committees. In addition, rTMS is under investigation as a potential treatment for various neurological and psychiatric disorders (George et al. 1999). Two large multicenter clinical trials in depression are currently under way.

Other chapters in this volume cover non-invasive ways for TMS to induce electrical currents in the outermost cortex (Cohen et al. 1990; Rothwell et al. 1991), as well as clinical and research applications of this technique. In this chapter we aim at detailing the practical use of TMS in research and, potentially, clinical settings by discussing various procedural steps. Such a discussion can serve as a general guide for safe and proper administration of this technology.

TMS MACHINES

All TMS machines share a common principle, although different manufacturers have implemented specifications that facilitate certain uses. As outlined in the discussion of the physics of TMS in Chapter 1, the console consists of a power supply, a single large capacitor for energy storage, and a triggering component that allows the charge stored on the capacitor to discharge. An inductive coil that receives the stored energy is attached to the console (Barker et al. 1985). There are two types of stimulators: single-pulse (primarily used for cortical mapping and electrophysiological studies) and rTMS devices that can deliver trains of stimuli to up to 60 hertz and rely on biphasic pulse of 200–300 microseconds in duration for rapid recharge of the capacitors. Because it is known that the frequency of stimulation can modulate the underlying activity of the stimulated brain region and its connected network, rTMS devices are the ones used in neuropsychiatric clinical research. The rapid discharge of close to 500 joules makes the coil casing expand and is responsible for the loud "popping" noise heard with each stimulus. The focality or precision of the magnetic field depends on the geometry and design of the coil. It is seldom less than 1 cm². The design of the coil also determines the degree of heat dissipation and thus the overheating of the coil itself. For the coil not to become a safety hazard, the temperature of the portion of the coil touching the scalp should not exceed 41°C. Repeated overheating could also lead to a rapid deterioration of the equipment. Most devices rely on built-in temperature sensors in the coil to interrupt the device in case of overheating. Some also use either air or liquid cooling to extend the length of the operation. Although such equipment is useful, it can also be cumbersome. One coil design, the iron core, is energy efficient and does not require any cooling.

As of November 2005, at least six companies manufacture TMS devices (Table 2–1). The Dantec and Magstim machines have add-on modules to their single-pulse devices that can be used to drive one coil with two to four pulses separated by 1 millisecond to 1 second. These devices are called *paired-pulse* or *quadruple-pulse* stimulators. In addition, two stimulator units can be used together to drive separate coils to stimulate different regions at the same time or in quick succession. This TMS mode is called *double-pulse* TMS. Not all manufacturers offer these options.

TMS PROTOCOLS

General Set-up

Unlike electroconvulsive therapy (Fink 1984), TMS and rTMS administration does not require general anesthesia. Absolute contraindications include the presence of ferromagnetic material anywhere in the head (excluding the mouth). This material includes, but is not limited to, devices such as cochlear implants, implanted brain stimulators or electrodes, aneurysm clips, and plates or screws. The presence of intracardiac lines also excludes subjects from receiving TMS because of the risk of creating a ground path for current produced by the stimulator.

In addition, increased intracranial pressure, severe cardiovascular disease, and other serious medical conditions require a careful assessment of the risk-benefit ratio given the potentially serious medical or neurological consequences in the event of seizure after rTMS.

Once subjects have signed informed consent and are carefully screened for any risks to undergo the procedure, sessions can be initiated according to specific protocols. A commonly used screening tool is the Transcranial Magnetic Stimulation Adult Safety Screen (TASS; Keel et al. 2000) (reproduced in the appendix to this chapter). There are, however, general guidelines that may be applicable in most

Table 2–1. Manufacturers of transcranial magnetic stimulation devices (as of November 2005)

- Magstim Company Ltd. (Whitland, Carmarthenshire, Wales, UK)
- Medtronic Dantec NeuroMuscular (Skovlunde, Denmark)
- Neuronetics Inc. (Malvern, PA)
- MAG&More GmbH (Munich, Germany)
- CR Tech (Haifa, Israel)
- Mcube Technology Co. Ltd. (Seoul, South Korea)

cases. It all starts with the manner by which the subject is greeted. In double-blind studies, it is advised that the TMS operator limit the initial interaction with the subject in order to minimize any subtle transferences and countertransferences that could ultimately influence the outcome of the study (Tetreault and Bordeleau 1971). The operator should start by asking about specific events that may affect the motor threshold (sleep hours, drinking of caffeinated beverage, taking of extra medications or new medications such as benzodiazepines, anticonvulsants, antipsychotics, or antidepressants). If a subject starts to discuss events related to his or her current condition and to explore social or psychological stressors, and the research protocol dictates it, the TMS operator will be empathic and refer the subject to the clinician assigned to his or her case. Otherwise, appropriate clinical management and attention to the subject's concerns and potential side effects take precedence over any procedure. Subjects are also asked to remove any ferromagnetic items that could come in close contact with the coil (particularly hair pins, clips, and earrings). These items are stored in a safe location away from the TMS coil until the end of the session.

When ready, the subject is then invited to sit in a chair. The back can be reclined for comfort. Some manufacturers have designed a special TMS chair with a headrest that is used for accurate repositioning of the TMS coil from session to session. The headrest also acts as a soft restraint that limits head movement. Other set-ups include a TMS coil holder that can be fixed in a rigid position and monitored to ensure continuous scalp-coil contact across long sessions. In settings where a stereotactic frame is used for immobilization of the head, the subject will rest his or her chin on the frame, with head and shoulders slightly leaning forward, and the height of the frame is adjusted so that the subject will be comfortable for the length of the session (see photo of subject in Figure 2–1, far right).

The subjects and TMS operators should wear earplugs of 30-decibel or greater noise reduction rating. In some settings, a swim cap can allow one to outline the TMS coil position and aid in its placement in each session for each subject.

Subjects undergoing the TMS procedure are alert and, depending on the type of study or treatment involved, can be instructed to perform a particular task during the session. Until now, there has been little experience in delivering TMS while subjects are asleep, with some researchers noting a possible change in cortical excitability during sleep (Salih et al. 2005). In treatment studies, subjects are often encouraged to relax but typically are prevented from falling asleep.

Motor Threshold Determination

When a TMS coil is discharged over the motor cortex, corticospinal neurons can be activated both pre- and (at higher stimulus intensity) postsynaptically (Hallett 2000; Ziemann and Hallett 2000). These neurons project directly to motor neurons, and the resulting descending volley can cause particular targeted muscles to twitch. The visible twitch is associated with a compound muscle action potential or *motor evoked potential* (MEP). The MEP can also be recorded by using surface electrodes applied to the skin overlying the muscle. The latency (time between TMS and onset of MEP), motor threshold (MT; the minimum TMS intensity necessary to evoke a MEP), and size of the MEP can be measured. The MEP size relates to the number of motor neurons activated in the muscle and, in turn, to the magnitude of the descending neuronal volley from the brain. The size can be affected by many factors, including the brain's excitability and the degree to which the descending pathways in the spinal cord are damaged.

Since few stimulated cortical areas other than motor cortex are associated with easily observable phenomena, it is the determination of the MT—the minimum energy needed to observe an abductor pollicis brevis (APB) contraction—that gives a relative indicator of the general cortical excitability and is used as a reference for subsequent applications. So, before any experiment or treatment session, an MT of the dominant hand should always be determined. Because it is believed that MT is relatively stable over time, it is customary to only do a full determination once every 1–2 weeks. The MT can be determined in two ways: 1) visual determination, in which the APB contraction is defined as a minimal twitch of the muscle (and not simply an overt movement of the thumb) and 2) MEP recording.

MEP Recording

Surface electromyographic activity is measured in the relaxed APB. To prepare the hand surface before electrodes are affixed, the skin surface is mildly abraded with alcohol wipes and allowed to dry. Disposable and pre-gelled electrodes (i.e.: Nicolet 20 × 25 mm Ag-AgCl) are used to record electromyographic activity and are placed over the region of the APB belly and associated tendon. A 40 × 50 mm pregelled Ag-AgCl ground electrode is also placed on the back of the hand and calf. The three-electrode leads measure 1 meter and are braided to reduce noise associated with lead movement. If other cortical excitability measures are to be obtained (see below), each subject will have the same electrodes for the full day to minimize variability in signal detection. The conversion of MEP signal from analog to digital requires a set of filters specific to each electromyographic device.

Motor Threshold Algorithms

Historically, MT is usually defined as the minimum TMS intensity needed to produce a peak-to-peak MEP of at least 50 μV, when measured by surface electromyography (EMG), during half of a specified number of trials. It is predominantly a measure of membrane excitability in cortical-cortical and thalamo-cortical fibers, yet it also involves other central fibers as well as peripheral fibers. As mentioned before, MT and cortical excitability are affected by medications that influence sodium and calcium channels.

Recently, measurement of MT has been automated and is determined by using a new procedure, the *best parameter estimation by sequential testing* (BEST PEST) method (Awiszus 2003). This method relies on an empirically supported and validated algorithm that was designed to determine MT more accurately and rapidly than do other existing methods. The BEST PEST algorithm can also be integrated into an interactive EMG computer software program using scripting language (Mishory et al. 2004). This program processes data from surface electromyographic recordings and instantaneously computes whether or not peak-to-peak electromyographic activity occurs within an acceptable latency post-TMS (i.e., not before 20 msec) and is of sufficient amplitude to qualify as a response (i.e., is greater than or equal to 50 μV (i.e., response). On the basis of this criterion, the intensity of TMS administration is automatically adjusted until MT is determined with the BEST PEST algorithm. This method does not rely on a criterion that requires that a response be obtained during half of a specified number of trials; rather, it is based on a mathematical function that describes the relationship between TMS intensity and probable MT values. Once the MT is determined, this information is used to administer TMS.

TMS Coil Placement

Before the MT determination proceeds, the optimal location for stimulus induction (the location that gives the maximum MEP amplitude for a specific muscle being investigated) should first be identified. At this location the TMS coil will be fixed firmly in place; the anterior pole of the TMS coil should be referenced with a mark on the scalp. It is important to note that moving the TMS coil slightly might still cause a depolarization of the APB area in the motor cortex but may not be the optimal spot with the minimal needed intensity.

To find the hand area of the motor cortex and to orient the figure-eight TMS coil optimally, the operator initially positions the center of the magnet 5 cm lateral to the vertex on the interauricular line and angles the handle 45 degrees away from the sagittal plane. An active muscle will have a lower MT, and so it may help initially to ask the subject to tense up his or her thumb while searching for the optimal location.

In some instances, the anterior tibialis muscle in the leg is used. Since the leg cortical representation is situated medially, it is often difficult to elicit a muscle contraction with regular figure-eight coils. In finding the leg area of the motor cortex, it is recommended that a double-cone TMS coil be used, with the center of the magnet initially positioned over the vertex on the interauricular line and the handle angled 0 degrees from the sagittal and coronal planes.

Once the subject is prepared and instructed to rest the arm on a flat surface at hip level, with the palm fully supported, the MT determination can proceed. The relaxed right index finger should be visible to the TMS operator.

Resting MT Determination

During determination of a resting MT (RMT) (Figure 2–1), the interpulse interval (IPI) is varied between 3 and 5 seconds to avoid conditioned responses to the sound of the TMS device. It is important to vary the IPI in this way because a continuous stimulation at a rate of 1 per second will increase the MT and thus falsely lead to a higher estimation (Fitzgerald et al. 2002). If the coil has to be moved away from the scalp, the TMS operator can use the mark on the scalp to relocate the exact position of the TMS coil. Once the RMT is calculated, the program pauses and waits for input from the experimenter to resume.

It should be noted that the MT will be markedly different if the studied muscle group is not at rest (Yahagi et al. 2003; Ziemann 2003). In fact, it is often easier, when looking for the optimal spot to induce contralateral muscle contraction, to ask the subject to "tense up your muscle." The threshold will be lower and the muscle contraction will be more visible. It has also been demonstrated that thinking on one's own about muscle movement also lowers the MT, as if the cortex were already primed and "ready to go."

Prefrontal rTMS for Clinical Treatments of Depression

Standard Method

The standard method adopted by many researchers in clinical trials originated back in 1994 (George and Wassermann 1994). Knowing that the prefrontal cortex is highly connected to limbic and mood regulating subcortical regions, George and Wasserman used a probabilistic brain atlas to determine an approximate method to reach the prefrontal cortex relative to the motor cortex where TMS can elicit an observable effect. This method has proven very practical, although, with different brain and skull sizes, it has been shown inadequate for at least one-third of stimulated subjects, in whom it leads to stimulating the frontal eye field or premotor associative area (Herwig et al. 2002). To define the left dorsolateral site of stimulation, the TMS operator measures 5 cm forward in a parasagittal plane from the motor threshold landmark. The TMS coil is then mounted on a TMS holder

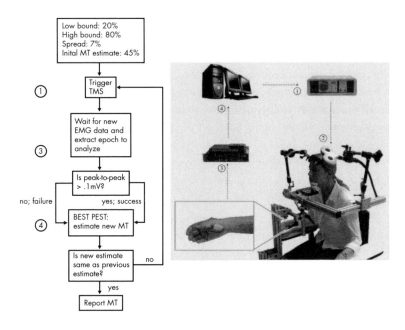

Figure 2–1. Setup for automated determination of resting motor threshold (RMT) by means of maximum-likelihood strategy using parameter estimation by sequential testing (MLS-PEST) and motor evoked potential–electromyography (MEP-EMG).

This flow diagram indicates the setup for determining motor threshold via MLS-PEST using automated electromyographic capture and analysis. Numbered steps in the control flow diagram (*left*) correspond to the hardware diagram (*right*). Initial parameters are fed into the control program and the TMS generator is triggered (1). The attached TMS coil is placed over the scalp position controlling movement in the contralateral dominant hand. (2) The subject pictured is a research assistant in the Medical University of South Carolina Brain Stimulation Laboratory. Electromyographic lead placement for the abductor pollicis brevis recording can be seen in the inset. The electromyography hardware (3) records muscle activity triggered by the TMS machine and records and processes the electromyographic data. The computer workstation (4) then calculates the peak-to-peak voltage of the MEP and passes the result to the MLS-PEST module, which determines a new TMS generator output on the basis of whether the current pulse produced a suprathreshold electromyogram. The cycle then repeats itself until the RMT is found—a process that typically takes less than 30 seconds.

Source. Reprinted from Mishory A, Molnar C, Koola J, et al.: "The Maximum-Likelihood Strategy for Determining Transcranial Magnetic Stimulation Motor Threshold, Using Parameter Estimation by Sequential Testing Is Faster Than Conventional Methods With Similar Precision." *Journal of ECT* 20:160–165, 2004. Copyright 2004 Lippincott Williams & Wilkins. Used with permission.

and positioned in place for stimulation, with the angles adjusted slightly to maintain good surface contact with the scalp while the coil's original anterior posterior orientation is maintained. The TMS machine is off during this time. The back of the TMS chair may be adjusted slightly to facilitate this maneuver. The use of a swim cap or other external markers may facilitate the set-up when subjects return for subsequent visits without having to reassess the motor threshold and remeasure this distance. It remains to be determined whether this variability in the prefrontal placement offers an advantage or disadvantage in the absence of an optimal cortical target for different treatment applications. Even when an external landmark is used, it is advised to repeat the whole procedure once every 1–2 weeks.

Before starting the treatment session, the TMS operator ensures that all the parameters and settings are correct. He or she then notifies the subject when the treatment will begin by indicating the time on the watch facing the TMS chair. The TMS operator also informs the subject of the frequency and duration of each train and how often it is repeated, then starts the session after a countdown. This helps reduce the anticipatory anxiety for each train. In research protocols, the TMS operator is advised to minimize any interactions with the subject. The operator should respond to questions about the pain perceived and explain that usually a tolerance is built to these sensations. Other chapters in this volume detail the current clinical findings on stimulation parameters, including session duration and length of treatments.

Stereotactic Positioning

To the extent that the TMS delivery needs to be individualized for each subject's own anatomy or underlying brain activity, the TMS coil placement can be guided stereotactically (Schonfeldt-Lecuona et al. 2005). This procedure, like the one used in neurosurgery but with accuracies not in the tenths-of-millimeter range and much more affordable, allows the registration of the subject's anatomy in space and a simultaneous display of the TMS coil and putative targeting site on a computer screen. The set-up utilizes a specially designed frame and an infrared-based tracking system with associated software (Figure 2–2). Brainsight software (Rogue Research Inc., Montreal, Quebec, Canada) allows registration and online monitoring of the head position with respect to the structural brain image and can track the position of the coil with respect to the underlying brain structures. Brain function, probed by means of imaging while the subject is performing a specific mental task or is at rest, can also be imported and merged onto a subject's own anatomical scan. This elaborate methodology is currently used in brain mapping and neuroscientific research (Paus 2001), but it has not yet been determined whether it yields higher efficacy when applied in the clinical treatment of depression.

Because the high variability of cortical anatomy among individuals makes it difficult to identify specific cortical structures on MRI scans with tools like Brain-

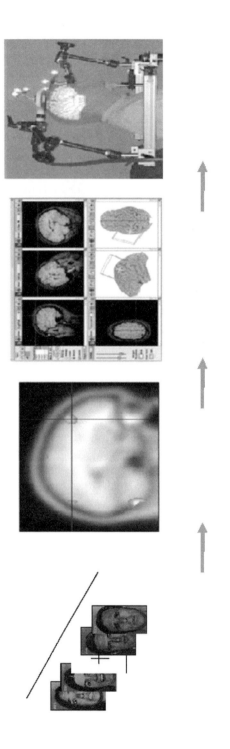

Figure 2–2. An illustration of using functional brain imaging results from an emotion-provocation paradigm and stereotactic transcranial magnetic stimulation (TMS).

The functional magnetic resonance imaging (MRI) individual statistical maps are imported and merged onto a high-resolution structural MRI scan with Brain-sight. After co-registration of the subject's images with his or her real location, a real-time visualization of TMS targets can be displayed, and the functional brain imaging results can be used to finalize the targeting location.

sight, we recently developed an automated method, Target-TMS, by which a structural brain MRI is piped through a local area network (LAN) and automatically transformed into a common brain space (Montreal Neurological Institute [MNI] template) based on normative data from 300 individuals (Figure 2–3). A reverse transformation is then applied to the MNI template, co-registered, and displayed via modified Register software (McGill University, Montreal, Quebec). A probabilistic tag of M1 cortical area (site for MT determination), along with other probabilistic Brodmann areas, is also displayed. A vector, with the shortest distance from cortex target to skull, is computed. Thus, for any given target, the coordinates are translated into a custom-built coil positioner or imported into Brainsight. Although this methodology is not solely based on individual anatomy, it allows one to reduce the error in coil placement and provides more likely accurate stimulation of an intended area as opposed to the 5-centimeter rule (see Chapter 9, "Transcranial Magnetic Stimulation and Brain Imaging," in this volume).

Electroencephalographic Method

TMS coil positioning can also utilize the International 10–20 system (Jasper 1958), which is commonly used for electroencephalographic electrode placement and for correlating external skull locations to underlying cortical areas. The system is based on the identification of anatomical landmarks such as nasion, inion, and preauricular points, with consecutive placement of the electrodes at fixed distances from these points in steps of 10% or 20%, to take into consideration variations of head size. The 10–20 system is easy and practical to use and is less expensive than the neuroimaging-based methodologies. F3 and F4 positions are thought to be landmarks for dorsolateral prefrontal cortex. But other landmarks can also help locate parietal, temporal, or other cortical regions. Herwig and colleagues (2003) suggest that this method yields about 20 mm in location variability, which may lead to targeting of neighboring Brodmann areas in about 10% of individuals with likely different functionality. It may still be a better approach to positioning the TMS than the "5-cm rule" but requires more preparation. In targeting the left dorsolateral prefrontal cortex, or Brodmann areas 9 and 46, respectively, Herwig et al. recommend guiding the coil placement by measuring from F3 (F4 right-sided) 1 cm in an anterolateral direction, or alternatively targeting the midpoint of the triangle between F3, F7, and Fp1.

Intensity Adjustments

In all TMS depression studies so far, the intensity of stimulation for each individual subject has been delivered on the basis of the individual subject's MT. With this approach it is also assumed that cortical areas other than motor cortex will respond similarly at a given MT. Our group has been invested in exploring the relationship among the distance from scalp to targeted cortical area, clinical response,

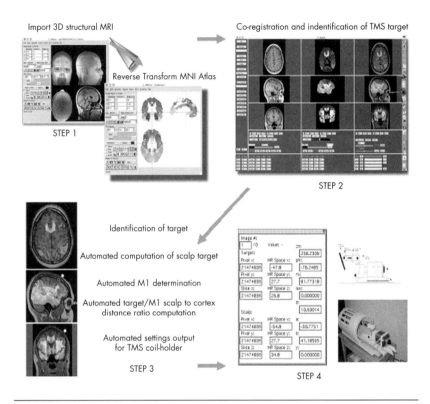

Import 3D structural MRI

Reverse Transform MNI Atlas

STEP 1

Co-registration and indentification of TMS target

STEP 2

Identification of target

Automated computation of scalp target

Automated M1 determination

Automated target/M1 scalp to cortex distance ratio computation

Automated settings output for TMS coil-holder

STEP 3

STEP 4

Figure 2–3.   Target-TMS, a method for final determination of target coordinates to be translated into a TMS-coil holder's articulations for accurate localization.

(1) A structural brain magnetic resonance image is piped through a local area network and automatically transformed into a common brain space (MNI template) based on normative data from 300 individuals. (2) A reverse transformation is then applied to the MNI template, co-registered, and displayed with modified Register software. (3) A probabilistic tag of M1 cortical area (site for motor threshold determination), along with other probabilistic Brodmann areas, is also displayed. A vector, with the shortest distance from cortex target to skull, is computed. (4) For any given target, the coordinates are translated into a custom-built coil positioner or imported into Brainsight.

and cortical excitability. This distance can be a major confound, since the intensity of the magnetic field drops off logarithmically as a function of distance from the coil and thus may lead to differential biological effects. We obtained brain magnetic resonance imaging (MRI) scans on subjects enrolled in rTMS clinical trials for depression and measured the distance from scalp to cortex at the site of stimulation (Kozel et al. 2000). We found that both motor and prefrontal cortex distance increased with age (as a function of atrophy), with prefrontal distance increasing at a faster rate. With adjunctive single-photon emission computed to-mography (SPECT) or interleaved TMS functional MRI scanning, we also found a negative correlation between regional cerebral activity underneath the TMS coil and prefrontal distance (Nahas et al. 2001) (i.e., the greater the distance from scalp to brain, the smaller the TMS-induced changes in blood flow). Another group has confirmed that increased prefrontal distance is associated with a poorer antidepressant response (Mosimann et al. 2002).

In measuring the relative distance from skull to motor cortex and skull to prefrontal cortex (or any other brain surface region) and possibly adjusting the stimulation intensity, different quantitative analysis methods can be used. One is based on the fiducial placement over the targeted area prior to obtaining the structural MRI scan, and the other on a standardized distance from the corpus callosum for each individual. A third method relies on the probabilistic Target-TMS placement method described earlier and an automated assessment of the shortest distance from skull to cortex. These measurements could later be used to determine the delivered TMS intensity. The formula used ($Sx = MT \cdot Exp[0.036 \cdot (dx - dm)]$, where dx is distance to target and dm is distance to motor, both in mm) assumes that the effective stimulation intensity (Sx) is proportional to the magnetic field measured at the center of the coil and has the same rate of exponential decrease with distance (Bohning 2000; Bohning et al. 1997).

It should be noted that because the average prefrontal-to-motor ratio rarely exceeds 1.2 (Nahas et al. 2001), it may be sufficient to stimulate the prefrontal cortex in depression trials at 120% of MT and assume that most of the subjects will receive a minimum intensity presumed adequate to depolarize underlying neurons.

Additional Measures of Nervous System Excitability

Aside from MT determination, other measures of motor cortex excitability can be used in a research setting using TMS and surface EMG. Measures include the cortical silent period (CSP) and the recruitment curve (RC) and paired-pulse (PP). Each measure of cortical excitability provides unique information about the neurophysiology associated with excitability of the central, and in some cases peripheral, nervous system (Ziemann and Hallett 2000; see Chapter 3, "Basic Neurophysiological Studies With Transcranial Magnetic Stimulation," in this volume) MT, as discussed earlier, is predominantly a measure of membrane excitability in cortico-cortical and thalamo-cortical fibers, yet it also involves other central as well as peripheral fibers. CSP is an interruption of voluntary activity that follows TMS that is delivered during a sustained contraction that is between 10% and 20% of a maximal contraction force. Intensity of TMS delivered to determine CSP is based on an individual's unique MT. CSP is a measure of exclusively cortico-cortical inhibition and can be influenced by factors that do not influence the

MT. RCs also rely on TMS that is based on an individual's MT and can be determined at rest and during voluntary muscle contraction. The RC is an index of the MEP facilitation that lowers MT values associated with muscle contraction. The RC is also an index of global corticospinal excitability that can be influenced by factors that do not influence the MT.

Cortical Silent Period

The subject is instructed to use the thumb and index finger to squeeze a dynamometer that records the maximum force of contraction. The dynamometer rests on a surface as this occurs. A visible needle that marks 30% of this force is set, and the participant is asked to deliver a constant 30% force while 10 TMS pulses are delivered at 120% of RMT with an IPI ranging from 3 to 5 seconds. This variable IPI is typically chosen to avoid conditioned responses and represents a further methodological refinement. The CSP region is marked on the electromyogram by activity in specific frequency bands that are prominent in the pre-trigger and post-CSP periods. Once the likely CSP region is identified, the slope of each segment of this region, and areas before and after it, are calculated, and when this slope exceeds a tolerable range, a marker is placed to mark the beginning and end of the CSP (Figure 2–4).

Recruitment Curve

Relaxation phase.   Typically RC data are acquired from use of six intensities of rTMS beginning at a setting 5% (of the maximal stimulator output of 100) below RMT and increasing in increments of 5% of maximal machine output until an intensity 20% above the RMT intensity setting is reached. At each intensity setting, six pulses are delivered consecutively, with an intertrain interval of 3–5 seconds, and then the next intensity setting is administered.

Contraction phase.   The subject is instructed to contract at 30% of maximal force, and six pulses are delivered at each of the same six TMS intensity levels, beginning 5% below RMT and ending 20% above RMT. The maximum peak-to-peak values for each pulse are often averaged across the six trials for each intensity setting and then plotted as a function of intensity and fit to a sigmoidal curve, from which is derived the slope, plateau, and other descriptive parameters.

Paired Pulse

With paired-pulse TMS, one delivers a normal TMS pulse preceded by a brief pre-pulse. This pre-pulse, depending on its intensity and timing relative to the later pulse, can either abolish or augment the normal motor response elicited by TMS (MEP). The MEP in this case is reduced when the interstimulus interval is 1–4 milliseconds and increased when it is 5–30 milliseconds, a pattern reflecting

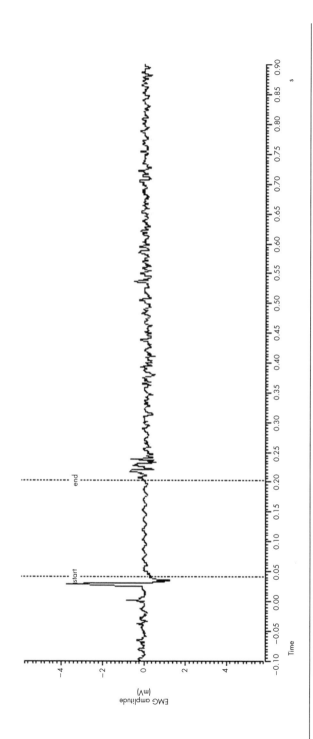

Figure 2–4. A cortical silent period (CSP) documented with electromyography.

Note the initial artifact generated by the TMS pulse, the active motor evoked potential shortly afterward, and the subsequent "quieting" of background activity recorded from the abductor pollicis brevis during active use of that muscle group.

intracortical inhibition and facilitation. Paired-pulse TMS is thus thought to be a tool for investigating local inhibition and excitation paths within motor cortex, often referred to as *intracortical inhibition* (ICI) and *intracortical facilitation* (ICF).

Seizure Management

It is of particular importance that sites in which rTMS is administered have a plan in place for the management of seizures. Until the safety of any specific stimulation regimen is firmly established, the plan should include the presence of medical personnel at all time with basic life support (BLS) or advanced cardiac life support (ACLS) accreditation, and the maintenance of emergency equipment and medication close by. This equipment should include a crash cart, an oxygen supply, and access to a phone to call for assistance if necessary.

Treatment of provoked seizures in otherwise healthy individuals should consist primarily of getting the patient onto his or her side on a flat surface away from sharp edges, managing the airway, gaining venous access, and providing oxygen. If the patient is having a grand mal seizure, the administering clinician should stand by him or her for a few minutes until the thrashing subsides, to guard against injury or airway obstruction. Usually only suctioning or turning the patient on his or her side is required, but breathing will be uncoordinated until the tonic-clonic phase is over. Once the patient is lying on the floor and is in a safe position, and if the clinician administering TMS is alone, the clinician should call for assistance. Each laboratory should have a number clearly posted. The clinician should watch the pattern of the seizure for clues to the etiology. Did a clonus start in one place and "march" out to the rest of the body? Did the eyes deviate one way throughout the seizure? Did the whole body participate? If the seizure lasts more than 2 minutes or recurs before the patient regains consciousness, drugs may be required to stop the seizure. (To the best of our knowledge, this has never happened in an accidental rTMS-induced seizure.) Such a seizure event, referred to as *status epilepticus,* is best treated with diazepam (Valium) 5-10 mg iv, followed by gradual loading with intravenous phenytoin.

After the seizure is over, the patient should be examined thoroughly for injuries, and a complete neurological examination should be done. Although the history of prior seizures is exclusionary, recheck with the patient for a previous history of seizure disorder, check old records, speak to his or her physician, find out whether he or she has been worked up for an etiology, and look for reasons for the relapse (e.g., infection, ethanol, lack of sleep). If the seizure is a new event, the clinician should make arrangements and consult with a neurologist to determine any need for further workup. It is important to remember not to stick anything in the mouth of a seizing patient. The ubiquitous padded throat sticks may serve as something for the patient to hold onto and bite on at the first sign of a seizure but do nothing to protect the airway and are ineffective when the jaw is clenched. Also, the clinician managing the adverse event should not rush to give intravenous diazepam to a seizing patient. Most seizures stop in a few minutes. It is diagnostically useful to see how the seizure resolves on its own. Also, the patient will awaken sooner if he or she has not been medicated. Diazepam should be reserved for genuine status epilepticus. Once the event has resolved, a seizure victim should not drive home. In addition, the seizure event should be reported to the local regulatory bodies and the TMS research community by contacting the ISTS.

REFERENCES

Awiszus F: TMS and threshold hunting. Suppl Clin Neurophysiol 56:13–23, 2003

Barker AT, Jalinous R, Freeston IL: Non-invasive magnetic stimulation of the human motor cortex. Lancet 1:1106–1107, 1985

Belmaker B, Fitzgerald P, George MS, et al: Managing the risks of repetitive transcranial stimulation. CNS Spectr 8:489, 2003

Bohning DE: Introduction and overview of TMS physics, in Transcranial Magnetic Stimulation in Neuropsychiatry. Edited by George MS, Belmaker RH. Washington, DC, American Psychiatric Press, 2000, pp 13–44

Bohning DE, Pecheny AP, Epstein CM, et al: Mapping transcranial magnetic stimulation (TMS) fields in vivo with MRI. Neuroreport 8:2535–2538, 1997

Cohen LG, Roth BJ, Nilsson J, et al: Effects of coil design on delivery of focal magnetic stimulation: technical considerations. Electroencephalo Clin Neurophysiol 75:350–357, 1990

Fink M: Meduna and the origins of convulsive therapy. Am J Psychiatry 141:1034–1141, 1984

Fitzgerald PB, Brown TL, Daskalakis ZJ, et al: Intensity-dependent effects of 1 Hz rTMS on human corticospinal excitability. Clin Neurophysiol 113:1136–1141, 2002

George MS, Wassermann EM: Rapid-rate transcranial magnetic stimulation (rTMS) and ECT. Convuls Ther 10:251–253, 1994

George MS, Lisanby SH, Sackeim HA: Transcranial magnetic stimulation: applications in neuropsychiatry. Arch Gen Psychiatry 56:300–311, 1999

Hallett M: Transcranial magnetic stimulation and the human brain. Nature 406(6792):147–150, 2000

Herwig U, Kolbel K, Wunderlich AP, et al: Spatial congruence of neuronavigated transcranial magnetic stimulation and functional neuroimaging. Clin Neurophysiol 113:462–468, 2002

Herwig U, Satrapi P, Schonfeldt-Lecuona C: Using the international 10–20 EEG system for positioning of transcranial magnetic stimulation. Brain Topogr 16(2):95–99, 2003

Jasper HH: The ten-twenty electrode system of the International Federation. Electroencephalogr Clin Neurophysiol 10:370–375, 1958

Keel JC, Smith MJ, Wassermann EM: A safety screening questionnaire for transcranial magnetic stimulation (letter). Clin Neurophysiol 112:720, 2000

Kozel FA, Nahas Z, deBrux C, et al: How coil-cortex distance relates to age, motor threshold, and antidepressant response to repetitive transcranial magnetic stimulation. J Neuropsychiatry Clin Neurosci 12:376–384, 2000

Mosimann UP, Marre SC, Werlen S, et al: Antidepressant effects of repetitive transcranial magnetic stimulation in the elderly: correlation between effect size and coil-cortex distance. Arch Gen Psychiatry 59:560–561, 2002

Mishory A, Molnar C, Koola J, et al: The maximum-likelihood strategy for determining transcranial magnetic stimulation motor threshold, using parameter estimation by sequential testing is faster than conventional methods with similar precision. J ECT 20:160–165, 2004

Nahas Z, Li X, Kozel FA, et al: Beneficial effects of distance-adjusted prefrontal TMS in geriatric depression. Presentation at the 14th annual meeting of the American Association of Geriatric Psychiatry, San Francisco, CA, February 2001

Paus T: Integration of transcranial magnetic stimulation and brain imaging (abstract). Biol Psychiatry 49(suppl):6s-#21, 2001

Rothwell JC, Thompson PD, Day BL, et al: Stimulation of the human motor cortex through the scalp. Exp Physiol 76:159–200, 1991

Salih F, Khatami R, Steinheimer S, et al: Inhibitory and excitatory intracortical circuits across the human sleep-wake cycle using paired-pulse transcranial magnetic stimulation. J Physiol 565 (pt 2):695–701, 2005

Schonfeldt-Lecuona C, Thielscher A, Freudenmann RW, et al: Accuracy of stereotaxic positioning of transcranial magnetic stimulation. Brain Topogr 17:253–259, 2005

Tetreault L, Bordeleau JM: On the usefulness of the placebo and of the double-blind technique in the evaluation of psychotropic drugs. Psychopharmacol Bull 7:44–64, 1971

Wassermann EM: Risk and safety of repetitive transcranial magnetic stimulation: report and suggested guidelines from the International Workshop in the Safety of Repetitive Transcranial Magnetic Stimulation, June 5–7, 1996. Electroencephalogr Clin Neurophysiol 108:1–16, 1998

Yahagi S, Ni Z, Takahashi M, et al: Excitability changes of motor evoked potentials dependent on muscle properties and contraction modes. Mot Control 7:328–345, 2003

Ziemann U: Pharmacology of TMS. Suppl Clin Neurophysiol 56:226–231, 2003

Ziemann U, Hallett M: Basic neurophysiological studies with TMS, in Transcranial Magnetic Stimulation in Neuropsychiatry. Edited by George MS, Belmaker RH. Washington, DC, American Psychiatric Press, 2000, pp 45–98

APPENDIX: TRANSCRANIAL MAGNETIC STIMULATION ADULT SAFETY SCREEN (TASS)

Form 32: Transcranial Magnetic Stimulation Adult Safety Screen (TASS)		Page 1 of 1
1	Have you ever had an adverse reaction to rTMS?	☐ No ☐ Yes
2	Have you ever had a seizure?	☐ No ☐ Yes
3	Have you ever had an EEG?	☐ No ☐ Yes
4	Have you ever had a stroke?	☐ No ☐ Yes
5	Have you ever had a head injury (including neurosurgery)?	☐ No ☐ Yes
6	Do you have any metal in your head (outside of the mouth) such as shrapnel, surgical clips, or fragments from welding or metalwork?	☐ No ☐ Yes
7	Do you have any implanted devices such as cardiac pacemakers, medical pumps, or intracardiac lines?	☐ No ☐ Yes
8	Do you suffer from frequent or severe headaches?	☐ No ☐ Yes
9	Have you ever had any other brain-related condition?	☐ No ☐ Yes
10	Have you ever had any illness that caused brain injury?	☐ No ☐ Yes
11	Are you taking any medications?	☐ No ☐ Yes
12	If you are woman of childbearing age, are you sexually active, and if so, are you *not using* a reliable method of birth control?	☐ No ☐ Yes
13	Does anyone in your family have epilepsy?	☐ No ☐ Yes
14	Do you need further explanation of rTMS and its associated risks?	☐ No ☐ Yes
15	If any item was marked 'yes', please provide a comment here:	

Source.   Keel et al. 2000.

3

BASIC NEUROPHYSIOLOGICAL STUDIES WITH TRANSCRANIAL MAGNETIC STIMULATION

Ulf Ziemann, M.D.
Mark Hallett, M.D.

Why is it important to provide an overview of basic neurophysiological studies with transcranial magnetic stimulation (TMS) in a book on TMS in neuropsychiatry? As we currently envisage it, the use of TMS in neuropsychiatry will take certain main routes, and, in particular, measurement of cortical connectivity or excitability and assessment of therapeutic intervention. For each of these routes, basic physiological knowledge of what can be measured and what can be affected with TMS is instrumental.

In this chapter, we survey the available single- and paired-pulse TMS techniques that allow quantitative measurements of cortical connectivity (discussed in the first part) and excitability (discussed in the second part). We focus on motor cortex, which has been studied much more extensively than other areas of the cerebral cortex. For each of the TMS measures, we briefly survey the definition, physiology, and clinical significance of TMS in the study of neuropsychiatric disease. Synoptic summaries are also provided in Tables 3–1 and 3–2 at the end of this chapter.

TMS MEASURES OF MOTOR CORTICAL CONNECTIVITY

Connection From Motor Cortex to Spinal Cord

Definition and General Findings

Measuring of the central motor conduction time (CMCT) to assess the integrity of the corticospinal tract was the first major clinical application of TMS (Barker et al. 1986). Several methods have been proposed for calculating CMCT. All of them use the difference between the onset latency of the motor evoked potential (MEP) elicited in the target muscle by TMS of the contralateral motor cortex and the peripheral motor conduction time (PMCT). PMCT can be measured by at least four different techniques: F-wave latency (Robinson et al. 1988), needle stimulation of the spinal roots (Evans et al. 1990), transcutaneous magnetic stimulation of the spinal roots (Epstein et al. 1991), or transcutaneous electrical stimulation of the spinal roots (Schmid et al. 1991). For the F-wave technique, PMCT is calculated by the formula $(F+M-1)/2$, where F is the shortest of usually 20 F-wave latencies, M is the M-wave latency, and 1 is the estimated delay (in milliseconds [msec]) for antidromic activation of the alpha-motoneuron. For all other techniques, PMCT is the onset latency of the compound muscle action potential evoked by stimulation of the spinal roots. CMCT includes the time to activate the corticospinal neurons in motor cortex, the conduction time along the corticospinal tract, and the summation time at the alpha-motoneuron to reach firing threshold.

For all techniques except the F-wave technique, CMCT is overestimated because it also includes the conduction time along the proximal segment of the spinal motor nerve down to region of the intervertebral foramen, where excitation takes place in the PMCT measurements (Epstein et al. 1991; Maccabee et al. 1991). This overestimation is, according to the distance of the proximal segment of the spinal motor nerve in the spinal canal, 0.5–1.4 msec for cervical roots (Chokroverty et al. 1991; Ugawa et al. 1989) and 3.0–4.1 msec for lumbo-sacral roots (Chokroverty et al. 1993; Ugawa et al. 1989). The CMCT is on average 2–3 msec shorter when measured during muscle activation compared with muscle rest (Hess et al. 1987). Normative CMCT data are available for many muscles of the upper and lower limbs and the axial and cranial muscles (Ziemann 2002).

Clinical Significance

Abnormal CMCT prolongation may be caused by demyelination or by ischemic or degenerative damage of the fastest-conducting corticospinal fibers. Accordingly, CMCT measurements are particularly useful in multiple sclerosis, cerebral stroke, myelopathy, and motor-degenerative diseases such as amyotrophic lateral sclerosis or multi-system atrophy. CMCT is usually normal in psychiatric disorders.

Connection Between the Two Motor Cortices

Definition and General Findings

The hand areas of the primary motor cortex in the two hemispheres are connected, although sparsely, by callosal fibers. This transcallosal connection can be tested by two TMS techniques: the ipsilateral silent period (ISP) (Meyer et al. 1995, 1998), and interhemispheric inhibition (IHI) and interhemispheric facilitation (IHF) measured with paired stimulation protocols (Ferbert et al. 1992; Hanajima et al. 2001). The ISP refers to an interruption of voluntary tonic activity in the electromyogram (EMG) after focal TMS of the motor cortex strictly ipsilateral to the target hand muscle. ISP onset is 10–15 msec later than the onset latency of MEPs elicited in the same muscle by TMS from the contralateral motor cortex. This matches closely the estimated conduction time through the corpus callosum (Cracco et al. 1989). The normal ISP duration is about 30 msec (Meyer et al. 1995, 1998). Although much of this effect is certainly transcallosal, some of the phenomenon may be mediated by ipsilateral descending pathways (Gerloff et al. 1998). The paired stimulation protocols use a conditioning stimulus over one motor cortex followed by a test stimulus over the other motor cortex. IHI of the test MEP by, on average, 50% occurs at interstimulus intervals of around 10 msec, if the intensity of both stimuli is clearly above MEP threshold (Ferbert et al. 1992). IHF occurs at shorter interstimulus intervals of 4–5 msec (Hanajima et al. 2001).

Clinical Significance

The usefulness of these measures for testing the integrity of the corpus callosum was demonstrated by a lack of an ISP in patients with surgical lesions or agenesis of the trunk of the corpus callosum (Meyer et al. 1995, 1998). The known reduction in corpus callosum size in patients with schizophrenia triggered several recent studies, which show consistently an ISP prolongation or an IHI reduction (Bajbouj et al. 2004; Boroojerdi et al. 1999; Daskalakis et al. 2002; Fitzgerald et al. 2002). These abnormalities are more pronounced in untreated patients compared with patients receiving antipsychotics (Daskalakis et al. 2002). Altered IHI was also observed in a proportion of first-degree relatives of patients with schizophrenia (Saka et al. 2005). Adolescent boys with attention-deficit/hyperactivity disorder (ADHD) show delayed maturation profiles for finger speed and age-dependent decrease of ISP onset latency—findings that suggest delayed or abnormal development of interhemispheric interactions in these patients (Garvey et al. 2005).

Connection From Cerebellum to Motor Cortex

Definition and General Findings

The cerebellar hemispheres can be activated with percutaneous electrical (Ugawa et al. 1991) or magnetic stimulation (Ugawa et al. 1995; Werhahn et al. 1996), leading to on average 50% inhibition of a test MEP elicited from the motor cortex contralateral to cerebellar conditioning stimulation at interstimulus intervals of 5–7 msec (Ugawa et al. 1995; Werhahn et al. 1996). It is thought that this cerebellar inhibition of the motor cortex (CBI) results from activation of Purkinje cells that inhibit the dentato-thalamo-motor cortical pathway.

Clinical Significance

CBI is reduced or absent in patients with lesions along the cerebello-dentato-thalamo-motor cortical pathway (Di Lazzaro et al. 1994; Ugawa et al. 1994, 1997). CBI is reduced in patients with schizophrenia, suggesting altered cerebellar inhibitory output or disrupted cerebellar-thalamo-cortical connectivity in this disease (Daskalakis et al. 2005).

Connections From Periphery to Motor Cortex

Definition and General Findings

Cutaneous and proprioceptive afferent information from the body can influence the excitability of corticospinal cells at short latency. TMS can be used to test these excitability changes of the corticospinal system after conditioning of afferent stimulation. Electrical stimulation of a mixed arm nerve below or at motor threshold results in short-latency afferent inhibition (SAI) of the MEP in muscles supplied by the stimulated nerve at interstimulus intervals around the N20-latency of the somatosensory evoked potential (Tokimura et al. 2000), and MEP facilitation at slightly longer interstimulus intervals (e.g., Mariorenzi et al. 1991). Cutaneous and muscle spindle afferents contribute to these effects. SAI is reduced by the anticholinergic scopolamine (Di Lazzaro et al. 2000b).

Clinical Significance

Patients with lesions of the central somato-sensory pathways lack a short-latency MEP modulation (Terao et al. 1999). In contrast, patients with certain forms of epilepsy, such as progressive myoclonic epilepsy, show a marked increase in short-latency MEP facilitation (Reutens et al. 1993), indicating motor cortical hyperexcitability time-locked to the afferent input. One of the hallmarks of Alzheimer's disease is a degeneration of the central cholinergic system. According to the prediction, SAI is abnormally reduced in Alzheimer's disease (Di Lazzaro et al. 2002b, 2004a, 2005a). This deficit in cholinergic inhibition is partially normalized by treatment with acetylcholinesterase inhibitors (Di Lazzaro et al. 2002b, 2004a), and the degree of normalization predicts the clinical response to this treatment (Di Lazzaro et al. 2005a).

TMS MEASURES OF MOTOR CORTICAL EXCITABILITY

Motor Threshold

Definition and General Findings

Motor threshold (MT) is commonly defined as the minimum TMS intensity that is necessary to produce a small MEP (>50 microvolts [μV]) in at least half of the trials (Rossini et al. 1999). Intersubject variability of MT is large, while, in a given individual, MT shows good reproducibility and small (<10% of the maximum stimulator output) interhemispheric difference (Cicinelli et al. 1997). MT is lowest in hand muscles and higher in proximal muscles of the arm, trunk, and lower limb (Chen et al. 1998). These differences most likely reflect the density of the cortico-motoneuronal projection, which is highest for intrinsic hand muscles. MT can be tested either during voluntary relaxation of the target muscle (resting motor threshold, or RMT) or during slight isometric muscle contraction (active motor threshold, or AMT). AMT is lower than RMT, usually by 5%–20% of the maximum stimulator output (Chen et al. 1998).

Physiology

Voltage-gated sodium channel–blocking drugs, such as carbamazepine, phenytoin, and lamotrigine, increase MT, whereas indirect enhancement of non–*N*-methyl-D-aspartate (NMDA) glutamatergic currents decreases MT (for review, see Ziemann 2004a). These findings suggest that MT tests membrane-related axon excitability (of cortical-cortical fibers) and excitability of fast ionotropic glutamatergic synapses from these fibers onto corticospinal neurons.

Clinical Significance

Neuropathological studies point to alterations in the glutamatergic system, such as a deficient glutamate reuptake by glutamate transporter proteins, in the brains of Alzheimer's disease patients. As a putative index of glutamatergic cortical hyperexcitability, most studies show an abnormally low MT in Alzheimer's disease patients (Alagona et al. 2001; de Carvalho et al. 1997; Di Lazzaro et al. 2002b, 2004a; Ferreri et al. 2003; Pennisi et al. 2002), which correlates with disease severity (Alagona et al. 2001; Pennisi et al. 2002). Current hypotheses favor excess activity at non-NMDA glutamatergic receptors in schizophrenia (Aghajanian and Marek 2000) and in psilocybin and ketamine models of psychosis (Aghajanian and Marek 1999). Accordingly, MT is reduced in drug-naive first-episode patients with schizophrenia (Eichhammer et al. 2004). MT data are less consistent in chronic patients with schizophrenia (Abarbanel et al. 1996; Daskalakis et al. 2002;

Fitzgerald et al. 2002, 2003; Pascual-Leone et al. 2002; Puri et al. 1996), and this inconsistency is most likely explained by treatment interactions.

Motor Evoked Potential Amplitude/ Intensity Curve

Definition and General Findings

MEP amplitude is usually measured peak to peak (Rossini et al. 1999) or as MEP area (Kiers et al. 1995). The ratio of MEP amplitude over the maximum M-wave (elicited by supra-maximal electrical stimulation of the peripheral nerve) provides an estimate of the portion of the pool of spinal motoneurons that is activated by TMS. MEP amplitude and MEP area increase with stimulation intensity (MEP intensity curve), usually in a nonlinear, sigmoid manner (Devanne et al. 1997). Voluntary activation of the target muscle facilitates MEP amplitude (Devanne et al. 1997; Hess et al. 1987). Cortical and spinal mechanisms contribute to this MEP facilitation (Di Lazzaro et al. 1998a). Measurements of MEP amplitude have two important limitations. One is a considerable trial-to-trial variability (Ellaway et al. 1998), the origins of which are poorly understood. The other one is that the portion of the corticospinal system activated by TMS is significantly underestimated. This is particularly true at high stimulus intensities, which lead to increasingly complex multiple corticospinal discharges (so-called D-waves and I-waves) (Di Lazzaro et al. 2004b; Ziemann and Rothwell 2000). In turn, activation of spinal motoneurons becomes increasingly desynchronized, leading to phase cancellation of action potentials in the MEP. This problem can be overcome by using either twitch force as the measure of TMS evoked motor output (Kiers et al. 1995) or the triple stimulation technique, which, through two collisions, links central to peripheral conduction and suppresses desynchronization of MEPs (Bühler et al. 2001; Magistris et al. 1998, 1999).

Physiology

The characteristics of the MEP intensity curve (threshold, slope, and plateau) depend on the excitability of the chain of neural elements activated by TMS (cortico-cortical fibers, corticomotoneuronal cells, spinal motoneurons). Therefore, MEP amplitude is a rather global measure of corticospinal excitability. Intrinsic hand muscles have significantly steeper intensity curves than proximal arm or lower limb muscles (Chen et al. 1998; Devanne et al. 1997). The steep part and the plateau of the MEP intensity curve reflect mainly recruitment of late I-waves (Di Lazzaro et al. 2004b). The late I-waves are easily suppressible by γ-aminobutyric acid (GABA)–ergic anesthetics (for review, see Ziemann 2004a). Accordingly, drugs that increase transmission through the $GABA_A$ receptor (e.g., benzodiazepines, barbiturates) flatten the MEP intensity curve. Furthermore, neuromodulators (e.g., dopamine, norepinephrine, serotonin, acetylcholine) may exert strong effects on the MEP intensity curve (Ziemann 2004a). These effects are mediated by hitherto only incompletely understood mechanisms that shift the balance between cortical inhibition and facilitation (Hasselmo 1995).

Clinical Significance

MEP amplitude is increased in patients with Alzheimer's disease (Alagona et al. 2001; de Carvalho et al. 1997), supporting the idea of a hyperexcitable motor cortex in this disorder (see discussion in subsection "Motor Threshold" earlier in this section). On the other hand, a lack of MEP facilitation by 5-Hz repetitive TMS (rTMS) suggests a deficient capability for short-term motor cortical plasticity in patients with this disorder (Inghilleri et al. 2006).

In patients with major depression, electroconvulsive therapy (ECT) results in an increase in the left-hemispheric MEP intensity curve in responders but not in nonresponders—suggesting that the antidepressant action of ECT occurs through increase of cortical excitability in the left hemisphere (Chistyakov et al. 2005)—while MEP intensity curves do not differ between patients with major depression and healthy control subjects (Grunhaus et al. 2003). MEP intensity curves were as of yet not studied in other neuropsychiatric disorders, although this would be of interest because many of these disorders are conceived as disorders of neurotransmitter systems that influence MEP amplitude.

MEP Maps

Definition and General Findings

An *MEP map* refers to the area on the scalp surface from which MEP in the target muscle can be obtained. A focal stimulating coil is moved along a grid to stimulate multiple scalp sites, usually 0.5–2 cm apart. The grid coordinates are referenced relative to standard landmarks, such as the vertex (C_z according to the International 10–20 electroencephalographic system). Measurements should continue until noneffective sites surround effective sites, and stimulus intensity should be 110%–120% above MT at the optimal site (Classen et al. 1998). With an optimal mapping technique, good reliability (Corneal et al. 2005; Mortifee et al. 1994) and a spatial resolution in the order of 0.5 cm (Brasil-Neto et al. 1992) can be achieved. Any map can be characterized by three properties: extent, location, and shape. The *extent* of a map is usually expressed as the number of effective stimulation sites. The definition of an effective stimulation site is necessarily arbitrary but can be reasonably related to an MT criterion (Wassermann et al. 1992) (see discussion in previous subsection). Map *location* is best expressed by the center of gravity (COG), which is calculated by weighting each effective stimulation site with its MEP amplitude divided by the total map volume (Wassermann et al. 1992). Map *shape* can be given only in descriptive terms. The combination of MEP mapping with functional neuroimaging studies demonstrated that the COG of the MEP maps projects onto the precentral gyrus and largely overlaps with the functional activation areas (e.g., Classen et al. 1998).

Physiology

Map location corresponds to the scalp site at which the greatest number of the most excitable corticospinal neurons can be stimulated (Classen et al. 1998; Thickbroom et al. 1998). Therefore, MEP mapping is the only TMS measure that explores the topographical organization of motor cortical representations. Map extent is more difficult to interpret because, in addition to reflecting excitability of the corticospinal system, it is confounded by current spread and the depth of the stimulated corticospinal neurons relative to the scalp surface (Thickbroom et al. 1998).

Clinical Significance

MEP mapping is time consuming and therefore not applicable to the clinical routine. The single available study in neuropsychiatric disease shows an anterior and medial shift of the hand representation in patients with mild Alzheimer's disease, which may indicate significant compensatory motor reorganization to preserve motor skill despite motor cortical degeneration (Ferreri et al. 2003).

Cortical Silent Period

Definition and General Findings

The *cortical silent period* (CSP) elicited by TMS refers to an interruption of voluntary activation of a target muscle, visible as a period of silence or decreased activity on the EMG. CSP onset often overlaps with the end of the preceding MEP. Therefore, CSP duration should be assessed by CSP offset only. This can be done by using a standardized mathematical approach, which compares the resumption of voluntary EMG at the end of the CSP with the prestimulus EMG (Daskalakis et al. 2003; Garvey et al. 2001). The CSP can be recorded in any target muscle but is longest in intrinsic hand muscles, where it may easily reach 200–300 msec (Cantello et al. 1992). CSP duration increases approximately linearly with stimulus intensity (Cantello et al. 1992). Increasing the level of voluntary muscle contraction has only a slight, if any, shortening effect on CSP duration (Cantello et al. 1992). CSP duration may be influenced significantly by motor task and motor attention (Classen et al. 1997; Mathis et al. 1999). Intersubject variability is high, while interhemispheric difference in homologous muscles is low (Cicinelli et al. 1997).

Physiology

CSP duration is independent of the amplitude of the preceding MEP (Cantello et al. 1992; Wassermann et al. 1993). CSP threshold is usually lower than MEP threshold (Cantello et al. 1992; Davey et al. 1994). The early part of the CSP is associated with inhibition of spinal motoneurons, whereas the late part of the CSP reflects long-lasting inhibition of motor cortex (Cantello et al. 1992; Fuhr et al. 1991; Inghilleri et al. 1993; Ziemann et al. 1993). It is thought that $GABA_B$ receptors mediate this cortical inhibition (Siebner et al. 1998; Werhahn et al. 1999). Dopaminergic drugs lengthen the CSP in healthy subjects (Priori et al. 1994; Ziemann et al. 1996a). Patients with a dopaminergic deficit, such as those with Parkinson's disease, show a shortened CSP (Cantello et al. 2002).

Clinical Significance

Although the CSP is technically easy to elicit, numerous factors may greatly influence CSP duration (see discussion in subsection "Definition and General Findings" earlier in this section). Therefore, it is indispensable to adhere strictly to a standardized stimulation and data analysis protocol. The CSP is abnormally short or even lacking in adult patients with Tourette's syndrome associated with tics in the EMG target muscle (Ziemann et al. 1997) and in children with tic disorder independent of tic location (Moll et al. 1999, 2001), whereas CSP duration is normal in children with ADHD without tics (Moll et al. 2001). These findings suggest uncontrolled (disinhibited) access of voluntary drive to the corticospinal system in tic disorders. CSP duration is also shortened in drug-naive patients with schizophrenia (Daskalakis et al. 2002)—a finding that fits to other evidence of reduced cortical inhibition in this disease. Drug-free patients with unipolar major depression also exhibit an abnormally short CSP duration (Bajbouj et al. 2006). This abnormality improves after ECT (Bajbouj et al. 2005b) and in patients who respond to 20-Hz rTMS of the left dorsolateral prefrontal cortex (Bajbouj et al. 2005a).

Long-Interval Intracortical Facilitation and Inhibition

Definition and General Findings

This protocol tests the effects of a conditioning TMS pulse (S1) on the amplitude of the MEP elicited by a test TMS pulse (S2) given 10–250 msec after S1 (Claus et al. 1992; Valls-Sole et al. 1992). Stimulus intensities of S1 and S2 are suprathreshold and usually set to 120%–150% of RMT. At interstimulus intervals of 10–40 msec, the test MEP is facilitated by S1 (long-interval intracortical facilitation, or LICF), whereas at intervals of 50–200 msec the test MEP is inhibited (long-interval intracortical inhibition, or LICI) (Claus et al. 1992; Valls-Sole et al. 1992). LICI seems to be related to the CSP, although these two forms of long-lasting cortical inhibition are not identical and sometimes can be dissociated in pathological conditions.

Physiology

LICF and LICI are caused mainly by intracortical mechanisms. This was proven by epidural recordings from the human spinal cord that showed facilitation of late I-waves when S1 was given 20–50 msec before S2, but inhibition of I-waves at intervals of 100–200 msec (Nakamura et al. 1997). LICI is mediated through activation of $GABA_B$ receptors (McDonnell et al. 2006).

Clinical Significance

LICI was reported to be normal in drug-free patients with schizophrenia (Fitzgerald et al. 2003). This finding contrasts with the finding of shortened CSP in schizophrenia (see discussion in subsection "Clinical Significance" in section on CSP), suggesting that, at least to some extent, different mechanisms are responsible for these two forms of inhibition.

Short-Interval Intracortical Inhibition

Definition and General Findings

SICI tests the inhibitory effects of a subthreshold first pulse (S1) on the amplitude of the test MEP elicited by a suprathreshold second pulse (S2) delivered at short interstimulus intervals of 1–5 msec through the same stimulating coil (Di Lazzaro et al. 1998b; Kujirai et al. 1993; Ziemann et al. 1996c). The intensity of S2 is usually adjusted to produce an unconditioned test MEP of about 1 mV in peak-to-peak amplitude in the target muscle. The intensity of S1 is set to 80% of the RMT (Kujirai et al. 1993) or to 90% of the active MT (Di Lazzaro et al. 1998b; Ziemann et al. 1996c). This intensity is too low to produce a corticospinal volley (Di Lazzaro et al. 1998b). Therefore, SICI takes place at the cortical and not at a subcortical or spinal level. SICI can be expressed by the ratio of the mean amplitude of the conditioned MEP at a given interstimulus interval over the mean unconditioned test MEP (Kujirai et al. 1993). Even minimal voluntary contraction of the target muscle leads to a significant reduction in SICI (Ridding et al. 1995). Therefore, testing of SICI requires continuous monitoring of the target muscle EMG. In patients who have difficulty fully relaxing, it is advisable to test SICI at a controlled level of target muscle contraction. SICI is usually tested in hand muscles, but similar SICI was found also in a wide range of other muscles (Chen et al. 1998). SICI develops gradually during the first two decades of life, is maximal in young adults, and declines again with age (Mall et al. 2004; Peinemann et al. 2001).

Physiology

Inhibition occurs in two phases, which differ in their physiological properties. SICI at an interstimulus interval of 1 msec is indicative of refractoriness and synaptic inhibition, whereas SICI at intervals of 2.5–4 msec reflects more purely $GABA_A$ receptor–

mediated synaptic inhibition (Fisher et al. 2002; Hanajima et al. 2003; Roshan et al. 2003). Increase of neurotransmission through the $GABA_A$ receptor (e.g., by benzodiazepines) results in an enhancement of SICI (Di Lazzaro et al. 2000a, 2005b; Ilic et al. 2002; Ziemann et al. 1996b). NMDA receptor blockers induce a similar increase in SICI (Schwenkreis et al. 1999, 2000; Ziemann et al. 1998a), suggesting that SICI is a net inhibition consisting of strong inhibition and weaker facilitation (Ilic et al. 2002). Neuromodulators (e.g., dopamine, norepinephrine, serotonin, acetylcholine) also modify SICI (for review see Ziemann 2004a). In summary, SICI tests mainly excitability of $GABA_A$-dependent inhibitory interneuronal circuits in motor cortex.

Clinical Significance

A reduction in SICI is a relatively nonspecific abnormality that is present in a variety of neurological disorders such as epilepsies, movement disorders, or motoneuron disease (for review, see Ziemann 1999). SICI is also reduced in Tourette's syndrome (Ziemann et al. 1997), obsessive-compulsive disorder (Greenberg et al. 1998, 2000), and ADHD (Moll et al. 2000, 2001). In Tourette's syndrome, the deficit in SICI shows a particularly strong correlation with the severity of ADHD comorbidity but less correlation with the severity of tics (Gilbert et al. 2004, 2005).

The deficit of SICI in these hyperkinetic disorders supports the pathogenetic model that afferent input into motor cortex results in excess excitation of motor output. Drug treatment may obscure SICI abnormality in these disorders (Moll et al. 2000; Ziemann et al. 1997).

SICI findings in Alzheimer's disease are inconsistent. Most studies show a normal or insignificantly reduced SICI (Di Lazzaro et al. 2002b, 2004a; Pepin et al. 1999), but two studies report a significant reduction in SICI (Liepert et al. 2001; Pierantozzi et al. 2004) that correlates with the severity of dementia (Liepert et al. 2001) and improves under treatment with acetylcholine esterase inhibitors (Liepert et al. 2001; Pierantozzi et al. 2004).

Disorders of cortical inhibitory interneurons have been implicated in schizophrenia. This view is supported by a finding of deficient SICI in one study (Daskalakis et al. 2002); however, SICI was not found to be deficient in two other studies (Eichhammer et al. 2004; Pascual-Leone et al. 2002). Drug-free patients with unipolar major depression also exhibit reduced SICI (Bajbouj et al. 2006) that improves after ECT (Bajbouj et al. 2005a) and in patients who respond to 20-Hz rTMS of the left dorsolateral prefrontal cortex (Bajbouj et al. 2005b).

Intracortical Facilitation

Definition and General Findings

ICF is measured with the same protocol as SICI (see discussion in previous section), except that longer interstimulus intervals of 7–20 msec are tested (Kujirai et al. 1993; Ziemann et al. 1996c).

Physiology

ICF originates at the level of motor cortex, not at a subcortical or spinal level (Na-kamura et al. 1997). ICF is not a mere rebound facilitation of SICI; rather, it underlies separate facilitatory mechanisms (Ziemann et al. 1996c). ICF is a net facilitation consisting of prevailing facilitation and weaker inhibition. The facilitation is most likely mediated by glutamatergic neurotransmission through the NMDA receptor. This idea is supported by the majority of the pharmacological studies, which shows a decrease of ICF by NMDA antagonists (Schwenkreis et al. 1999; Ziemann et al. 1998a). The inhibition probably comes from the tail of the $GABA_A$-mediated SICI that has a duration of approximately 20 msec (Hanajima et al. 1998). Accordingly, $GABA_A$ agonists also decrease ICF (Ziemann et al. 1995, 1996b). The pharmacological profiles of ICF and SICI are similar though not identical (for review, see Ziemann 2004a). In summary, ICF tests mainly excitability of NMDA receptor–dependent excitatory interneuronal circuits in motor cortex.

Clinical Significance

Altered glutamatergic neurotransmission through the NMDA receptor has been advocated to contribute to neuropsychiatric disorders, including Alzheimer's disease and schizophrenia. However, ICF is normal in patients with Alzheimer's disease (Di Lazzaro et al. 2002b; Liepert et al. 2001; Pepin et al. 1999; Pierantozzi et al. 2004) and medication-free patients with schizophrenia (Daskalakis et al. 2002; Eichhammer et al. 2004; Pascual-Leone et al. 2002). ICF is also normal in drug-free patients with unipolar major depression (Bajbouj et al. 2006).

Short-Interval Intracortical Facilitation

Definition and General Findings

SICF (I-wave faciliation) is measured in a paired-pulse protocol using two pulses of equal intensity just above motor threshold, or a suprathreshold first pulse (S1) followed by a subthreshold second pulse (S2) at short interstimulus intervals of 0.5–6 msec delivered through the same stimulating coil (Tokimura et al. 1996; Ziemann et al. 1998b). S2 facilitates the MEP elicited by S1 at discrete ranges of interstimulus intervals of 1.1–1.5 msec, 2.3–2.9 msec, and 4.1–4.5 msec, separated by intervals during which S2 has no effect (Tokimura et al. 1996; Ziemann et al. 1998b).

Physiology

The site of SICF is in motor cortex, not at a subcortical or the spinal level (Di Lazzaro et al. 1999). The interval between successive SICF peaks is approximately

1.5 msec, which closely matches the interval between successive I-waves of the corticospinal volley (Patton and Amassian 1954). It is therefore thought that SICF tests excitability of those excitatory interneurons in motor cortex, which are responsible for the generation of I-waves (Hanajima et al. 2002; Ilic et al. 2002). SICF is controlled by $GABA_A$-dependent inhibition (Ilic et al. 2002; Ziemann et al. 1998c).

Clinical Significance

SICF is exaggerated in medicated and medication-free patients with schizophrenia (Fitzgerald et al. 2003). Given the control of SICF by $GABA_A$–dependent inhibition, this was interpreted as supporting the concept of cortical disinhibition in schizophrenia.

Repetitive TMS and Measures of Motor Excitability

Definition and General Findings

The information in this subsection is at the intersection between the measures of motor cortical connectivity and excitability by single-pulse and paired-pulse TMS and applications of rTMS. Usually, the intention of using rTMS is to alter excitability and function of the stimulated cortex. rTMS is divided into low-frequency rTMS (≤ 1 Hz) and high-frequency rTMS (> 1 Hz) (Wassermann 1998). This distinction is based on the general finding that low-frequency rTMS tends to reduce excitability of excitatory neural elements of the stimulated cortex (Boroojerdi et al. 2000; Chen et al. 1997; Maeda et al. 2000b; Muellbacher et al. 2000; Ziemann 2004b), whereas high-frequency rTMS tends to increase it (Di Lazzaro et al. 2002a; Maeda et al. 2000b; Pascual-Leone et al. 1994; Ziemann 2004b).

With particular rTMS protocols, it is possible to affect selectively particular inhibitory or excitatory neural circuits (Berardelli et al. 1999; Wu et al. 2000). The rTMS effects can outlast the rTMS train by up to many minutes. However, rTMS effects depend not only on the rTMS frequency but also on the number of pulses in the stimulus train, stimulus intensity, total number of stimuli (if there is more than one train), the inter-train interval, and the time when cortical excitability is measured after rTMS (Modugno et al. 2001; Ziemann 2004b). Furthermore, there exists a substantial inter-individual variability of rTMS effects (Maeda et al. 2000a; Sommer et al. 2002).

Finally, rTMS effects are not limited to the stimulated cortex but can be measured also in connected cortical areas (Gerschlager et al. 2001; Gilio et al. 2003; Münchau et al. 2002; Rizzo et al. 2004). The internationally accepted safety guidelines (Wassermann 1998) should be followed. rTMS can result in spread of excitation and even induction of seizure activity if the safety limits are exceeded.

Physiology

Relatively little is known about the mechanisms underlying lasting rTMS effects. Various mechanisms have been advocated, including neurotransmitter depletion and short-term and long-term synaptic plasticity (for review, see Ziemann 2004b). Recent evidence supports the view that the long-lasting depression of MEP size by low-frequency rTMS is a phenomenon similar to long-term depression (Iyer et al. 2003; Siebner et al. 2004).

Clinical Findings

Treatment effects of rTMS in patients with neuropsychiatric disorders are dealt with extensively in other chapters of this book. Conceptually, rTMS may be used to disrupt unwanted brain activity (e.g., auditory hallucinations in schizophrenia), enhance desired activity (e.g., dopamine release in the striatum in patients with Parkinson's disease), increase low cortical activity (e.g., in the left dorsolateral prefrontal cortex of patients with major depression), or decrease high cortical activity (e.g., right dorsolateral prefrontal cortex of patients with mania). rTMS- or ECT-induced normalization of altered motor cortical excitability can be monitored with the various TMS protocols described earlier and may be associated with or predict a favorable response to treatment (Bajbouj et al. 2005a; Chistyakov et al. 2005)

SUMMARY

In this chapter, we have presented an overview of how transcranial magnetic stimulation can be used to measure connectivity and excitability of human cerebral cortex. The content is basic and possibly beyond the scope and interest of most clinical psychiatrists. Our primary intention was for the chapter to serve as a reference whenever there is the need for looking up basic neurophysiological TMS studies.

We first surveyed the *TMS measures of motor cortical connectivity.* The connections that can be studied at present are the crossed corticospinal projection (connection from motor cortex to spinal cord), the transcallosal connection between the two motor cortices, connections from cerebellum to the motor cortex, and connections (afferents) from periphery to motor cortex. The physiology and clinical significance of these measures are summarized in Table 3–1. Probing cortical connectivity is developing into an interesting field in neuropsychiatry because disordered cortical connectivity appears to contribute to disease (e.g., in schizophrenia).

We then described the currently available *TMS measures of motor cortical excitability,* including resting and active motor threshold, motor evoked potential intensity curve, motor evoked potential intensity curve map, cortical silent period,

Table 3–1. Transcranial magnetic stimulation (TMS) measures of motor cortical connectivity

Measure	Definition	Purpose and physiological interpretation
Central motor conduction time (CMCT)	Difference between corticomuscular latency (MEP onset latency) and peripheral motor conduction time	Assessment of functional integrity of the fastest conducting fibers of the corticospinal tract
Connections between the two primary motor cortices: —ipsilateral silent period (ISP) —interhemispheric inhibition (IHI)	ISP: Interruption of voluntary tonic electromyographic activity in a target muscle ipsilateral to the stimulated motor cortex IHI: Inhibitory effect of conditioning TMS over one motor cortex on the amplitude of the test MEP elicited with TMS over the other motor cortex (ISI = ~10 msec)	Assessment of functional integrity of interhemispheric (mainly transcallosal) connections between homologous representations of the two motor cortices
Connections from cerebellum to motor cortex (CBI)	Inhibitory effect of conditioning stimulation over one cerebellar hemisphere on the amplitude of the test MEP elicited by TMS over the contralateral motor cortex (ISI = 5–7 msec)	Assessment of the inhibitory effects of Purkinje cells on the dentato–thalamo–motor cortical pathway
Connections from the periphery to the motor cortex: —short-interval afferent inhibition (SAI)	Modulatory effect of peripheral conditioning stimulation (of motor, mixed, or sensory nerves) on the amplitude of the test MEP elicited by TMS over the contralateral motor cortex (SAI: ISI = ~20 msec)	Assessment of the functional integrity of somatosensory afferents into motor cortex (SAI: cholinergic inhibition)

Note. ISI = interstimulus interval; MEP = motor evoked potential.

Table 3–2. Transcranial magnetic stimulation (TMS) measures of motor cortical excitability

Measure	Definition	Purpose and physiological interpretation
Motor threshold (MT)	Minimum TMS intensity that is necessary to produce a small MEP (> 50 μV) in at least half of the trials	Reflects membrane-related neuronal excitability, primarily of cortico-cortical fibers, and excitability of their glutamatergic synapses with corticospinal neurons
MEP input-output curve	MEP amplitude (peak-to-peak, or area) as a function of TMS intensity; the usually sigmoid function is characterized by threshold, slope, and plateau	Measure of corticospinal excitability; slope and plateau of the MEP input-output curve are modifiable by changes in GABAergic and glutamatergic neurotransmission, and neuromodulators
MEP map	Area on the scalp surface from which MEP in the target muscle can be obtained; a map is characterized by its extent (number of effective stimulation sites), location (center of gravity), and shape	Map extent is a measure of the density and excitability of the corticospinal projection to the target muscle (confounded by current spread and the depth of corticospinal neurons relative to the scalp surface); map location assesses the location of the corticospinal neurons activated by TMS
Cortical silent period (CSP)	Interruption of voluntary tonic electromyographic activity of the target muscle contralateral to the stimulated motor cortex	Assessment of long-lasting cortical inhibition, most likely mediated through the $GABA_B$ receptor

Table 3–2. Transcranial magnetic stimulation (TMS) measures of motor cortical excitability *(continued)*

Measure	Definition	Purpose and physiological interpretation
Long-interval intracortical inhibition (LICI)	Inhibition of a test MEP by a suprathreshold conditioning pulse delivered through the same stimulating coil (ISI=50–250 msec)	Assessment of long-lasting cortical inhibition, most likely mediated through the $GABA_B$ receptor
Short-interval intracortical inhibition (SICI)	Inhibition of a test MEP by a subthreshold conditioning pulse delivered through the same stimulating coil (ISI=1–5 msec)	Assessment of short-lasting cortical inhibition, mediated through the $GABA_A$ receptor
Intracortical facilitation (ICF)	Facilitation of a test MEP by a subthreshold conditioning pulse delivered through the same stimulating coil (ISI=7–20 msec)	Assessment of cortical facilitation, most likely mediated through the NMDA receptor
Short-interval intracortical facilitation (SICF, I-wave facilitation)	Facilitation of a test MEP by a subthreshold pulse given through the same stimulating coil 0.5–6 msec after the first stimulus; MEP facilitation at 1.1–1.5 msec, 2.3–2.9 msec, and 4.1–4.5 msec	Assessment of excitability of the neuronal structures in the motor cortex that are responsible for the generation of I-waves; control by $GABA_A$-dependent inhibition

Note.   ISI=interstimulus interval; MEP=motor evoked potential.

long-interval intracortical facilitation and inhibition, short-interval intracortical inhibition, intracortical facilitation, and short-interval intracortical facilitation. The physiology and clinical significance of these measures are summarized in Table 3–2. TMS measures of cortical excitability are of importance to the psychiatrist for at least three reasons. First, they are valuable as diagnostic tools, since there is increasing evidence of altered motor cortical excitability in many psychiatric disorders. Second, it is a safety requirement to adjust stimulus parameters (in particular stimulus intensity) in repetitive transcranial magnetic stimulation treatment protocols to the patient's individual motor excitability. Therefore, knowledge of the methods and meaning of TMS measures of motor cortical excitability is indispensable. Third, there is evidence that various rTMS protocols can increase or decrease cortical excitability. This effect may be used therapeutically to normalize altered excitability in psychiatric disease. TMS measures of cortical excitability may be applied to monitor the rTMS effects on cortical excitability in the therapeutic setting.

REFERENCES

Abarbanel JM, Lemberg T, Yaroslavski U, et al: Electrophysiological responses to transcranial magnetic stimulation in depression and schizophrenia. Biol Psychiatry 40:148–150, 1996

Aghajanian GK, Marek GJ: Serotonin and hallucinogens. Neuropsychopharmacology 21 (2, suppl):16S–23S, 1999

Aghajanian GK, Marek GJ: Serotonin model of schizophrenia: emerging role of glutamate mechanisms. Brain Res Brain Res Rev 31:302–312, 2000

Alagona G, Bella R, Ferri R, et al: Transcranial magnetic stimulation in Alzheimer disease: motor cortex excitability and cognitive severity. Neurosci Lett 314:57–60, 2001

Bajbouj M, Gallinat J, Lang UE, et al: Abnormalities of inhibitory neuronal mechanisms in the motor cortex of patients with schizophrenia. Pharmacopsychiatry 37:74–80, 2004

Bajbouj M, Brakemeier EL, Schubert F, et al: Repetitive transcranial magnetic stimulation of the dorsolateral prefrontal cortex and cortical excitability in patients with major depressive disorder. Exp Neurol 196:332–338, 2005a

Bajbouj M, Lang UE, Niehaus L, et al: Effects of right unilateral electroconvulsive therapy on motor cortical excitability in depressive patients. J Psychiatr Res 40:322–327, 2005b

Bajbouj M, Lisanby SH, Lang UE, et al: Evidence for impaired cortical inhibition in patients with unipolar major depression. Biol Psychiatry 59:395–400, 2006

Barker AT, Freeston IL, Jalinous R, et al: Clinical evaluation of conduction time measurements in central motor pathways using magnetic stimulation of human brain (letter). Lancet 1:1325–1326, 1986

Berardelli A, Inghilleri M, Gilio F, et al: Effects of repetitive cortical stimulation on the silent period evoked by magnetic stimulation. Exp Brain Res 125:82–86, 1999

Boroojerdi B, Topper R, Foltys H, et al: Transcallosal inhibition and motor conduction studies in patients with schizophrenia using transcranial magnetic stimulation. Br J Psychiatry 175:375–379, 1999

Boroojerdi B, Prager A, Muellbacher W, et al: Reduction of human visual cortex excitability using 1-Hz transcranial magnetic stimulation. Neurology 54:1529–1531, 2000

Brasil-Neto JP, McShane LM, Fuhr P, et al: Topographic mapping of the human motor cortex with magnetic stimulation: factors affecting accuracy and reproducibility. Electroencephalogr Clin Neurophysiol 85:9–16, 1992

Bühler R, Magistris MR, Truffert A, et al: The triple stimulation technique to study central motor conduction to the lower limbs. Clin Neurophysiol 112:938–949, 2001

Cantello R, Gianelli M, Civardi C, et al: Magnetic brain stimulation: the silent period after the motor evoked potential. Neurology 42:1951–1959, 1992

Cantello R, Tarletti R, Civardi C: Transcranial magnetic stimulation and Parkinson's disease. Brain Res Brain Res Rev 38:309–327, 2002

Chen R, Classen J, Gerloff C, et al: Depression of motor cortex excitability by low-frequency transcranial magnetic stimulation. Neurology 48:1398–1403, 1997

Chen R, Tam A, Butefisch C, et al: Intracortical inhibition and facilitation in different representations of the human motor cortex. J Neurophysiol 80:2870–2881, 1998

Chistyakov AV, Kaplan B, Rubichek O, et al: Effect of electroconvulsive therapy on cortical excitability in patients with major depression: a transcranial magnetic stimulation study. Clin Neurophysiol 116:386–392, 2005

Chokroverty S, Picone MA, Chokroverty M: Percutaneous magnetic coil stimulation of human cervical vertebral column: site of stimulation and clinical application. Electroencephalogr Clin Neurophysiol 81:359–365, 1991

Chokroverty S, Flynn D, Picone MA, et al: Magnetic coil stimulation of the human lumbosacral vertebral column: site of stimulation and clinical application. Electroencephalogr Clin Neurophysiol 89:54–60, 1993

Cicinelli P, Traversa R, Bassi A, et al: Interhemispheric differences of hand muscle representation in human motor cortex. Muscle Nerve 20:535–542, 1997

Classen J, Schnitzler A, Binkofski F, et al: The motor syndrome associated with exaggerated inhibition within the primary motor cortex of patients with hemiparetic stroke. Brain 120:605–619, 1997

Classen J, Knorr U, Werhahn KJ, et al: Multimodal output mapping of human central motor representation on different spatial scales. J Physiol 512:163–179, 1998

Claus D, Weis M, Jahnke U, et al: Corticospinal conduction studied with magnetic double stimulation in the intact human. J Neurol Sci 111:180–188, 1992

Corneal SF, Butler AJ, Wolf SL: Intra- and intersubject reliability of abductor pollicis brevis muscle motor map characteristics with transcranial magnetic stimulation. Arch Phys Med Rehabil 86:1670–1675, 2005

Cracco RQ, Amassian VE, Maccabee PJ, et al: Comparison of human transcallosal responses evoked by magnetic coil and electrical stimulation. Electroencephalogr Clin Neurophysiol 74:417–424, 1989

Daskalakis ZJ, Christensen BK, Chen R, et al: Evidence for impaired cortical inhibition in schizophrenia using transcranial magnetic stimulation. Arch Gen Psychiatry 59:347–354, 2002

Daskalakis ZJ, Molnar GF, Christensen BK, et al: An automated method to determine the transcranial magnetic stimulation-induced contralateral silent period. Clin Neurophysiol 114:938–944, 2003

Daskalakis ZJ, Christensen BK, Fitzgerald PB, et al: Reduced cerebellar inhibition in schizophrenia: a preliminary study. Am J Psychiatry 162:1203–1205, 2005

Davey NJ, Romaiguere P, Maskill DW, et al: Suppression of voluntary motor activity revealed using transcranial magnetic stimulation of the motor cortex in man. J Physiol (Lond) 477:223–235, 1994

de Carvalho M, de Mendonca A, Miranda PC, et al: Magnetic stimulation in Alzheimer's disease. J Neurol 244:304–307, 1997

Devanne H, Lavoie BA, Capaday C: Input-output properties and gain changes in the human corticospinal pathway. Exp Brain Res 114:329–338, 1997

Di Lazzaro V, Molinari M, Restuccia D, et al: Cerebro-cerebellar interactions in man: neurophysiological studies in patients with focal cerebellar lesions. Electroencephalogr Clin Neurophysiol 93:27–34, 1994

Di Lazzaro V, Restuccia D, Oliviero A, et al: Effects of voluntary contraction on descending volleys evoked by transcranial magnetic stimulation in conscious humans. J Physiol 508:625–633, 1998a

Di Lazzaro V, Restuccia D, Oliviero A, et al: Magnetic transcranial stimulation at intensities below active motor threshold activates intracortical inhibitory circuits. Exp Brain Res 119:265–268, 1998b

Di Lazzaro V, Rothwell JC, Oliviero A, et al: Intracortical origin of the short latency facilitation produced by pairs of threshold magnetic stimuli applied to human motor cortex. Exp Brain Res 129:494–499, 1999

Di Lazzaro V, Oliviero A, Meglio M, et al: Direct demonstration of the effect of lorazepam on the excitability of the human motor cortex. Clin Neurophysiol 111:794–799, 2000a

Di Lazzaro V, Oliviero A, Profice P, et al: Muscarinic receptor blockade has differential effects on the excitability of intracortical circuits in human motor cortex. Exp Brain Res 135:455–461, 2000b

Di Lazzaro V, Oliviero A, Berardelli A, et al: Direct demonstration of the effects of repetitive transcranial magnetic stimulation on the excitability of the human motor cortex. Exp Brain Res 144:549–553, 2002a

Di Lazzaro V, Oliviero A, Tonali PA, et al: Noninvasive in vivo assessment of cholinergic cortical circuits in AD using transcranial magnetic stimulation. Neurology 59:392–397, 2002b

Di Lazzaro V, Oliviero A, Pilato F, et al: Motor cortex hyperexcitability to transcranial magnetic stimulation in Alzheimer's disease. J Neurol Neurosurg Psychiatry 75:555–559, 2004a

Di Lazzaro V, Oliviero A, Pilato F, et al: The physiological basis of transcranial motor cortex stimulation in conscious humans. Clin Neurophysiol 115:255–266, 2004b

Di Lazzaro V, Oliviero A, Pilato F, et al: Neurophysiological predictors of long term response to AChE inhibitors in AD patients. J Neurol Neurosurg Psychiatry 76:1064–1069, 2005a

Di Lazzaro V, Pilato F, Dileone M, et al: Dissociated effects of diazepam and lorazepam on short latency afferent inhibition. J Physiol 569:315–323, 2005b

Eichhammer P, Wiegand R, Kharraz A, et al: Cortical excitability in neuroleptic-naive first-episode schizophrenic patients. Schizophr Res 67:253–259, 2004

Ellaway PH, Davey NJ, Maskill DW, et al: Variability in the amplitude of skeletal muscle responses to magnetic stimulation of the motor cortex in man. Electroencephalogr Clin Neurophysiol 109:104–113, 1998

Epstein CM, Fernandez-Beer E, Weissman JD, et al: Cervical magnetic stimulation: the role of the neural foramen. Neurology 41:677–680, 1991

Evans BA, Daube JR, Litchy WJ: A comparison of magnetic and electrical stimulation of spinal nerves. Muscle Nerve 13:414–420, 1990

Ferbert A, Priori A, Rothwell JC, et al: Interhemispheric inhibition of the human motor cortex. J Physiol 453:525–546, 1992

Ferreri F, Pauri F, Pasqualetti P, et al: Motor cortex excitability in Alzheimer's disease: a transcranial magnetic stimulation study. Ann Neurol 53:102–108, 2003

Fisher RJ, Nakamura Y, Bestmann S, et al: Two phases of intracortical inhibition revealed by transcranial magnetic threshold tracking. Exp Brain Res 143:240–248, 2002

Fitzgerald PB, Brown TL, Daskalakis ZJ, et al: A study of transcallosal inhibition in schizophrenia using transcranial magnetic stimulation. Schizophr Res 56:199–209, 2002

Fitzgerald PB, Brown TL, Marston NA, et al: A transcranial magnetic stimulation study of abnormal cortical inhibition in schizophrenia. Psychiatry Res 118:197–207, 2003

Fuhr P, Agostino R, Hallett M: Spinal motor neuron excitability during the silent period after cortical stimulation. Electroencephalogr Clin Neurophysiol 81:257–262, 1991

Garvey MA, Ziemann U, Becker DA, et al: New graphical method to measure silent periods evoked by transcranial magnetic stimulation. Clin Neurophysiol 112:1451–1460, 2001

Garvey MA, Barker CA, Bartko JJ, et al: The ipsilateral silent period in boys with attention-deficit/hyperactivity disorder. Clin Neurophysiol 116:1889–1896, 2005

Gerloff C, Cohen LG, Floeter MK, et al: Inhibitory influence of the ipsilateral motor cortex on responses evoked by transcranial stimulation of the human cortex and pyramidal tract. J Physiol 510:249–259, 1998

Gerschlager W, Siebner HR, Rothwell JC: Decreased corticospinal excitability after sub-threshold 1 Hz rTMS over lateral premotor cortex. Neurology 57:449–455, 2001

Gilbert DL, Bansal AS, Sethuraman G, et al: Association of cortical disinhibition with tic, ADHD, and OCD severity in Tourette syndrome. Mov Disord 19:416–425, 2004

Gilbert DL, Sallee FR, Zhang J, et al: Transcranial magnetic stimulation-evoked cortical inhibition: a consistent marker of attention-deficit/hyperactivity disorder scores in tourette syndrome. Biol Psychiatry 57:1597–1600, 2005

Gilio F, Rizzo V, Siebner HR, et al: Effects on the right motor hand-area excitability produced by low-frequency rTMS over human contralateral homologous cortex. J Physiol 551:563–573, 2003

Greenberg BD, Ziemann U, Harmon A, et al: Decreased neuronal inhibition in cerebral cortex in obsessive-compulsive disorder on transcranial magnetic stimulation. Lancet 352:881–882, 1998

Greenberg BD, Ziemann U, Cora-Locatelli G, et al: Altered cortical excitability in obsessive-compulsive disorder. Neurology 54:142–147, 2000

Grunhaus L, Polak D, Amiaz R, et al: Motor-evoked potential amplitudes elicited by transcranial magnetic stimulation do not differentiate between patients and normal controls. Int J Neuropsychopharmacol 6:371–378, 2003

Hanajima R, Ugawa Y, Terao Y, et al: Paired-pulse magnetic stimulation of the human motor cortex: differences among I waves. J Physiol 509:607–618, 1998

Hanajima R, Ugawa Y, Machii K, et al: Interhemispheric facilitation of the hand motor area in humans. J Physiol 531:849–859, 2001

Hanajima R, Ugawa Y, Terao Y, et al: Mechanisms of intracortical I-wave facilitation elicited with paired-pulse magnetic stimulation in humans. J Physiol 538:253–261, 2002

Hanajima R, Furubayashi T, Iwata NK, et al: Further evidence to support different mechanisms underlying intracortical inhibition of the motor cortex. Exp Brain Res 151:427–434, 2003

Hasselmo ME: Neuromodulation and cortical function: modeling the physiological basis of behavior. Behav Brain Res 67:1–27, 1995

Hess CW, Mills KR, Murray NM: Responses in small hand muscles from magnetic stimulation of the human brain. J Physiol 388:397–419, 1987

Ilic TV, Meintzschel F, Cleff U, et al: Short-interval paired-pulse inhibition and facilitation of human motor cortex: the dimension of stimulus intensity. J Physiol 545:153–167, 2002

Inghilleri M, Berardelli A, Cruccu G, et al: Silent period evoked by transcranial stimulation of the human cortex and cervicomedullary junction. J Physiol 466:521–534, 1993

Inghilleri M, Conte A, Frasca V, et al: Altered response to rTMS in patients with Alzheimer's disease. Clin Neurophysiol 117:103–109, 2006

Iyer MB, Schleper N, Wassermann EM: Priming stimulation enhances the depressant effect of low-frequency repetitive transcranial magnetic stimulation. J Neurosci 23:10867–10872, 2003

Kiers L, Clouston P, Chiappa KH, et al: Assessment of cortical motor output: compound muscle action potential versus twitch force recording. Electroencephalogr Clin Neurophysiol 97:131–139, 1995

Kujirai T, Caramia MD, Rothwell JC, et al: Corticocortical inhibition in human motor cortex. J Physiol 471:501–519, 1993

Liepert J, Bar KJ, Meske U, et al: Motor cortex disinhibition in Alzheimer's disease. Clin Neurophysiol 112:1436–1441, 2001

Maccabee PJ, Amassian VE, Eberle LP, et al: Measurement of the electric field induced into inhomogeneous volume conductors by magnetic coils: application to human spinal neurogeometry. Electroencephalogr Clin Neurophysiol 81:224–237, 1991

Maeda F, Keenan JP, Tormos JM, et al: Interindividual variability of the modulatory effects of repetitive transcranial magnetic stimulation on cortical excitability. Exp Brain Res 133:425–430, 2000a

Maeda F, Keenan JP, Tormos JM, et al: Modulation of corticospinal excitability by repetitive transcranial magnetic stimulation. Clin Neurophysiol 111:800–805, 2000b

Magistris MR, Rosler KM, Truffert A, et al: Transcranial stimulation excites virtually all motor neurons supplying the target muscle: a demonstration and a method improving the study of motor evoked potentials. Brain 121:437–450, 1998

Magistris MR, Rosler KM, Truffert A, et al: A clinical study of motor evoked potentials using a triple stimulation technique. Brain 122:265–279, 1999

Mall V, Berweck S, Fietzek UM, et al: Low level of intracortical inhibition in children shown by transcranial magnetic stimulation. Neuropediatrics 35:120–125, 2004

Mariorenzi R, Zarola F, Caramia MD, et al: Non-invasive evaluation of central motor tract excitability changes following peripheral nerve stimulation in healthy humans. Electroencephalogr Clin Neurophysiol 81:90–101, 1991

Mathis J, de Quervain D, Hess CW: Task-dependent effects on motor-evoked potentials and on the following silent period. J Clin Neurophysiol 16:556–565, 1999

McDonnell MN, Orekhov Y, Ziemann U: The role of GABA(B) receptors in intracortical inhibition in the human motor cortex. Exp Brain Res, February 18, 2006 (Epub ahead of print)

Meyer B-U, Röricht S, Gräfin von Einsiedel H, et al: Inhibitory and excitatory interhemispheric transfers between motor cortical areas in normal humans and patients with abnormalities of the corpus callosum. Brain 118:429–440, 1995

Meyer B-U, Röricht S, Woiciechowsky C: Topography of fibers in the human corpus callosum mediating interhemispheric inhibition between the motor cortices. Ann Neurol 43:360–369, 1998

Modugno N, Nakamura Y, MacKinnon CD, et al: Motor cortex excitability following short trains of repetitive magnetic stimuli. Exp Brain Res 140:453–459, 2001

Moll GH, Wischer S, Heinrich H, et al: Deficient motor control in children with tic disorder: evidence from transcranial magnetic stimulation. Neurosci Lett 272:37–40, 1999

Moll GH, Heinrich H, Trott G, et al: Deficient intracortical inhibition in drug-naive children with attention-deficit hyperactivity disorder is enhanced by methylphenidate. Neurosci Lett 284:121–125, 2000

Moll GH, Heinrich H, Trott GE, et al: Children with comorbid attention-deficit-hyperactivity disorder and tic disorder: evidence for additive inhibitory deficits within the motor system. Ann Neurol 49:393–396, 2001

Mortifee P, Stewart H, Schulzer M, et al: Reliability of transcranial magnetic stimulation for mapping the human motor cortex. Electroencephalogr Clin Neurophysiol 93:131–137, 1994

Muellbacher W, Ziemann U, Boroojerdi B, et al: Effects of low-frequency transcranial magnetic stimulation on motor excitability and basic motor behavior. Clin Neurophysiol 111:1002–1007, 2000

Münchau A, Bloem BR, Irlbacher K, et al: Functional connectivity of human premotor and motor cortex explored with repetitive transcranial magnetic stimulation. J Neurosci 22:554–561, 2002

Nakamura H, Kitagawa H, Kawaguchi Y, et al: Intracortical facilitation and inhibition after transcranial magnetic stimulation in conscious humans. J Physiol 498:817–823, 1997

Pascual-Leone A, Valls-Sole J, Wassermann EM, et al: Responses to rapid-rate transcranial magnetic stimulation of the human motor cortex. Brain 117:847–858, 1994

Pascual-Leone A, Manoach DS, Birnbaum R, et al: Motor cortical excitability in schizophrenia. Biol Psychiatry 52:24–31, 2002

Patton HD, Amassian VE: Single- and multiple-unit analysis of cortical stage of pyramidal tract activation. J Neurophysiol 17:345–363, 1954

Peinemann A, Lehner C, Conrad B, et al: Age-related decrease in paired-pulse intracortical inhibition in the human primary motor cortex. Neurosci Lett 313:33–36, 2001

Pennisi G, Alagona G, Ferri R, et al: Motor cortex excitability in Alzheimer disease: one year follow-up study. Neurosci Lett 329:293–296, 2002

Pepin JL, Bogacz D, de Pasqua V, et al: Motor cortex inhibition is not impaired in patients with Alzheimer's disease: evidence from paired transcranial magnetic stimulation. J Neurol Sci 170:119–123, 1999

Pierantozzi M, Panella M, Palmieri MG, et al: Different TMS patterns of intracortical inhibition in early onset Alzheimer dementia and frontotemporal dementia. Clin Neurophysiol 115:2410–2418, 2004

Priori A, Berardelli A, Inghilleri M, et al: Motor cortical inhibition and the dopaminergic system: pharmacological changes in the silent period after transcranial brain stimulation in normal subjects, patients with Parkinson's disease and drug-induced parkinsonism. Brain 117:317–323, 1994

Puri BK, Davey NJ, Ellaway PH, et al: An investigation of motor function in schizophrenia using transcranial magnetic stimulation of the motor cortex. Br J Psychiatry 169:690–695, 1996

Reutens DC, Puce A, Berkovic SF: Cortical hyperexcitability in progressive myoclonus epilepsy: a study with transcranial magnetic stimulation. Neurology 43:186–192, 1993

Ridding MC, Taylor JL, Rothwell JC: The effect of voluntary contraction on corticocortical inhibition in human motor cortex. J Physiol 487:541–548, 1995

Rizzo V, Siebner HR, Modugno N, et al: Shaping the excitability of human motor cortex with premotor rTMS. J Physiol 554:483–495, 2004

Robinson LR, Jantra P, MacLean IC: Central motor conduction times using transcranial stimulation and F wave latencies. Muscle Nerve 11:174–180, 1988

Roshan L, Paradiso GO, Chen R: Two phases of short-interval intracortical inhibition. Exp Brain Res 151:330–337, 2003

Rossini PM, Berardelli A, Deuschl G, et al: Applications of magnetic cortical stimulation. Electroencephalogr Clin Neurophysiol Suppl 52:171–185, 1999

Saka MC, Atbasoglu EC, Ozguven HD, et al: Cortical inhibition in first-degree relatives of schizophrenic patients assessed with transcranial magnetic stimulation. Int J Neuropsychopharmacol 8:595–599, 2005

Schmid UD, Walker G, Schmid-Sigron J, et al: Transcutaneous magnetic and electrical stimulation over the cervical spine: excitation of plexus roots-rather than spinal roots. Electroencephalogr Clin Neurophysiol Suppl 43:369–384, 1991

Schwenkreis P, Witscher K, Janssen F, et al: Influence of the N-methyl-D-aspartate antagonist memantine on human motor cortex excitability. Neurosci Lett 270:137–140, 1999

Schwenkreis P, Liepert J, Witscher K, et al: Riluzole suppresses motor cortex facilitation in correlation to its plasma level. Exp Brain Res 135:293–299, 2000

Siebner HR, Dressnandt J, Auer C, et al: Continuous intrathecal baclofen infusions induced a marked increase of the transcranially evoked silent period in a patient with generalized dystonia. Muscle Nerve 21:1209–1212, 1998

Siebner HR, Lang N, Rizzo V, et al: Preconditioning of low-frequency repetitive transcranial magnetic stimulation with transcranial direct current stimulation: evidence for homeostatic plasticity in the human motor cortex. J Neurosci 24:3379–3385, 2004

Sommer M, Wu T, Tergau F, et al: Intra- and interindividual variability of motor responses to repetitive transcranial magnetic stimulation. Clin Neurophysiol 113:265–269, 2002

Terao Y, Ugawa Y, Hanajima R, et al: Air-puff-induced facilitation of motor cortical excitability studied in patients with discrete brain lesions. Brain 122:2259–2277, 1999

Thickbroom GW, Sammut R, Mastaglia FL: Magnetic stimulation mapping of motor cortex: factors contributing to map area. Electroencephalogr Clin Neurophysiol 109:79–84, 1998

Tokimura H, Ridding MC, Tokimura Y, et al: Short latency facilitation between pairs of threshold magnetic stimuli applied to human motor cortex. Electroencephalogr Clin Neurophysiol 101:263–272, 1996

Tokimura H, Di Lazzaro V, Tokimura Y, et al: Short latency inhibition of human hand motor cortex by somatosensory input from the hand. J Physiol 523:503–513, 2000

Ugawa Y, Rothwell JC, Day BL, et al: Magnetic stimulation over the spinal enlargements. J Neurol Neurosurg Psychiatry 52:1025–1032, 1989

Ugawa Y, Day BL, Rothwell JC, et al: Modulation of motor cortical excitability by electrical stimulation over the cerebellum in man. J Physiol 441:57–72, 1991

Ugawa Y, Hanajima R, Kanazawa I: Motor cortex inhibition in patients with ataxia. Electroencephalogr Clin Neurophysiol 93:225–229, 1994

Ugawa Y, Uesaka Y, Terao Y, et al: Magnetic stimulation over the cerebellum in humans. Ann Neurol 37:703–713, 1995

Ugawa Y, Terao Y, Hanajima R, et al: Magnetic stimulation over the cerebellum in patients with ataxia. Electroencephalogr Clin Neurophysiol 104:453–458, 1997

Valls-Sole J, Pascual-Leone A, Wassermann EM, et al: Human motor evoked responses to paired transcranial magnetic stimuli. Electroencephalogr Clin Neurophysiol 85:355–364, 1992

Wassermann EM: Risk and safety of repetitive transcranial magnetic stimulation: report and recommendations from the International Workshop on the Safety of Repetitive Transcranial Magnetic Stimulation June 5–7, 1996. Electroencephalogr Clin Neurophysiol 108:1–16, 1998

Wassermann EM, McShane LM, Hallett M, et al: Noninvasive mapping of muscle representations in human motor cortex. Electroencephalogr Clin Neurophysiol 85:1–8, 1992

Wassermann EM, Pascual-Leone A, Valls-Sole J, et al: Topography of the inhibitory and excitatory responses to transcranial magnetic stimulation in a hand muscle. Electroencephalogr Clin Neurophysiol 89:424–433, 1993

Werhahn KJ, Taylor J, Ridding M, et al: Effect of transcranial magnetic stimulation over the cerebellum on the excitability of human motor cortex. Electroencephalogr Clin Neurophysiol 101:58–66, 1996

Werhahn KJ, Kunesch E, Noachtar S, et al: Differential effects on motorcortical inhibition induced by blockade of GABA uptake in humans. J Physiol 517:591–597, 1999

Wu T, Sommer M, Tergau F, et al: Lasting influence of repetitive transcranial magnetic stimulation on intracortical excitability in human subjects. Neurosci Lett 287:37–40, 2000

Ziemann U: Intracortical inhibition and facilitation in the conventional paired TMS paradigm. Electroencephalogr Clin Neurophysiol Suppl 51:127–136, 1999

Ziemann U: Assessment of motor cortex and descending motor pathways, in Neuromuscular Function and Disease: Basic, Clinical, and Electrodiagnostic Aspects. Edited by Brown WF, Bolton CF, Aminoff MJ. Philadelphia. PA, WB Saunders, 2002, pp 189–221

Ziemann U: TMS and drugs. Clin Neurophysiol 115:1717–1729, 2004a

Ziemann U: TMS induced plasticity in human cortex. Rev Neurosci 15:252–266, 2004b

Ziemann U, Rothwell JC: I-waves in motor cortex. J Clin Neurophysiol 17:397–405, 2000

Ziemann U, Netz J, Szelenyi A, et al: Spinal and supraspinal mechanisms contribute to the silent period in the contracting soleus muscle after transcranial magnetic stimulation of human motor cortex. Neurosci Lett 156:167–171, 1993

Ziemann U, Lönnecker S, Paulus W: Inhibition of human motor cortex by ethanol: a transcranial magnetic stimulation study. Brain 118:1437–1446, 1995

Ziemann U, Bruns D, Paulus W: Enhancement of human motor cortex inhibition by the dopamine receptor agonist pergolide: evidence from transcranial magnetic stimulation. Neurosci Lett 208:187–190, 1996a

Ziemann U, Lönnecker S, Steinhoff BJ, et al: The effect of lorazepam on the motor cortical excitability in man. Exp Brain Res 109:127–135, 1996b

Ziemann U, Rothwell JC, Ridding MC: Interaction between intracortical inhibition and facilitation in human motor cortex. J Physiol 496:873–881, 1996c

Ziemann U, Paulus W, Rothenberger A: Decreased motor inhibition in Tourette disorder: evidence from transcranial magnetic stimulation. Am J Psychiatry 154:1277–1284, 1997

Ziemann U, Chen R, Cohen LG, et al: Dextromethorphan decreases the excitability of the human motor cortex. Neurology 51:1320–1324, 1998a

Ziemann U, Tergau F, Wassermann EM, et al: Demonstration of facilitatory I-wave interaction in the human motor cortex by paired transcranial magnetic stimulation. J Physiol 511:181–190, 1998b

Ziemann U, Tergau F, Wischer S, et al: Pharmacological control of facilitatory I-wave interaction in the human motor cortex: a paired transcranial magnetic stimulation study. Electroencephalogr Clin Neurophysiol 109:321–330, 1998c

4

TRANSCRANIAL MAGNETIC STIMULATION IN EPILEPSY, MOVEMENT DISORDERS, AND PAIN

Charles M. Epstein, M.D.

Transcranial magnetic stimulation (TMS) has been used extensively in attempts to induce and inhibit seizures and to investigate their pathophysiology. TMS has also been applied to studying the effects and mechanisms of anticonvulsants. Finally, TMS has been used in localizing language and memory, with the aim of simplifying evaluation for epilepsy surgery. In this chapter, I summarize the literature for these uses of TMS and discuss further applications under investigation.

INDUCTION AND INHIBITION OF SEIZURES

The simplest and most obvious effect of TMS is the production of contralateral limb movement. The lowest stimulus level at which single TMS pulses produce detectable muscle activity is called the *motor threshold* (MT). MT is commonly used in setting the intensity of TMS for other applications and in estimating its safety. Because single TMS pulses appear to be excitatory in the production of movement, it is easy to assume that a train of TMS pulses will be excitatory as well.

Such an assumption was made in the earliest TMS studies in epilepsy. However, as discussed more extensively in Chapter 3 ("Basic Neurophysiological Studies With Transcranial Magnetic Stimulation") in this volume, extensive evidence suggests that long pulse trains at 1 Hz or below tend to have overall inhibitory effects on visual, motor, and sensory cortex (Boroojerdi et al. 2000; Chen et al. 1997; Knecht et al. 2003). There is also increasing evidence of effects on cortical areas remote from stimulation (Gorsler et al. 2003; Plewnia et al. 2003). Most of these remote effects are inhibitory, but some may be excitatory (Gilio et al. 2003; Plewnia et al. 2003). With repetitive TMS (rTMS) above 1 Hz, higher-frequency trains are increasingly excitatory (Wassermann 1998).

One theoretical risk of TMS is *kindling*— a process in which the daily administration of an apparently innocuous cerebral stimulus eventually produces increasing afterdischarges, triggered seizures, and finally spontaneous epileptic seizures (Goddard et al. 1969). Hippocampus and amygdala are the areas most easily kindled in rodents; neocortical regions are more resistant than limbic areas, and primate brains are more resistant to kindling than brains of smaller animals. The classic kindling preparation uses brief trains of pulses delivered from electrodes implanted in gray matter. Both the kindling process and the subsequent induction of triggered seizures are easiest at frequencies around 60 Hz but substantially more difficult to produce at 10 Hz or below. The possible relationship of kindling to long-term potentiation and its role in human epilepsy remain provocative but unconfirmed.

Although kindling has been accomplished with intracranial *electrical* stimulation as slow as 1 Hz, pulse trains at this frequency or lower often produce long-term depression of synaptic transmission—a finding consistent with the suspected effect of TMS at similar frequencies.

Low-Frequency TMS

Hufnagel and colleagues (1990a) first used long trains of slow TMS in attempts to activate known epileptic foci. With the equipment then available, the maximum repetition rate at 100% output was 0.3 Hz or less, and the round magnetic coils were not highly localizing. Recording from subdural electrodes in patients with intractable temporal lobe epilepsy, the authors believed that they had activated increased spikes at the epileptiform focus in 12 of 13 patients, and they later reported the induction of characteristic seizures in several subjects (Hufnagel and Elger 1991). However, subsequent studies cast doubt on this conclusion. Tassinari and colleagues (1990) concluded that slow TMS neither induced the characteristic seizures of subjects with intractable epilepsies nor produced electroencephalographic changes. Several other groups reported similarly disappointing results, even using fast rTMS in subjects with subdural electrodes (Dhuna et al.

1991; Jennum et al. 1994b; Schuler et al. 1993). In many of these patients, the rate of epileptiform discharges actually decreased after rTMS. These and other results are consistent with the concept that trains of stimulation at 1 Hz and below may have an inhibitory effect on cortical excitability.

This hypothesis was strengthened by animal research, in which 0.5-Hz rTMS prolonged the latency to development of pentylenetetrazol-induced seizures (Akamatsu et al. 2001). Another study investigated whether the cerebrospinal fluid (CSF) of humans exposed to 1- or 10-Hz rTMS might inhibit kindling: Anschel and colleagues (2003) found that in a rat seizure model, the kindling rate was significantly decreased by intraventricular injection of CSF from depressed patients exposed to 1-Hz rTMS. The CSF from patients that underwent 10-Hz rTMS produced a trend toward an increased kindling rate.

Subsequent human treatment studies have therefore focused on inhibiting seizures with slow rTMS. In a small series, Wedegaertner and colleagues (1997) found that 1-Hz pulse trains reduce action myoclonus in human subjects. Action myoclonus is a consequence of anoxic cortical injury and is not considered a form of epilepsy; nonetheless this work represented a potential model for other possible applications of TMS. However, a larger sham-controlled series involving 10 days of treatment reportedly produced no benefit (Wassermann and Lisanby 2001). Several later uncontrolled studies reported improvement in epileptic seizures or interictal epileptiform discharges following trains of slow rTMS (Menkes and Gruenthal 2000; Steinhoff et al. 2002; Tergau et al. 1999b). Sites of stimulation were not necessarily related to the regions of seizure onset. Again, however, a larger controlled trial showed no benefit (Theodore et al. 2002). There was a nonsignificant trend toward improvement in the patients with neocortical epilepsy—for whom the coil could be placed more directly above a known focus. Even 3 months of more modest rTMS (three times a week, 95% of MT) failed to produce substantial improvement (Brasil-Neto et al. 2004). Subsequent uncontrolled studies in several patients appeared to show improvement with slow rTMS in patients with refractory epilepsy or epilepsia partialis continua (EPC) when due to cortical dysplasia (Fregni et al. 2005; Misawa et al. 2005; Rossi et al. 2004).

Only one patient has been reported in whom seizures could be triggered repeatedly by focal single-pulse TMS (Classen et al. 1995). This patient had an epileptic focus in the left supplementary motor cortex. The semiology of seizures triggered by TMS was the same as that of spontaneous seizures. Seizures could be triggered only when a figure-eight coil was located at a specific angle and position over the interhemispheric sulcus. Across many thousands of patients receiving diagnostic TMS, the rate of seizure induction has in fact turned out to be remarkably low (Michelucci et al. 1996; Reutens et al. 1993b; Tassinari et al. 1990).

A recent report describes a psychiatry patient who was being used as a pilot subject in a MT study and experienced a secondarily generalized seizure 1 minute after receiving his third single pulse (Tharayil et al. 2005). The description of this episode is fairly convincing. However, the patient was acutely manic at the time he received TMS and was receiving lithium and chlorpromazine. Subsequently, the investigators learned that a sibling had a history of suspected epilepsy. With such a combination of risk factors, this patient probably should not have received TMS; nor should he be considered a "normal" subject. Other rare reported cases of seizures occurring near the time of slow TMS involved preexisting brain lesions, making the association of seizure with TMS difficult to distinguish with certainty from coincidence (Fauth et al. 1992; Homberg and Netz 1989).

Fast Repetitive TMS

The first reported series of fast rTMS in humans described a known epileptic subject who experienced a clinical seizure during stimulation. The seizure began focally on the side of stimulation but contralateral to his characteristic focus (Dhuna et al. 1991). This worrisome finding was soon replicated in a "normal" volunteer (Wassermann 1998). Both of these subjects were receiving 100% output from the Cadwell High-Speed Stimulator, but several subsequent "normal" subjects had seizures with lower intensities of stimulation. As discussed in Chapter 1 ("Overview of Transcranial Magnetic Stimulation") in this volume, available evidence suggests that the ability of fast rTMS to induce seizures goes up with stimulation rate, intensity, and train duration, and it also rises as the intertrain interval falls below several seconds.

The present safety guidelines for fast rTMS are enormously valuable but should not be misinterpreted as absolute. Stimulation parameters *approaching* the proposed limits are likely to carry a small though presently unquantified risk of seizure induction. The presence of cerebral lesions or the use of medications known to lower seizure thresholds now appears very likely to increase the risk (Fauth et al. 1992; Homberg and Netz 1989).

Yet even fast rTMS in long trains at high frequencies has shown little ability to produce "seizures on demand" with conventional technology (Dhuna et al. 1991; Jennum et al. 1994b). Electroconvulsive therapy (ECT) and electrical stimulation of the human brain may represent models for potential long-term effects of TMS, such as kindling; so it is noteworthy that no evidence for the induction of an epileptic focus has been found in patients undergoing prolonged electrical cortical stimulation or large numbers of ECT treatments (Goldensohn 1984; Krueger et al. 1993). And despite multiple studies and the recent advent of magnetic seizure therapy (MST), no model of spontaneously recurrent seizures has been reported in rodents or in nonhuman primates. This lack of an animal model for spontaneously recurrent seizures may be due in part to the inefficiency of human-sized coils when used with very small brains and in part to the ethical need to anesthetize primates in studies designed to induce seizures. Jennum and Klitgaard (1996) reported that chronic rTMS for 30 days at 50 Hz in rats failed to produce seizures directly but did shorten the time to onset of seizures that were subsequently induced with pentylenetetrazole. At present this is the only evidence for a process related to kindling with TMS.

As elsewhere in medicine, apparent seizures in proximity to TMS have a differential diagnosis. Clinical phenomena reported with rTMS include syncope (Figiel et al. 1998; Wassermann 1998), induction of limb jerking, and transient homonymous hemianopia (Michelucci et al. 1994). We have witnessed recurrence of long-standing motor tics in the midst of fast rTMS and the evolution of psychogenic pseudoseizures during a prolonged course of fast rTMS treatment (Figiel et al. 1998). Differentiation of such events from true or incipient epileptic seizures may be difficult. An example is the case reported by Conca and colleagues (2000), in which the authors noted that fast rTMS *may* have induced a frontal lobe complex partial seizure during treatment for depression. As described, the episode sounds equally compatible with syncope. Notably, however, the patient was also receiving antidepressant medications along with rTMS.

NEUROPHYSIOLOGY OF EPILEPSY

Although the biophysical properties of TMS are most consistent with depolarization of myelinated axons, the production of motor evoked potentials (MEPs) usually appears to be transsynaptic. This mode of activation, and the availability of paired-pulse stimulation, provide abundant opportunities to use TMS in exploring aspects of epilepsy through excitation and inhibition in the motor cortex.

Primary generalized epilepsy (PGE) is a genetic condition with incomplete penetrance and is associated with seizures beginning in childhood or adolescence. Subsets of PGE include juvenile myoclonic epilepsy, true petit mal with three-per-second spike-wave on the electroencephalogram (EEG), most cases of photosensitive epilepsy, and primary generalized convulsions. Using TMS of motor areas to assess general properties of the cerebral cortex, Reutens and colleagues (1993a) showed that mean MT in untreated patients with PGE was lower than in normal control subjects. Treatment with valproic acid, the classic drug of choice for PGE, raised mean MT above that of normal control subjects (Figure 4–1). Assuming that a lower MT reflects a more excitable cortex, these results are consistent with animal studies indicating that widespread cortical hyperexcitability is a central feature of PGE, and are supported by increases in the cortical silent period (Macdonell et al. 2001). Valproic acid may specifically reverse the diffuse hyperexcitable state.

Using paired-pulse stimulation, Caramia and colleagues (1996) found that patients with juvenile myoclonic epilepsy lack the normal motor inhibition to paired stimuli. Interestingly, if TMS is triggered during the slow wave portion of a spike-

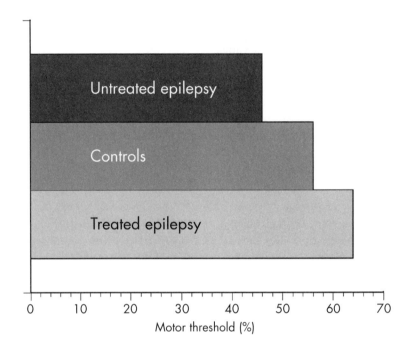

Figure 4-1. Mean transcranial magnetic stimulation motor thresholds for patients with primary generalized epilepsy before and after treatment with valproic acid, compared with control subjects.

Source. Adapted from Reutens DC, Berkov SF, Macdonell RA, et al.: "Magnetic Stimulation of the Brain in Generalized Epilepsy: Reversal of Cortical Hyperexcitability by Anticonvulsants." *Annals of Neurology* 34:351–355, 1993. Used with permission.

and-wave complex, the size of the MEPs decreases (Gianelli et al. 1994). This is consistent with the concept of the aftercoming slow wave as a state of inhibitory hyperpolarization that follows the epileptic spike. Following an initial generalized convulsive seizure, 18 patients studied for MT and cortical excitability had markedly reduced intracortical facilitation (ICF) (Delvaux et al. 2001). The authors speculated that these changes might represent post-ictal protective mechanisms.

Patients with progressive myoclonus epilepsies apparently have not undergone TMS testing while not taking anticonvulsants, so possible effects of their condition on MT are unknown. However, two patients who had conditioning stimuli with peripheral nerve shocks delivered 20–60 milliseconds (msec) prior to TMS had a markedly augmented facilitatory effect on motor responses (Reutens et al. 1993b). This result suggested that the excitability of the sensorimotor cortex was abnormally enhanced by peripheral afferent input.

In focal epilepsies, Werhahn and colleagues (2000) found that over the hemisphere of seizure origin (the "abnormal" side) there was a reduction of ICF and normal intracortical inhibition (ICI), whereas in the "normal" hemisphere there was a reduced ICI and a slight reduction of ICF. ICF on the "abnormal" side was reduced ($P < 0.05$) compared with the "normal" hemisphere. However, other studies in patients with focal epilepsy have failed to show consistent results. Varrasi and colleagues (2004) found disrupted cortical inhibition in only one-third of drug-naive patients and correlated this finding with interictal epileptiform discharges.

Epilepsia partialis continua is a state of continuous muscle activity due to sustained seizure activity in an area of motor cortex. Cockerell and colleagues (1996) reported a variety of abnormalities in MEPs from six patients with EPC; however, they did not test MT. Epstein (1998) measured MT in the involved limbs of four patients with EPC. All had marked asymmetry of MTs between involved and normal limbs. The two with spasticity and hyperreflexia had elevated MTs on the involved side; the others, without spasticity or reflex change, had lowered thresholds in the symptomatic limbs. Elevated MT and the upper motor neuron syndrome may both reflect a state of increased neuronal inhibition at the focus, whereas reduced MT may indicate a condition of local hyperexcitability.

EFFECTS OF ANTICONVULSANTS

As noted earlier, therapeutic levels of valproic acid have a prominent effect in elevating TMS MT, and this property is shared by other anticonvulsants that act at the voltage-dependent sodium channel in neuronal membranes (Boroojerdi et al. 2001; Hufnagel et al. 1990b, Ziemann et al. 1996b). This class of drugs includes phenytoin, carbamazepine, lamotrigine, and valproic acid. All these agents appear to hold sodium channels in an inactive configuration, raising the threshold to action potentials and especially to repetitive firing at high frequencies. The more antiepileptic drugs taken, the higher the threshold to TMS (Cantello et al. 2000).

In contrast, other antiepileptic drugs, such as vigabatrin and tiagabine, appear to augment the effect of the neurotransmitter γ-aminobutyric acid (GABA)—and thus to facilitate the opening of inhibitory chloride channels in neuronal membranes. Although the final effects of both anticonvulsant classes are mediated through membrane ion channels, the latter are often described as *neuromodulators* because their influence is indirect. In some studies, the GABAergic neuromodulators fail to affect MT at therapeutic levels. Instead, when studied with paired-pulse TMS paradigms, they were shown to increase ICI and reduce ICF (Ziemann et al. 1996b). Other reports, however, described measurable elevations in MT (Palmieri et al. 1999) or failed to find short-latency changes. Instead, they pointed to alterations in stimulus-response curves as a common feature of drug effects on TMS measures (Boroojerdi et al. 2001). The direction of excitability changes with TMS may be a complicated function of differential effects on type A ($GABA_A$) and type B ($GABA_B$) GABA receptors (Werhahn et al. 1999).

Despite these complications, TMS studies may help to clarify mechanisms of anticonvulsant action. For example, gabapentin, a drug whose mode of action was initially uncertain, clearly segregates with the agents known to operate at the GABAergic chloride channel (Rizzo et al. 2001; Ziemann et al. 1996b). Levetiracetam, whose mechanism of action remains poorly understood, shows only changes in recruitment curves (Sohn et al. 2001).

Epstein and colleagues (1997) followed MT over time in patients undergoing acute taper of anticonvulsants during inpatient epilepsy monitoring. For 7 of 10 patients, a fall in MT showed correlations of 90%–99% with daily dose or blood levels (Figure 4–2). It is possible that the patients with refractory epilepsy who showed little change in MT harbor genetic polymorphisms that influence the sodium channel, or have active transport systems that reduce the intracellular accumulation of anticonvulsants (Tishler et al. 1995). Lee and colleagues (2005) administered carbamazepine and lamotrigine to normal volunteers for 5 weeks while tracking MT and ICI; they found that abrupt withdrawal of carbamazepine was followed by persistent drug effects in some subjects and a decrease in MT below the original level in others.

MAPPING OF SPEECH, LANGUAGE, AND MEMORY

The *intracarotid amobarbital test,* or *Wada test,* is widely used in planning surgery for intractable epilepsy. Although amobarbital injection was originally introduced only for the lateralization of language, additional testing for the possibility of unilateral memory impairment has long been a standard part of the procedure. Because the Wada test is cumbersome and expensive and requires the risk of arteriography, the idea of supplementing or replacing it was one of the earliest goals for TMS in cognitive testing. However, initial attempts using single-pulse stimulation over Broca's and Wernicke's areas produced no obvious effects. In the first successful protocol, Pascual-Leone and colleagues (1991) used fast rTMS rates from 8 to 25 Hz for 10 seconds and output intensities up to 80% of full scale with the Cadwell High Speed Stimulator. The subjects were six patients with intractable epilepsy who were undergoing presurgical evaluation. At sufficiently high intensities all subjects had total anarthria with fast rTMS over the left frontotemporal region but not the right. Speech arrest took 4–6 seconds to develop, and it ceased as soon as stimulation was stopped. Wada tests confirmed language lateralization to the left hemisphere in all cases.

Other studies of fast rTMS and speech have produced more equivocal results.

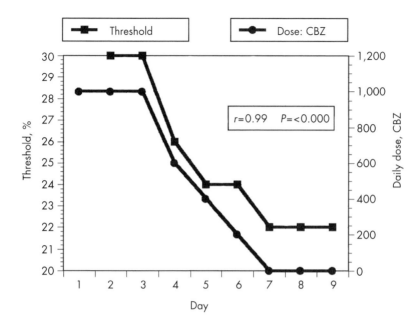

Figure 4–2. Transcranial magnetic stimulation motor threshold in the left hand versus total daily dose of carbamazepine (CBZ).

The patient was undergoing rapid withdrawal of carbamazepine monotherapy. The graphs are vertically offset for clarity. The physician making motor threshold measurements was blinded to anticonvulsant dose.

Source. Epstein CM, He L, Henry TR, et al.: "Alterations to Motor Threshold in Transcranial Magnetic Stimulation During Anticonvulsant Withdrawal." *Journal of Clinical Neurophysiology* 14:446, 1997. Copyright 1997 Lippincott Williams & WIlkins. Used with permission.

Jennum and colleagues (1994a) studied epilepsy patients by using rTMS at 30 Hz and a system from Dantec Medical (Medtronic Dantec NeuroMuscular, Skovlunde, Denmark). Stimulus trains lasted 1 or 2 seconds. Total speech arrest occurred in 14 of 21 subjects; in the 7 other subjects, the stronger stimulation was found to be too painful or the stimulator lacked sufficient output. When the results (including effects that were less than total speech arrest) were compared with those of the Wada test, the concordance was 95%. One patient who was left-dominant on Wada testing had greater speech inhibition over the right hemisphere with fast rTMS. The authors also noted that "rTMS might have over-diagnosed bilateral language representation."

Using the Cadwell High Speed Stimulator, Michelucci and colleagues (1994) studied 14 epilepsy patients. Stimulation frequencies were 16–25 Hz, with pulse trains of 7–10 seconds. Even at 100% stimulator output, these authors were able to demonstrate clear-cut speech arrest in only 7 of 14 subjects. The positive results showed high concordance with handedness, though Wada tests were not performed.

Using a more focal and powerful stimulation coil, Epstein and colleagues (1996) found that speech arrest could be obtained with a repetition rate as low as 2 Hz, an intensity of 150% of MT or less, and pulse trains of no more than 5 seconds. In a comparison of multiple stimulus rates and intensities, rTMS at lower rates required higher stimulator output but produced significantly less discomfort and less prominent contraction of oral-facial musculature. For several of these subjects the first reaction to speech arrest was laughter. With 4-Hz rTMS, six of six normal subjects had complete, reproducible speech arrest with stimulation over one hemisphere but not the other. However, this series was surprising for implying 33% right hemisphere dominance in a small, unselected sample. In direct comparison with the Wada test, a series of 17 patients showed a significant excess of apparent bilateral and right hemisphere language dominance by rTMS (Epstein et al. 2000). Although speech arrest by fast rTMS is highly correlated with handedness and with results of the Wada test, it also produces inflated estimates of bilateral and right-sided language dominance, which substantially diminishes its clinical utility.

Epstein and colleagues (1999) mapped sites of speech arrest in normal subjects. The site of speech arrest by 4 Hz rTMS appeared congruous with the facial motor cortex, and the function most impaired was the de novo assembly of spontaneous speech. In this series, magnetic speech arrest did not represent Broca's aphasia. Stewart and colleagues (2001) described a second, more anterior site of speech arrest in the vicinity of Broca's area. However, extensive language testing was not performed.

At present, none of the classic aphasias have been reproduced with TMS. Thus far, the effects of rTMS on language, as compared with motor speech output, have been modest. True aphasic errors are infrequent. Reported findings include increased verbal comprehension errors when right-handed subjects were stimulated over the left hemisphere (Claus et al. 1993) and increased picture-word identification errors with left-sided rTMS (Flitman et al. 1998). Demonstrating these effects required multiple stimulus trains plus pooling of data across several subjects.

Grafman and colleagues (1994) used trains of fast rTMS lasting 500 milliseconds during presentation of word lists, attempting to disrupt verbal memory. They found that rTMS significantly impaired word recall at left midtemporal and bilateral frontal sites.

More recently, it has become apparent that granular prefrontal cortex, known to subserve working memory, also plays an important role in encoding novel stimuli. Floel and colleagues (2004) showed that encoding of verbal material was disrupted by left prefrontal TMS, whereas encoding of nonverbal material was disrupted by right prefrontal stimulation. Since the prefrontal cortex is much more accessible to TMS than the mesial temporal lobe, such findings raise the possibility of a procedure robust enough for clinical use.

FURTHER CONSIDERATIONS ON CURRENT USES

Applications of TMS in epilepsy continue to evolve. Conventional rTMS can induce seizures often enough to raise concerns about safety but not frequently enough to be reliable in producing seizures even at known epileptic foci. The use of slow rTMS to suppress some focal epilepsies remains promising, although thus far this effect has been unconfirmed by controlled trials. Because slow rTMS is extremely safe, it should be considered in refractory neocortical seizures, especially those associated with cortical dysplasias.

TMS demonstrates alterations in cortical excitability with the use of anticonvulsants and is likely to become more useful in analyzing anticonvulsant effects. rTMS can block speech output reliably and safely; but at present the apparent lateralization of rTMS speech arrest fails to correlate completely with the results of Wada tests.

FURTHER APPLICATIONS UNDER DEVELOPMENT

Movement Disorders

Paired-pulse studies in a variety of movement disorders have shown a general tendency toward decreased ICI in Parkinson's disease, Huntington's disease, Tourette's syndrome, task-specific dystonia, Wilson's disease, corticobasal degeneration (CBD), and progressive supranuclear palsy (Abbruzzese et al. 1997; Hanajima et al. 1996; Kleine et al. 2001; Ridding et al. 1995a, 1995b; Rona et al. 1998; Ziemann et al. 1996a, 1997). ICF in the same series was more likely to be normal, although it was reported to be increased in Huntington's disease and CBD. Younger children with Tourette's syndrome showed only a decrease in cortical silent period (Moll et al. 1999). Across this group of disorders, changes in MT were not seen. Since the pathophysiologies of movement disorders are predominantly subcortical, the changes in intracortical inhibition are considered to reflect alterations in cortical-basal ganglia loops; but they are obviously not specific, and their clinical significance is unclear.

The rationales for possible benefit of TMS in movement disorders include increased release of dopamine, altered release of other neurotransmitters, and modulation of activity in cerebral cortex. The most common serious movement disorder, Parkinson's disease, has been the main focus of research.

Keck and colleagues (2002) used intracerebral microdialysis in Wistar rats to monitor the effects of acute 20-Hz rTMS on the intrahippocampal, intraaccumbal, and intrastriatal release patterns of dopamine and its metabolites. A round coil (winding diameter 6–57 mm) was activated in 20 trains at 130% of MT. In the dorsal hippocampus, the shell of the nucleus accumbens, and the dorsal striatum, the extracellular concentration of dopamine was significantly elevated in response to rTMS. This study was intended to model antidepressant effects and not the treatment of disorders such as Parkinson's disease.

Kanno and colleagues (2004) carried out a similar rat study, using a full-size figure-eight coil with outer diameter 70 mm. The frontal area of each rat received 500 rTMS stimuli from 20 trains in one day. A stimulation intensity of close to 110% of MT markedly increased extracellular dopamine concentrations in the rat dorsolateral striatum. In contrast, no increase occurred at higher or lower stimulus intensities. There was no significant difference in concentrations of serotonin (5-hydroxytryptamine [5-HT]). (Kole et al. [1999] had previously found that a single treatment with rTMS in rats significantly increased 5-HT binding sites in the frontal cortex, the cingulate cortex, and the anterior olfactory nucleus.)

There is some question whether a round or figure-eight coil many times larger than a rat brain can induce truly focal stimulation equivalent to that of a figure-eight coil in a human. However, human studies show similar results. Strafella and colleagues (2001) used ^{11}C-labeled raclopride and positron emission tomography (PET) to measure changes in extracellular dopamine concentration in vivo after rTMS of the dorsolateral prefrontal cortex in healthy human subjects. (Binding of ^{11}C]raclopride is inversely proportional to levels of extracellular dopamine.) Repetitive TMS was performed with a round coil over the left dorsolateral prefrontal cortex or the left occipital cortex. Three rTMS blocks of 10-Hz rTMS were delivered before the start of PET acquisition. Left prefrontal rTMS caused a reduction in ^{11}C]raclopride binding in the left dorsal caudate nucleus. The authors concluded that rTMS of the prefrontal cortex induces the release of endogenous dopamine in the ipsilateral caudate nucleus.

These studies leave little doubt that under some conditions rTMS induces dopamine release in the basal ganglia and other regions. However, it is not clear that inducing greater release of dopamine from striatal cells that are already depleted and dying is likely to be an effective long-term treatment strategy in Parkinson's disease. In theory, effects involving other neurotransmitters and other brain regions might be preferable.

Parkinson's Disease

Acute effects.   The earliest positive results for Parkinson's disease were reported by Pascual-Leone and colleagues (1994), who applied rTMS at 5 Hz and 90% of resting motor threshold (RMT) to the motor cortex while the subject carried out the Grooved Pegboard Test (Lezak 1995) with the opposite hand. Parkinson's disease patients had significantly improved task performance in the unmedicated state, when they were clinically "off" and maximally symptomatic, whereas healthy control subjects showed no change. However, when the same experiment was repeated by Ghabra and colleagues (1999), stimulation at 90% of RMT produced overt movements of the tested hand, which severely impaired task performance. At lower stimulus intensities, stimulus-induced movements were avoided, but no benefit was obtained during or after rTMS.

Siebner and colleagues (1999a, 1998b) used similar parameters in Parkinson's disease patients, applying 2,250 stimuli over the motor cortex at 90% of RMT and 5 Hz; rTMS was broken up into five trains of 30-second duration. They reported improved movement time in a ballistic arm pointing task. In addition, movement became measurably smoother. Sham stimulation with the coil applied at 45 degrees over the midfrontal cortex produced no benefit. Unfortunately, sham stimulation in this study differed from real stimulation both in coil tilt and coil placement.

Exploring a wider range of stimuli, Tergau and colleagues (1999a) applied rTMS at 90% of RMT and 1, 5, 10, and 20 Hz on different days. Responses in treated patients were evaluated before and after with motor tests from the Unified Parkinson's Disease Rating Scale (UPDRS). After 500 pulses, the authors found no change in performance in walking or in a simple reaction time.

Boylan and colleagues (2001) targeted the supplementary motor area at a midsagittal location, applying 10-Hz rTMS at 150% of RMT for a total of 50 pulse trains lasting 5 seconds each. None of the eight patients improved after stimulation; instead, they experienced worsening of reaction time and spiral drawing.

Ikeguchi and colleagues (2003) studied the effects of 0.2-Hz rTMS performed six times for 2 weeks in 12 patients with idiopathic Parkinson's disease. Ten patients received rTMS to the bilateral frontal cortex, and 6 patients received stimulation to the bilateral occipital cortex. Both frontal and occipital rTMS *reduced* rCBF in the cortical areas around the stimulated site. Several activity and motor scores improved; in contrast, occipital rTMS had no benefit.

Lefaucheur and colleagues (2004b) performed 10-Hz rTMS on the left motor cortical area in 12 "off-drug" patients with Parkinson's disease. "Real" rTMS at 10 or 0.5 Hz, but not "sham" stimulation, improved motor performance. High-frequency rTMS decreased rigidity and bradykinesia in the upper limb contralateral to the stimulation, while low-frequency rTMS reduced upper limb rigidity bilaterally and improved walking. Clinical improvement induced by rTMS was too short-lasting to consider therapeutic application.

Chronic effects.   Mally and Stone (1999) and Shimamoto and colleagues (2001) employed a variety of stimulus rates, intensities, and number of stimuli given through a round coil to patients with Parkinson's disease. The authors reported substantial improvements that persisted for weeks or months after the end of treatment. A collaborative study group using the 0.2-Hz parameters advocated by Shimamoto et al. subsequently enrolled 85 patients and used an advanced sham with electrical scalp stimulation (Okabe et al. 2003). They found no benefit of rTMS over the sham. Mally and colleagues (2004) later reported sustained benefit over

3 years, using near-homeopathic doses of TMS (a total of 700 pulses over 7 days at 0.6 tesla, repeated "at least twice a year"). Controlled replication of these astonishing open-label results would seem highly desirable, especially since Parkinson's disease patients are known to show prominent placebo responses in blinded trials (Goetz et al. 2000), and since a highly realistic sham appeared to nullify the apparent benefits of the Shimamoto technique.

Other Movement Disorders

Münchau and colleagues (2002) performed a single-blind, placebo-controlled, crossover trial of rTMS in 16 patients with Tourette's syndrome. Patients received, in random sequence, 1-Hz motor, premotor, and sham rTMS, which each consisted of two 20-minute rTMS sessions applied on two consecutive days. The rTMS intensity was 80% of active MT. In the 12 patients who completed the trial, there was no significant improvement of symptoms after any of the rTMS conditions. Stimulation at 80% of active MT had been chosen to avoid excess activation of neighboring structures. The authors noted that this level of stimulation might simply have been too modest to produce any effect, especially as they did not use precise neuronavigation techniques to locate the premotor area. There is some indication that their speculation may have been correct; in a preliminary study, Karp and colleagues (1997) found that 1-Hz rTMS of motor cortex may reduce the frequency of tics.

Siebner and colleagues (1999b) applied 1-Hz rTMS at 90% of RMT to the motor cortices of patients with writer's cramp and healthy controls. Twenty minutes after treatment with 1,800 pulses, the authors found reduced paired-pulse cortical excitability, prolonged cortical silent period, and decreased measures of writing pressure. They reported transient clinical improvement in some subjects. There was, however, no change in normal control subjects.

Shimizu and colleagues (1999) gave single-pulse TMS to four patients with hereditary spinocerebellar degeneration through a circular coil, using 30 pulses/day at 100% of MT and less than 0.2 Hz for 21 consecutive days. They reported improvements in gait and balance for all four subjects. The same group subsequently described a total of 74 patients treated in the same fashion, with almost half receiving sham stimulation (Shiga et al. 2002). Again the treatment group improved significantly, along with mean regional blood flow in the cerebellum and pons. These results are remarkable, not merely for the small number of pulses but for the modest stimulus intensity, considering that even the surface of the cerebellum is relatively distant from the scalp surface compared with the cerebral cortex. Replication by other laboratories would be an exciting development.

Discussion

Decreased ICI across many movement disorders is striking but not specific. Attempts at alleviating Parkinson's disease and other conditions have shown little reproducible benefit, although a few studies have described prolonged improvement. At times similar treatment parameters have given opposite results. Placebo effects in Parkinson's disease may be substantial and insidious; replication of apparent positive results, rigorous controls, and realistic shams are urgently needed.

Pain

Electrical stimulation has been widely applied for pain relief in both the peripheral and central nervous systems. The number of potential treatment sites is large: pain-related increases of cerebral blood flow have been reported in primary somatosensory cortex, second somatosensory cortex, parietal operculum, insular cortex, anterior cingulate cortex, orbitofrontal cortex, ipsilateral thalamus, upper brain stem, and cerebellum (Garcia-Larrea et al. 1999; Peyron et al. 1995). All these sites might be considered potential targets for TMS, although some are obviously more approachable by external magnetic fields than others. But the best-established model for the use of rTMS to control pain turns out to be electrical stimulation of the motor cortex (MCS) with epidural electrodes (Garcia-Larrea et al. 1999; Katayama et al. 1998; Meyerson et al. 1993; Nguyen et al. 1997; Tsubokawa et al. 1991, 1993). In MCS, stimulation settings vary widely but might typically involve monophasic pulses with duration of 0.1 to 0.5 milliseconds, adjusted to just below the threshold for inducing movement. Pulse trains are delivered at 25–50 Hz for 5–20 minutes (Katayama et al. 1998; Tsubokawa et al. 1993). Most of these parameters can be approximated with TMS. However, rTMS at 25 Hz and above would be difficult because of system heating, the risk of inducing seizures, and increased local pain induced by rapid rTMS itself. An easier approach is to use low-frequency rTMS, with the anticipation that the decrease in cortical excitability produced by slow rTMS might result in reduced pain perception.

Slow Motor Cortex Stimulation

The first description of rTMS over the primary motor cortex (M1) for pain was given by Migita and colleagues (1995). They administered low-frequency, monophasic TMS to the motor cortex in two patients, producing 30% pain relief in one patient and no relief in the other.

Tamura and colleagues (2004) studied slow rTMS over the left motor cortex following contralateral injections of capsaicin into the right volar forearm of healthy volunteers. The intensity of stimulation was fixed at 1.3 times active MT. Following the administration of capsaicin, 300 stimuli of 1-Hz rTMS were applied over the left motor cortical area for 5 minutes. Pain was estimated with 10-point visual-analog scales.

This study included an unusually comprehensive approach to sham stimulation, including scalp contact, sound, and weak electrical stimulation. Compared

with pain intensity ratings for both sham and control conditions, the pain intensity ratings with rTMS were significantly lower—by an average of about
2 points—from 2 to 7 minutes after capsaicin injection (Figure 4–3). The lack of
a significant difference after 7 minutes may have been due, in part, to a ceiling effect, with pain ratings in all conditions falling into a similar range. Single-photon
emission computed tomography scans following M1 rTMS showed cerebral blood
flow changes in areas remote from the motor cortex.

Rapid Motor Cortex Stimulation

Rollnik and colleagues (2002) studied a mixed population of 12 patients with
therapy-resistant chronic pain, which involved multiple areas, including face and
limbs. Rapid-rate rTMS was targeted at the motor cortex contralateral to the pain
site by means of a circular coil over the vertex. A double-cone coil was used to stimulate the corresponding leg area. The investigators performed twenty 2-second,
20-Hz stimulations with 80% of MT intensity over 20 minutes. Sham stimulation
occurred in the same manner, except that the angle of the coil was at 45 degrees
off the skull. Sham and active treatment were given in random order on different
days. Six of 12 patients experienced an analgesic effect, but the analgesia remitted
within 5 minutes of ending stimulation. For the whole group, however, the difference between active and sham did not reach significance. Despite the lack of overall significant benefit, this study was notable for improvement in some patients
with use of rapid rTMS, even at the modest intensity of 80% of MT.

Summers and colleagues (2004) examined whether a session of rTMS would
produce sensory threshold changes in 40 healthy individuals. Detection and pain
thresholds for cold sensations were compared following low-frequency (1-Hz) and
high-frequency (20-Hz) repetitive TMS over the left motor cortex. Although cold
detection threshold was significantly lowered by both rTMS rates, only high-
frequency rTMS produced a significant change in cold pain threshold. In contrast,
sham rTMS did not alter thresholds for cold stimuli. At 95% of MT, the effect size
was relatively small.

Pleger and colleagues (2004) investigated the analgesic efficacy of 10-Hz
rTMS applied to the motor cortex in 10 patients with complex regional pain syndrome type I involving the hand. Pulse intensity was 110% of RMT, applied con-
tralaterally to the side affected by the pain syndrome in 10 trains of 1.2-second
duration. Seven of 10 patients reported decreased pain intensities. Pain relief began 30 seconds after stimulation, reaching a maximum 15 minutes later. Pain returned 45 minutes later. Sham rTMS with the coil tilted 45 degrees did not alter
pain perception.

Lefaucheur and colleagues (2001a) studied 18 patients with intractable, unilateral neurogenic pain of various origins, predominantly in the hand. The patients underwent real and sham rTMS sessions with twenty 10-Hz trains at 80%

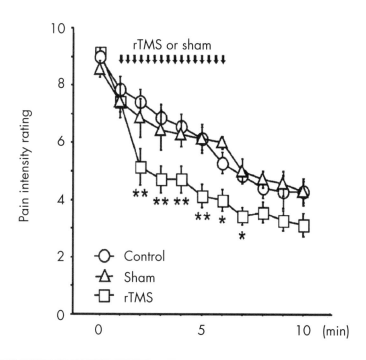

Figure 4–3. Time course of pain intensity ratings after slow repetitive transcranial magnetic stimulation (rTMS) over the left motor cortex following contralateral injections of capsaicin into the right volar forearm of healthy volunteers.

Source. Reprinted from Tamura Y, Okabe S, Ohnishi T, et al.: "Effects of 1-Hz Repetitive Transcranial Magnetic Stimulation on Acute Pain Induced by Capsaicin." *Pain* 107:107–115, 2004. Copyright 2004 International Association of the Study of Pain. Used with permission.

of MT, and also a 20-minute treatment at 0.5 Hz and 80% of RMT. Pain intensity was assessed by means of visual-analog scales 5–10 minutes after the end of each rTMS session. A significant decrease in the mean pain level was obtained only after 10-Hz real rTMS. In terms of individual results, effects on pain level were classified as good or excellent in only two patients. The duration of benefit was brief, although not precisely delineated. In another report, however, Lefaucheur and colleagues (2001b) described significant pain decrease up to 8 days after a single "real" rTMS session, in which 10-Hz stimulation was used. This series included 14 patients with intractable pain due to thalamic stroke or trigeminal neuropathy. As noted below, these patients may represent relatively favorable groups for rTMS response.

In a subsequent study, the same group (Lefaucheur et al. 2004a) treated 60 right-handed patients with intractable, unilateral neuropathic pain of different etiologies. Treatment was 10-Hz rTMS. Pain reduction was significantly greater following real than sham rTMS (−22.9% vs. −7.8%; $P=0.0002$.) Results were worse in patients with brain stem stroke, whatever the site of pain. Better results were obtained for facial pain, although stimulation was targeted on the hand cortical area. The degree of sensory loss did not influence TMS effects, but the benefit remained transient.

Subsequently, Khedr and colleagues (2005) reported that in patients with trigeminal neuralgia and poststroke pain syndrome, rTMS over the hand area of motor cortex at 20 Hz and 80% of MT for 5 days produced benefit that was superior to sham. Improvement was still evident 2 weeks after the end of treatment.

TMS at Nonmotor Sites

Kanda and colleagues (2003) applied weak CO_2 laser stimuli, at an intensity around the threshold for pain, to the dorsum of the left hand in nine normal subjects. At variable delays after the onset of the laser stimulus, pairs of TMS pulses were applied in separate blocks of trials over either the right sensorimotor cortex, midline occipital cortex, second somatosensory cortex, or medial frontal cortex—near the area of anterior cingulate cortex that is associated with pain on cerebral blood flow studies. The intensity of TMS was set at 1.2 times the RMT. The CO_2 laser stimuli were delivered to the dorsum of the left hand at intervals of 4–6 seconds, occasionally followed by TMS. Subjects judged that the stimulus was more painful when TMS was delivered over sensorimotor areas at 150–200 milliseconds after the laser stimulus; the opposite occurred when TMS was delivered over medial frontal cortex at 50–100 milliseconds.

Kanda et al. hypothesized that TMS might reduce effective pain sensation at the medial frontal cortex site by affecting the emotional aspect of pain. There is, however, substantial uncertainty about how selectively the anterior cingulate cortex can be activated by TMS; models of the induced electric field suggest that it may be difficult to stimulate sites in the medial wall of the hemisphere without also involving more widespread areas of superficial cortex. The anatomic area involved in pain relief is therefore unresolved.

Töpper and colleagues (2003) studied two patients with a long-standing unilateral avulsion of the lower cervical roots and chronic pain in the arm. Multiple cortical sites were stimulated with a figure-eight coil, using 10- to 15-Hz trains of 2-second duration at 110% of MT. Stimulation of the contralateral parietal cortex led to a reproducible reduction in pain intensity lasting up to 10 minutes. Relief started 20–30 seconds after the completion of stimulation and lasted up to 10 minutes. The maximal mean pain reduction was 75%–88% (Figure 4–4). The degree of pain relief achieved with this method was considered to be superior to various

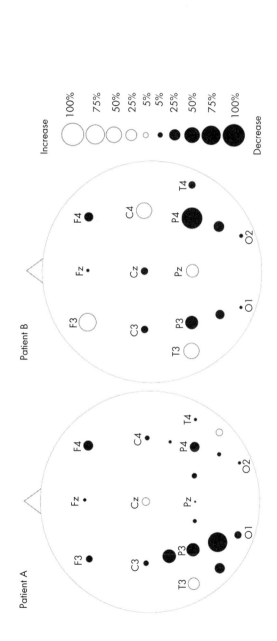

Figure 4–4.   Changes in pain intensity following repetitive transcranial magnetic stimulation (rTMS) of various cortical sites in two patients.

Size of the circles is an index of the degree of change in pain severity compared with the baseline pain intensity before rTMS. Each circle represents the mean change of pain following three different stimulation trains. Shaded circles indicate a decrease in pain intensity; light circles indicate an increase. Stimulation of the contralateral parietal cortex (left hemisphere in patient A and right hemisphere in patient B) was followed by a marked decrease in pain intensity.

Source.   Töpper R, Foltys H, Meister IG, et al.: "Repetitive Transcranial Magnetic Stimulation of the Parietal Cortex Transiently Ameliorates Phantom Limb Pain-Like Syndrome." Clinical Neurophysiology 114:1521–1530, 2003, copyright 2003. Used by permission of the International Federation of Clinical Neurophysiology.

previous anaesthesiological blockades. Both 1- and 10-Hz rTMS trains applied to the contralateral parietal cortex on weekdays for three consecutive weeks failed to produce permanent changes in pain intensity.

Amassian and colleagues (1997) had previously suggested that rTMS over the parietal cortex could produce analgesic effects through induction of endorphin release. However, in the Töpper et al. (2003) study, the opiate antagonist naloxone failed to prevent rTMS-induced pain reduction. Although responses to rTMS in this study were striking, the authors concluded that their results did not favor the use of rTMS in the treatment of deafferentation pain because the effects could not be sustained.

Although the pain relief from rTMS has thus far been brief, it may be useful for predicting benefit from the more invasive technique of MCS. Canavero and colleagues (2002) delivered slow rTMS trains over the motor cortex contralateral to the side of chronic neurogenic pain. Two patients were temporarily worsened by TMS, but three had transient improvement of both spontaneous pain and allodynia. These outcomes had a high correlation with the results of an IV propofol test. One patient who obtained no improvement from rTMS and one who had fair relief underwent implantation of MCS systems; only the latter benefited from MCS. Although this result is tantalizing, larger numbers are clearly needed.

DISCUSSION

Although caution is advisable in mixing results from chronic pain patients and healthy volunteers, doing so permits some tentative conclusions about TMS and pain. First, TMS at multiple sites is capable of providing substantial pain relief in many subjects. Effective locations include contralateral motor cortex, contralateral parietal cortex, and medial frontal cortex. At motor cortex, slow rTMS produced benefit only at intensities well above MT (which give repeated movement of the limb) and not at 80% of MT. Fast rTMS did produce benefit at 80% of MT, a level low enough that induced movement should not be a problem. Paired pulses of TMS, precisely timed with respect to a CO_2 laser, were sufficient to reduce the sensation of pain at medial frontal cortex, perhaps through emotional mechanisms. rTMS over contralateral parietal cortex led to striking benefit in patients with chronic neurogenic pain but not in normal subjects. Facial pain may be a relatively favorable finding for rTMS response, and brain stem stroke may be a relatively unfavorable finding.

At present, the greatest limitation of TMS for pain relief is the short duration of the effect. In only one study has benefit persisted after repeated treatments. Expectations of prolonged benefit from TMS were based on much longer responses in other conditions; reasons for the difference are unknown. True clinical utility is likely to depend on development of methods to sustain the treatment response.

REFERENCES

Abbruzzese G, Buccolieri A, Marchese R, et al: Intracortical inhibition and facilitation are abnormal in Huntington's disease: a paired magnetic stimulation study. Neurosci Lett 228:87–90, 1997

Akamatsu N, Fueta Y, Endo Y, et al: Decreased susceptibility to pentylenetetrazol-induced seizures after low-frequency transcranial magnetic stimulation in rats. Neurosci Lett 310:153–156, 2001

Amassian VE, Vergara MS, Somasundaram M, et al: Induced pain is relieved by repetitive stimulation (rTMS) of human parietal lobe through endorphin release (abstract). Electroencephalogr Clin Neurophysiol 103:179, 1997

Anschel DJ, Pascual-Leone A, Holmes GL: Anti-kindling effect of slow repetitive transcranial magnetic stimulation in rats. Neurosci Lett 351:9–12, 2003

Boroojerdi B, Prager A, Muellbacher W, et al: Reduction of human visual cortex excitability using 1-Hz transcranial magnetic stimulation. Neurology 54:1529–1531, 2000

Boroojerdi B, Battaglia F, Muellbacher W, et al: Mechanisms influencing stimulus-response properties of the human corticospinal system. Clin Neurophysiol 112:931–937, 2001

Boylan LS, Pullman SL, Lisanby SH, et al: Repetitive transcranial magnetic stimulation worsens complex movements in Parkinson's disease. Clin Neurophysiol 112:259–264, 2001

Brasil-Neto JP, de Araujo DP, Teixeira WA, et al: Experimental therapy of epilepsy with transcranial magnetic stimulation: lack of additional benefit with prolonged treatment. Arq Neuropsiquiatr 62:21–25, 2004

Canavero S, Bonicalzi V, Dotta M, et al: Transcranial magnetic cortical stimulation relieves central pain. Stereotact Funct Neurosurg 78:192–196, 2002

Cantello R, Civardi C, Cavalli A, et al: Cortical excitability in cryptogenic localization-related epilepsy: interictal transcranial magnetic stimulation studies. Epilepsia 41:694–704, 2000

Caramia MD, Gigli G, Iani C, et al: Distinguishing forms of generalized epilepsy using magnetic brain stimulation. Electroencephalogr Clin Neurophysiol 98:14–19, 1996

Chen R, Classen J, Gerloff C, et al: Depression of motor cortex excitability by low-frequency transcranial magnetic stimulation. Neurology 48:1398–1403, 1997

Classen J, Witte OW, Schlaug G, et al: Epileptic seizures triggered directly by focal transcranial magnetic stimulation. Electroencephalogr Clin Neurophysiol 94:19–25, 1995

Claus D, Weis M, Treig T, et al: Influence of repetitive magnetic stimuli on verbal comprehension. J Neurol 240:149–150, 1993

Cockerell OC, Rothwell J, Thompson PD, et al: Clinical and physiological features of epilepsia partialis continua: cases ascertained in the UK. Brain 119:393–407, 1996

Conca A, Konig P, Hausmann A: Transcranial magnetic stimulation induces "pseudo-absence seizure." Acta Psychiatr Scand 101:246–248, 2000

Delvaux V, Alagona G, Gerard P, et al: Reduced excitability of the motor cortex in untreated patients with de novo idiopathic "grand mal" seizures. J Neurol Neurosurg Psychiatry 71:772–776, 2001

Dhuna A, Gates J, Pascual-Leone A: Transcranial magnetic stimulation in patients with epilepsy. Neurology 41:1067–1071, 1991

Epstein CM: Motor evoked potential thresholds in epilepsia partialis continua. Epilepsia 39:201–202, 1998

Epstein CM, Lah JJ, Meador K, et al: Optimum stimulus parameters for lateralized suppression of speech with magnetic brain stimulation. Neurology 47:1590–1593, 1996

Epstein CM, He L, Henry TR, et al: Alterations in motor threshold to transcranial magnetic stimulation during anticonvulsant withdrawal. J Clin Neurophysiol 14:446, 1997

Epstein CM, Meador K, Loring DR, et al: Localization and characterization of speech arrest during transcranial magnetic stimulation. Clin Neurophysiol 110:1073–1079, 1999

Epstein CM, Woodard JL, Stringer AY, et al: Repetitive transcranial magnetic stimulation does not replicate the Wada test. Neurology 55:1025–1027, 2000

Fauth C, Meyer B-U, Prosiegel M, et al: Seizure induction and magnetic brain stimulation after stroke. Lancet 339(8789):362, 1992

Figiel GS, Epstein C, McDonald WM, et al: The use of rapid-rate transcranial magnetic stimulation (rTMS) in refractory depressed patients. J Neuropsychiatr Clin Neurosci 10:20–25, 1998

Flitman SS, Grafman J, Wassermann EM, et al: Linguistic processing during repetitive transcranial magnetic stimulation. Neurology 50:175–181, 1998

Floel A, Poeppel D, Buffalo EA, et al: Prefrontal cortex asymmetry for memory encoding of words and abstract shapes. Cereb Cortex 14:404–409, 2004

Fregni F, Thome-Souza S, Bermpohl F, et al: Antiepileptic effects of repetitive transcranial magnetic stimulation in patients with cortical malformations: an EEG and clinical study. Stereotact Funct Neurosurg 83:57–62, 2005

Garcia-Larrea L, Peyron R, Mertens P, et al: Electrical stimulation of motor cortex for pain control: a combined PET-scan and electrophysiological study. Pain 83:259–273, 1999

Ghabra MB, Hallett M, Wassermann EM: Simultaneous repetitive transcranial magnetic stimulation does not speed fine movement in PD. Neurology 52:768–770, 1999

Gianelli M, Cantello R, Civardi C, et al: Idiopathic generalized epilepsy: magnetic stimulation of motor cortex time-locked and unlocked to 3-Hz spike-and-wave discharges. Epilepsia 35:53–60, 1994

Gilio F, Rizzo V, Siebner HR, et al: Effects on the right motor hand-area excitability produced by low-frequency rTMS over human contralateral homologous cortex. J Physiol 551:563–573, 2003

Goddard GV, McIntyre PC, Leech CK: A permanent change in brain function resulting from daily electrical stimulation. Exp Neurol 25:295–330, 1969

Goetz CG, Leurgans S, Raman R, et al: Objective changes in motor function during placebo treatment in Parkinson's disease. Neurology 54:710–714, 2000

Goldensohn ES: The relevance of secondary epileptogenesis to the treatment of epilepsy: kindling and the mirror focus. Epilepsia 25 (suppl 2):S156-S168, 1984

Gorsler A, Baumer T, Weiller C, et al: Interhemispheric effects of high and low frequency rTMS in healthy humans. Clin Neurophysiol 114:1800–1807, 2003

Grafman J, Pascual-Leone A, Alway D, et al: Induction of a recall deficit by rapid-rate transcranial magnetic stimulation. Neuroreport 5:1157–1160, 1994

Hanajima R, Ugawa Y, Terao Y, et al: Ipsilateral cortico-cortical inhibition of the motor cortex in various neurological disorders. J Neurol Sci 140:109–116, 1996

Homberg V, Netz J: Generalised seizures induced by transcranial magnetic stimulation of motor cortex. Lancet 2(8763):1223, 1989

Hufnagel A, Elger CE: Responses of the epileptic focus to transcranial magnetic stimulation. Electroencephalogr Clin Neurophysiol Suppl 43:86–99, 1991

Hufnagel A, Elger CE, Durwen HF, et al: Activation of the epileptic focus by transcranial magnetic stimulation of the human brain. Ann Neurol 27:49–60, 1990a

Hufnagel A, Elger CE, Marx W, et al: Magnetic motor-evoked potentials in epilepsy: effects of the disease and of anticonvulsant medication. Ann Neurol 28:680–686, 1990b

Ikeguchi M, Tougea T, Nishiyama Y, et al: Effects of successive repetitive transcranial magnetic stimulation on motor performances and brain perfusion in idiopathic Parkinson's disease. J Neurol Sci 209:41– 46, 2003

Jennum P, Klitgaard H: Repetitive transcranial magnetic stimulations of the rat: effect of acute and chronic stimulations on pentylenetetrazole-induced clonic seizures. Epilepsy Res 23:115–122, 1996

Jennum P, Friberg L, Fuglsang-Frederiksen A, et al: Speech localization using repetitive transcranial magnetic stimulation. Neurology 44:269–273, 1994a

Jennum P, Winkel H, Fuglsang-Frederiksen A, et al: EEG changes following repetitive transcranial magnetic stimulation in patients with temporal lobe epilepsy. Epilepsy Res 18:167–173, 1994b

Kanda M, Mima T, Oga T, et al: Transcranial magnetic stimulation (TMS) of the sensorimotor cortex and medial frontal cortex modifies human pain perception. Clin Neurophysiol 114:860–866, 2003

Kanno M, Matsumoto M, Togashi H, et al: Effects of acute repetitive transcranial magnetic stimulation on dopamine release in the rat dorsolateral striatum. J Neurol Sci 217:73–81, 2004

Karp BI, Wassermann EM, Porter S, et al: Transcranial magnetic stimulation acutely decreases motor tics (abstract). Neurology 48:A397, 1997

Katayama Y, Fukaya C, Yamamoto T. Poststroke pain control by chronic motor cortex stimulation: neurological characteristics predicting a favorable response. J Neurosurg 89:585–591, 1998

Keck ME, Welt T, Müller MB, et al: Repetitive transcranial magnetic stimulation increases the release of dopamine in the mesolimbic and mesostriatal system. Neuropharmacology 43:101–109, 2002

Khedr EM, Kotb H, Kamel NF, et al: Longlasting antalgic effects of daily sessions of repetitive transcranial magnetic stimulation in central and peripheral neuropathic pain. J Neurol Neurosurg Psychiatry 76:833–838, 2005

Kleine BU, Praamstra P, Stegeman DF, et al: Impaired motor cortical inhibition in Parkinson's disease: motor unit responses to transcranial magnetic stimulation. Exp Brain Res 138:477–483, 2001

Knecht S, Ellger T, Breitenstein C, et al: Changing cortical excitability with low frequency transcranial magnetic stimulation can induce sustained disruption of tactile perception. Biol Psychiatry 53:175–179, 2003

Kole HP, Fuchs E, Ziemann U, et al: Changes in 5HT1A and NMDA binding sites by a single rapid transcranial magnetic stimulation procedure in rats. Brain Res 826:309–312, 1999

Krueger RB, Fama JM, Devanand DP, et al: Does ECT permanently alter seizure threshold? Biol Psychiatry 33:272–276, 1993

Lee HW, Seo HJ, Cohen LG, et al: Cortical excitability during prolonged antiepileptic drug treatment and drug withdrawal. Clin Neurophysiol 116:1105–1112, 2005

Lefaucheur J-P, Drouot X, Keravel Y, et al: Pain relief induced by repetitive transcranial magnetic stimulation of precentral cortex. Neuroreport 12:2963–2965, 2001a

Lefaucheur JP, Drouot X, Nguyen JP: Interventional neurophysiology for pain control: duration of pain relief following repetitive transcranial magnetic stimulation of the motor cortex. Clin Neurophysiol 31:247–252, 2001b

Lefaucheur JP, Drouot X, Menard-Lefaucheur I, et al: Neurogenic pain relief by repetitive transcranial magnetic cortical stimulation depends on the origin and the site of pain. J Neurol Neurosurgery Psychiatry 75:612–616, 2004a

Lefaucheur J-P, Drouot X, Von Raison F, et al: Improvement of motor performance and modulation of cortical excitability by repetitive transcranial magnetic stimulation of the motor cortex in Parkinson's disease. Clin Neurophysiol 115:2530–2541, 2004b

Lezak MD: Neuropsychological Assessment, 3rd Edition. New York, NY, Oxford University Press, 1995

Macdonell RA, King MA, Newton MR, et al: Prolonged cortical silent period after transcranial magnetic stimulation in generalized epilepsy. Neurology 57:706–708, 2001

Mally J, Stone TW: Improvement in parkinsonian symptoms after repetitive transcranial magnetic stimulation. J Neurol Sci 162:179–184, 1999

Mally J. Farkas R, Tothfalusi L, et al: Long-term follow-up study with repetitive transcranial magnetic stimulation (rTMS) in Parkinson's disease. Brain Res Bull 64:259–263, 2004

Menkes DL, Gruenthal M: Slow-frequency repetitive transcranial magnetic stimulation in a patient with focal cortical dysplasia. Epilepsia 41:240–242, 2000

Meyerson BA, Lindblom U, Linderoth B, et al: Motor cortex stimulation as treatment of trigeminal neuropathic pain. Acta Neurochir Suppl 58:150–153, 1993

Michelucci R, Valzania F, Passarelli D, et al: Rapid-rate transcranial magnetic stimulation and hemispheric language dominance: usefulness and safety in epilepsy. Neurology 44:1697–1700, 1994

Michelucci R, Passarelli D, Riguzzi P, et al: Transcranial magnetic stimulation in partial epilepsy: drug-induced changes of motor excitability. Acta Neurol Scand 94:24–30, 1996

Migita K, Uozumi T, Arita K, et al: Transcranial magnetic coil stimulation of motor cortex in patients with central pain. Neurosurgery 36:1037–1039, 1995

Misawa S, Kuwabara S, Shibuya K, et al: Low-frequency transcranial magnetic stimulation for epilepsia partialis continua due to cortical dysplasia. J Neurol Sci 234:37–39, 2005

Moll GH, Wischer S, Heinrich H, et al: Deficient motor control in children with tic disorder: evidence from transcranial magnetic stimulation. Neurosci Lett 272:37–40, 1999

Münchau A, Bloem BR, Thilo KV, et al: Repetitive transcranial magnetic stimulation for Tourette syndrome. Neurology 59:1789–1791, 2002

Nguyen JP, Keravel Y, Feve A, et al: Treatment of deafferentation pain by chronic stimulation of the motor cortex: report of a series of 20 cases. Acta Neurochir Suppl 68:54–60, 1997

Okabe S, Ugawa Y, Kanazawa I: 0.2-Hz Repetitive transcranial magnetic stimulation has no add-on effects as compared to a realistic sham stimulation in Parkinson's disease. Mov Disord 18:382–388, 2003

Palmieri MG, Iani C, Scalise A, et al: The effect of benzodiazepines and flumazenil on motor cortical excitability in the human brain. Brain Res 815:192–199, 1999

Pascual-Leone A, Gates JR, Dhuna A: Induction of speech arrest and counting errors with rapid-rate transcranial magnetic stimulation. Neurology 41:697–702, 1991

Pascual-Leone A, Valls-Sole J, Brasil-Neto JP, et al: Akinesia in Parkinson's disease, II: shortening of choice reaction time and movement time with subthreshold repetitive transcranial motor cortex stimulation. Neurology 44:892–898, 1994

Peyron R, Garcia-Larrea L, Deiber MP, et al: Electrical stimulation of precentral cortical area in the treatment of central pain: electrophysiological and PET study. Pain 62:275–286, 1995

Pleger B, Janssen F, Schwenkreis P, et al: Repetitive transcranial magnetic stimulation of the motor cortex attenuates pain perception in complex regional pain syndrome type I. Neurosci Lett 356:87–90, 2004

Plewnia C, Lotze M, Gerloff C: Disinhibition of the contralateral motor cortex by low-frequency rTMS. Neuroreport 14:609–612, 2003

Reutens DC, Berkovic SF, Macdonell RA, et al: Magnetic stimulation of the brain in generalized epilepsy: reversal of cortical hyperexcitability by anticonvulsants. Ann Neurol 34:351–355, 1993a

Reutens DC, Puce A, Berkovic SF: Cortical hyperexcitability in progressive myoclonus epilepsy: a study with transcranial magnetic stimulation. Neurology 43:186–92, 1993b

Ridding MC, Inzelberg R, Rothwell JC: Changes in excitability of motor cortical circuitry in patients with Parkinson's disease. Ann Neurol 37:181–188, 1995a

Ridding MC, Sheean G, Rothwell JC, et al: Changes in the balance between motor cortical excitation and inhibition in focal, task specific dystonia. J Neurol Neurosurg Psychiatry 59:493–498, 1995b

Rizzo V, Quartarone A, Bagnato S, et al: Modification of cortical excitability induced by gabapentin: a study by transcranial magnetic stimulation. Neurol Sci 22:229–232, 2001

Rollnik JD, Wustefeld S, Dauper J, et al: Repetitive transcranial magnetic stimulation for the treatment of chronic pain: a pilot study. Eur Neurol 48:6–10, 2002

Rona S, Berardelli A, Vacca L, et al: Alterations of motor cortical inhibition in patients with dystonia. Mov Disord 13:118–124, 1998

Rossi S, Ulivelli M, Bartalini S, et al: Reduction of cortical myoclonus-related epileptic activity following slow-frequency rTMS. Neuroreport 15:293–296, 2004

Schuler P, Claus D, Stefan H: Hyperventilation and transcranial magnetic stimulation: two methods of activation of epileptiform EEG activity in comparison. J Clin Neurophysiol 10:111–115, 1993

Shiga Y, Tsuda T, Itoyama Y, et al: Transcranial magnetic stimulation alleviates truncal ataxia in spinocerebellar degeneration. J Neurol Neurosurg Psychiatry 72:124–126, 2002

Shimamoto H, Takasaki K, Shigemori M, et al: Therapeutic effect and mechanism of repetitive transcranial magnetic stimulation in Parkinson's disease. J Neurol 248:48–52,
2001

Shimizu H, Tsuda T, Shiga Y, et al: Therapeutic efficacy of transcranial magnetic stimulation for hereditary spinocerebellar degeneration. Tohoku J Exp Med 189:203–211,
1999

Siebner HR, Mentschel C, Auer C, et al: Repetitive transcranial magnetic stimulation has
a beneficial effect on bradykinesia in Parkinson's disease. Neuroreport 10:589–594,
1999a

Siebner HR, Tormos JM, Ceballos-Baumann AO, et al: Low frequency repetitive transcranial magnetic stimulation of the motor cortex in writers' cramp. Neurology 52:529–
537, 1999b

Sohn YH, Kaelin-Lang A, Jung HY, et al: Effect of levetiracetam on human corticospinal
excitability. Neurology 57:858–863, 2001

Steinhoff BJ, et al: Transcranial magnetic stimulation for therapy of refractory epilepsy (abstract). Epilepsia 43(suppl 8):12, 2002

Stewart L, Walsh V, Frith U, et al: TMS produces two dissociable types of speech disruption. Neuroimage 13:472–478, 2001

Strafella AP, Paus T, Barrett J, et al: Repetitive transcranial magnetic stimulation of the human prefrontal cortex induces dopamine release in the caudate nucleus. J Neurosci
21(15):RC157, 2001

Summers J, Johnson S, Pridmore S, et al: Changes to cold detection and pain thresholds
following low and high frequency transcranial magnetic stimulation of the motor cortex. Neurosci Lett 368:197–200, 2004

Tamura Y, Okabe S, Ohnishi T, et al: Effects of 1-Hz repetitive transcranial magnetic stimulation on acute pain induced by capsaicin. Pain 107:107–115, 2004

Tassinari CA, Michelucci R, Forti A, et al: Transcranial magnetic stimulation in epileptic
patients: usefulness and safety. Neurology 40:1132–1133, 1990

Tergau F, Naumann U, Paulus W, et al: Low-frequency repetitive transcranial magnetic
stimulation improves intractable epilepsy. Lancet 353:2209, 1999a

Tergau F, Wassermann EM, Paulus W, et al: Lack of clinical improvement in patients with
Parkinson's disease after low and high frequency repetitive transcranial magnetic stimulation. Electroencephalogr Clin Neurophysiol Suppl 51:281–288, 1999b

Tharayil BJ, Gangadhar BN, Jagadisha AL: Seizure risk with TMS: should we take a second
look? J ECT 21:188–189, 2005

Theodore WH, Hunter K, Chen R, et al: Transcranial magnetic stimulation for the treatment of seizures: a controlled study. Neurology 59:560–562, 2002

Tishler DM, Weinberg KI, Hinton DR, et al: MDR1 gene expression in brain of patients
with medically intractable epilepsy. Epilepsia 36:1–6, 1995

Töpper R, Foltys H, Meister IG, et al: Repetitive transcranial magnetic stimulation of the
parietal cortex transiently ameliorates phantom limb pain-like syndrome. Clin Neurophysiol 114:1521–1530, 2003

Tsubokawa T, Katayama Y, Yamamoto T, et al: Chronic motor cortex stimulation for the
treatment of central pain. Acta Neurochir Suppl (Wien) 52:137–139, 1991

Tsubokawa T, Katayama Y, Yamamoto T, et al: Chronic motor cortex stimulation in patients with thalamic pain. J Neurosurg 78:393–401, 1993

Varrasi C, Civardi C, Boccagni C, et al: Cortical excitability in drug-naive patients with partial epilepsy: a cross-sectional study. Neurology 63:2051–2055, 2004

Wassermann EM: Risk and safety of repetitive transcranial magnetic stimulation: report and suggested guidelines from the International Workshop on the Safety of Repetitive Transcranial Magnetic Stimulation, June 5–7, 1996. Electroencephalogr Clin Neurophysiol 108:1–16, 1998

Wassermann EM, Lisanby SH: Therapeutic application of repetitive transcranial magnetic stimulation: a review. Clin Neurophysiol 112:1367–1377, 2001

Wedegaertner FR, Garvey MA, Cohen LG, et al: Low frequency repetitive transcranial magnetic stimulation can reduce action myoclonus. Neurology 48:A119, 1997

Werhahn KJ, Kunesch E, Noachtar S, et al: Differential effects on motorcortical inhibition induced by blockade of GABA uptake in humans. J Physiol (Lond) 517:591–597, 1999

Werhahn KJ, Lieber J, Classen J, et al: Motor cortex excitability in patients with focal epilepsy. Epilepsy Res 41:179–189, 2000

Ziemann U, Bruns D, Paulus W: Impaired motor cortex inhibition in patients with Parkinson's disease and other parkinsonian syndromes: a transcranial magnetic stimulation study. Mov Disord 11 (suppl 1):72, 1996a

Ziemann U, Lonnecker S, Steinhoff BJ, et al: Effects of antiepileptic drugs on motor cortex excitability in humans: a transcranial magnetic stimulation study. Ann Neurol 40:367–378, 1996b

Ziemann U, Paulus W, Rothenberger A. Decreased motor inhibition in Tourette's disorder: evidence from transcranial magnetic stimulation. Am J Psychiatry 154:1277–1284, 1997

5

TRANSCRANIAL MAGNETIC STIMULATION IN MAJOR DEPRESSION

Antonio Mantovani, M.D.

Sarah H. Lisanby, M.D.

Since its introduction roughly 20 years ago, use of transcranial magnetic stimulation (TMS) in major depression remains the most studied clinical application in psychiatry. Studies have ranged from uncontrolled clinical observations of therapeutic effects to randomized, controlled clinical trials (Table 5–1). Taken together, the findings are promising, as well as controversial. Effect sizes vary considerably, and some, but not all, major findings have not yet been systematically replicated. In this chapter, we present a critical review of the work to date on the use of TMS as a therapeutic intervention and a neurophysiological probe in major depression.

Table 5–1. Clinical trials of TMS in depression

Study	N	Mean age	Design	Sham	Depression subtype	Medication resistance?	Site	TMS type	Coil	Frequency (Hz)	Intensity	Train duration (sec)	ITI (sec)	Trains	Sessions	Total pulses
												Stimulation parameters				
Hoflich et al. 1993	2	42	Open	None	Psychotic	Yes	Vertex	SP	14 cm, round	<0.3	105%–130% MT	—a	—a	—a	10	2,500
George et al. 1995	6	46	Open	None	—a	Yes	Left DLPFC	rTMS	Figure 8	20	80% MT	2	60	20	≥5	≥4,000
Grisaru et al. 1995	10	39	Open	None	Psychotic (n=3)	—a	Vertex and bilateral frontal	SP	14 cm, round	0.3	Maximum output	—a	—a	—a	1	30
Kolbinger et al. 1995	15	49	Open	None	—a	—a	Vertex	SP	14 cm, round	<0.5	0.3 above and below MT	—a	—a	—a	5	1,250
Catalá et al. 1996	7	—a	O+C	None	Psychotic	Yes	Left+right DLPFC	rTMS	Figure 8	10	110% MT	5	25	20	10	10,000
Conca et al. 1996	24	42	Open	None	Nonpsychotic	No	Multiple sites	SP	Round	0.17	1.9 tesla	—a	—a	—a	10	400
Pascual-Leone et al. 1996b	17	49	B+C	1-wing, 90°	Psychotic	Yes	Left+right DLPFC and vertex	rTMS	Figure 8	10	90% MT	10	50	20	5	10,000

Table 5–1. Clinical trials of TMS in depression *(continued)*

Study	N	Mean age	Design	Sham	Depression subtype	Medication resistance?	Site	TMS type	Coil	Frequency (Hz)	Intensity	Train duration (sec)	ITI (sec)	Trains	Sessions	Total pulses
George et al. 1997	12	42	B+C	1-wing, 45°	—[a]	—[a]	Left DLPFC	rTMS	Figure 8	20	80% MT	2	>58	20	10	8,000
Epstein et al. 1998	32	40	Open	None	Psychotic (n=2)	Yes, in at least 1 trial	Left DLPFC	rTMS	Custom	10	110% MT	5	30	10	5	2,500
Feinsod et al. 1998	14	58	Open	None	—[a]	—[a]	Right DLPFC	rTMS	9 cm, round	1	1	60	180	2	10	12,000
Figiel et al. 1998	56	60	Open	None	Comorbid dementia (n=4)	Yes, in most patients	Left DLPFC	rTMS	Custom	10	110% MT	5	30	10	5	2,500
Grunhaus et al. 1998	16	62	Open	None	Psychotic (n=8)	—[a]	Left DLPFC	rTMS	14 cm, figure 8	10	90% MT	2–6	—[a]	≤20	20	8,000–24,000
Menkes et al. 1998	5	—[a]	Open	None	—[a]	—[a]	Right frontal cortex	SP	—[a]	0.5	—[a]				8	800
Nahas et al. 1998	30	49	B+P	1-wing, 45°	—[a]	—[a]	Left DLPFC	rTMS	Figure 8	5 / 20	100% MT	8 / 2	28 / 22	40	10	16,000
Padberg et al. 1998	18	51	B+P	1-wing, 90°	—[a]	Yes	Left DLPFC	SP / rTMS	Figure 8	0.3 / 10	90% MT	5		5	5 / 5	1,250 / 1,250

Table 5–1. Clinical trials of TMS in depression *(continued)*

Study	N	Mean age	Design	Sham	Depression subtype	Medication resistance?	Site	TMS type	Coil	Frequency (Hz)	Intensity	Train duration (sec)	ITI (sec)	Trains	Sessions	Total pulses
Klein et al. 1999	71	59	B+P	90°, coil off the scalp	Nonpsychotic	–a	Right DLPFC	rTMS	9 cm, round	1	1 tesla	60	180	2	10	1,200
Tormos et al. 1999	45	53	B+P	1-wing, 90°	Nonpsychotic	–a	Left+right DLPFC	rTMS	Figure 8	10 / 1	110% MT	8 / 1,600		20	10	16,000
Kimbrell et al. 1999	13	42	B+P	1-wing, 45°	–a	–a	Left+right DLPFC	rTMS	Figure 8	1	80% MT	2 / 1,200	60	20 / 1	10	8,000
Menkes et al. 1999	14	33	O+P	None	Nonpsychotic vs. healthy	No	Right DLPFC	SP	–a	0.5	100% MT		60	20	8	160
Triggs et al. 1999	10	52	Open	None	Nonpsychotic	Yes	Left DLPFC	rTMS	7 cm, figure 8	20	80% MT	2	28	50	10	20,000
Pridmore et al. 1999	12	57	Open	None	Nonpsychotic	Yes	Left DLPFC	rTMS	7 cm, figure 8	10	90%–100% MT	5	25	20	10 or 14	10,000
Loo et al. 1999	18	48	B+P	2-wing, 45°	–a	Yes	Left DLPFC	rTMS	7 cm, figure 8	10	110% MT	5	30	30	10	15,000
George et al. 2000	30	45	B+P	1-wing, 45°	Nonpsychotic	–a	Left DLPFC	rTMS	7 cm, figure 8	20 / 5	100% MT	2 / 8	28 / 22	40	10	16,000

Stimulation parameters (columns: Frequency, Intensity, Train duration, ITI, Trains, Sessions, Total pulses)

Table 5–1. Clinical trials of TMS in depression *(continued)*

Study	N	Mean age	Design	Sham	Depression subtype	Medication resistance?	Site	TMS type	Coil	Frequency (Hz)	Intensity	Train duration (sec)	ITI (sec)	Trains	Sessions	Total pulses
Berman et al. 2000	20	42	B+P	2-wing, 45°	—[a]	Yes	Left DLPFC	rTMS	Figure 8	20	80% MT	2	58	20	10	8,000
Manes et al. 2001	20	60	B+P	—[a]	—[a]	Yes	Left DLPFC	rTMS	—[a]	20	80% MT	2	—[a]	20	5	4,000
Garcia-Toro et al. 2001a	35	50	B+P	2-wing, 90°	—[a]	Yes	Left DLPFC	rTMS	8.5 cm, figure 8	20	90% MT	2	20–40	30	20	24,000
Garcia-Toro et al. 2001b	22	44	B+P	2-wing, 90°	Nonpsychotic	Add-on	Left DLPFC	rTMS	8.5 cm, figure 8	20	90% MT	2	20–40	30	10	12,000
Lisanby et al. 2001c	36		B+P			Add-on	Left DLPFC Right DLPFC	rTMS	7 cm, figure 8	10 1	—[a]	—[a]	—[a]	—[a]	—[a]	—[a]
Hoppner et al. 2003	30	56	B+P	—[a]	—[a]	—[a]	Left DLPFC Right DLPFC	rTMS	Figure 8	20 1	90% MT 120% MT	2 60	60 180	20 2	10	8,000 1,200
Herwig et al. 2003	25	45	B+P	Midline	—[a]	—[a]	Left DLPFC	rTMS	Figure 8	15	110% MT	2	4	100	10	30,000

Table 5–1. Clinical trials of TMS in depression *(continued)*

Study	N	Mean age	Design	Sham	Depression subtype	Medication resistance?	Site	TMS type	Coil	Frequency (Hz)	Intensity	Train duration (sec)	ITI (sec)	Trains	Sessions	Total pulses
Fitzgerald et al. 2003	60	45	B+P	1-wing, 45°	—a	Yes	Left DLPFC	rTMS	7 cm, figure 8	10 1	100% MT	5 60	25 60	20 5	20	20,000 6,000
Schule et al. 2003	26	52	Open	None	—a	Yes	Left DLPFC	rTMS	7 cm, figure 8	10	100% MT	10	30	15	10 or 13	15,000 19,500
Mosimann et al. 2004	24	62	B+P	2-wing, 90°	—a	Yes	Left DLPFC	rTMS	Figure 8	20	100% MT	2	28	40	10	16,000
Hausmann et al. 2004	41	46	B+P	Coil off the scalp	Nonpsychotic	Add-on	Left DLPFC Left+right DLPFC	rTMS	Figure 8	20 20 + 1	100% MT 100%– 120% MT	10 10+ 600	90	10 10 + 1	10	20,000 26,000
Koerselman et al. 2004	55	55	B+P		—a		Left DLPFC	rTMS	Figure 8	20	80% MT	2	58	20	10	8,000
Kauffmann et al. 2004	12	52	B+P	1-wing, 45°	—a	Yes	Right DLPFC	rTMS	9 cm, round	1	110% MT	60	180	2	10	1,200
Fujita and Koga 2005	23	60	Open	None	—a	—a	Multiple sites	SP	9 cm, round	—a	2 tesla	5	6–10	4	5	
Rumi et al. 2005	46	39	B+P	Iron- ferrit	Nonpsychotic	Add-on	Left DLPFC	rTMS	Figure 8	5	120% MT	10	20	25	20	25,000

Table 5–1. Clinical trials of TMS in depression *(continued)*

Study	N	Mean age	Design	Sham	Depression subtype	Medication resistance?	Site	TMS type	Coil	Frequency (Hz)	Intensity	Train duration (sec)	ITI (sec)	Trains	Sessions	Total pulses
Avery et al. 2006	68	44	B+P	2-wing, 90°	Nonpsychotic	Yes	Left DLPFC	rTMS	Figure 8	10	110% MT	5	25	32	15	24,000
Fitzgerald et al. 2006	50	46	B+P	1-wing, 45°	—[a]	Yes	Left+Right DLPFC	rTMS	Figure 8	1 + 10	110% MT / 100% MT	140 / 5	30 / 25	3 / 15	30	12,600 / 22,500

Note. B+C=blind, crossover; B+P=blind, parallel; DLPFC=dorsolateral prefrontal cortex; ITI=intertrain interval; MT=motor threshold; O+C=open, crossover; O+P=open, parallel; rTMS=repetitive transcranial magnetic stimulation; SP=single pulse; TMS=transcranial magnetic stimulation.
[a]Not reported.
[b]See also Geller et al. 1997.

BACKGROUND SUPPORTING THE USE OF TMS IN DEPRESSION

Theoretical Challenges to the Potential Antidepressant Action of TMS

Initial skepticism about the potential utility of TMS in depression was based on the fact that the stimulation is subconvulsive and the direct effects of TMS are limited to a relatively focal region of superficial cortex.

Subconvulsive Stimulation

Although studies of TMS in depression are now proliferating, the initial idea that this intervention might be effective in major depression went against clinical dogma in the field of electroconvulsive therapy (ECT). The tenet that a seizure is necessary but not sufficient for ECT to exert antidepressant effects is now widely accepted (Sackeim et al. 1993). Subconvulsive electrical stimulation has long been known to be ineffective in depression (Fink et al. 1958), and thus it seemed unlikely that electrical stimulation induced in the brain via TMS would behave differently than the direct application of electricity transcranially. On closer investigation, however, TMS and subconvulsive ECT bear little resemblance to each other as somatic interventions. Studies of subconvulsive stimulation with ECT used a single train of electrical stimuli, whereas the therapeutic use of TMS involves repeated trains (repetitive TMS or rTMS). The transcranial application of electricity is impeded by the scalp and skull, resulting in a substantial dropoff in amplitude and loss of focal precision. The transcranial induction of electricity via an alternating magnetic field avoids these drawbacks and may, at least in part, explain why these two modalities may behave differently.

Focal Stimulation

Depression is thought to involve dysregulation in a collection of brain structures, some of which are deep and not directly accessible to the TMS coil. Some postulate that diencephalic stimulation is necessary for the clinical benefits of ECT (Abrams and Taylor 1976; Fink and Ottosson 1980). Two points mitigate this objection to the potential utility of TMS in depression. First, more recent work has challenged the view that diencephalic stimulation is necessary for the clinical benefits of ECT by demonstrating that neuroendocrine measures of diencephalic stimulation do not correlate with the therapeutic properties of ECT (Devanand et al. 1998; Lisanby et al. 1998). Second, functional neuroimaging studies with TMS have consistently demonstrated that this focal cortical intervention alters activity in remote brain structures through transsynaptic effects (e.g., Fox et al. 1997; Paus et al. 1997).

TMS as a Probe of Mood Circuits via Action at Dorsolateral Prefrontal Cortex

As a relatively focal intervention, TMS holds the potential of being able to modulate activity selectively in brain areas involved in mood circuits. One such candidate brain area that has been the focus of much work with TMS in depression as well as mania is the dorsolateral prefrontal cortex (DLPFC). Located on the lateral aspect of the middle frontal gyrus, this brain area is readily accessible to the TMS coil and is highly interconnected with limbic structures implicated in functional neuroimaging studies to play a role in mood modulation and major depression (Soares and Mann 1997). Indeed, rTMS has been shown to affect neural activity at the site of stimulation as well as in distal regions that are richly interconnected with the DLPFC and highly implicated in mood, motivation, and arousal such as the striatum, thalamus, and the anterior cingulate cortex (Barbas 2000; Paus et al. 2001; Petrides and Pandya 1999). It has also been shown to exert cortical blood flow and glucose metabolism changes in the same direction as found after both antidepressant drug treatments (Kennedy et al. 2001) and ECT (Nobler et al. 2001).

As reviewed below, rTMS has been applied to the DLPFC to manipulate mood-related circuits with varying degrees of success in healthy volunteers and patients with depression (George et al. 1999; Martin et al. 2003; Post et al. 1999). In taking advantage of the differential physiological effects of high and low frequency stimulation (Chen et al. 1997), rTMS has been used in an attempt to normalize prefrontal hypo- or hyperperfusion and hemispheric asymmetries seen in depression (Davidson et al. 2002; Drevets 2000; Mayberg 2003), with some evidence of success as evidenced by clinical improvement and as visualized by functional imaging (Mottaghy et al. 2002).

TMS-Induced Mood Modulation in Normal Volunteers

Several findings early in the research with TMS were suggestive that TMS may possess mood-altering properties. Bickford and colleagues (1987) observed transient mood elevation in several normal volunteers receiving single-pulse TMS to the motor cortex. Later, acute crying was noted in a few of the early studies that used rTMS to produce speech arrest (Michelucci et al. 1994; Pascual-Leone et al. 1991). Using a within-subject crossover design, Pascual-Leone and colleagues (1996a) reported that a single session of high-frequency rTMS to the left DLPFC produced transient sadness, whereas right-sided stimulation produced transient happiness in normal volunteers as measured on visual-analog rating scales. Conditions were separated by 30 minutes, and this raised the possibility of carry-over effects. George and colleagues (1996) replicated this finding in a within-subject crossover study with each condition administered on separate days, and George's group further noted that the effect was dependent on the type of coil used (Dearing et al. 1996). More recent work has failed to replicate mood effects in normal volunteers. Using twice as many pulses per day, Mosimann and colleagues (2000) failed to find significant mood effects in a sham-controlled trial; however, they stimulated a lateral prefrontal cortex site 2 cm inferior to the DLPFC and studied only men.

Grisaru and colleagues (2001) were the first to examine the mood effects of slow rTMS applied to the DLPFC. One-hertz rTMS was applied to the left and right DLPFC in a sham-controlled crossover trial that used the same number of pulses as used in the George et al. (1996) and Pascual-Leone et al. (1996a) studies. No effects on mood or sleep, assessed by questionnaire, were found. Using twice as many pulses, Schutter and colleagues (2001) reported a reduction in anxiety, but Jenkins and colleagues (2002) failed to replicate this effect.

Research into emotion and emotional disorders by rTMS has largely been restricted to the prefrontal regions. However, the parietal cortex has also been implicated in emotional functioning. Van Honk and colleagues (2003) used rTMS to investigate the role of the right parietal cortex in mood regulation. In a placebo-controlled design, 2-Hz rTMS at 90% of the individual motor threshold (MT) was applied over the right parietal cortex of eight healthy subjects for 20 minutes continuously. Effects on mood, autonomic activity, and motivated attention were investigated. Significant reductions in depressive mood were observed immediately following and 30 minutes after stimulation. Moreover, these findings were objectified by a concurring pattern of autonomically mediated changes in the attentional processing of angry facial expressions. These data suggest a role for the right parietal cortex in affective brain circuits regulating phenomenological, physiological, and attentional aspects of mood functioning, confirming the theoretical notion of a dyscommunication between the right parietal and left prefrontal cortex in mood regulation. To investigate the neural substrates of rTMS-induced changes in the affective state of healthy volunteers, Barrett and colleagues (2004) combined 10-Hz and 1-Hz rTMS applied over the left DLPFC with 1) a speech task to examine rTMS-induced changes in paralinguistic aspects of speech production and 2) positron emission tomography (PET) to examine rTMS-induced changes in the functional connectivity of the DLPFC. The results of the two experiments revealed that high-frequency rTMS decreased affect and pitch variation in speech and increased the functional connectivity between the site of stimulation and other brain areas associated with affect, such as the anterior cingulate gyrus, insula, thalamus, parahippocampal gyrus, and caudate nucleus. No robust changes in behavior or brain activity were observed following low-frequency rTMS. Taken together, their results suggest that changes in affect and affect-relevant behavior following 10-Hz rTMS applied over the left DLPFC may be related to changes in neural activity in brain regions that are widely implicated in affective states, including a frontocingulate circuit.

While these findings may be relevant to theories regarding the lateralization of emotion regulation, it is important to note that the magnitude of these mood effects was small and the changes were often not clinically apparent to the investigators or to the subjects themselves. A. Pascual-Leone (personal communication, 1996) has observed that the mood effect of left DLPFC rTMS in normal volunteers is highly dependent on the instruction given to the subjects. When subjects were told the purpose of the study was to assay memory effects, no significant change in mood was found. Another study (Hajak et al. 1999) on the effects of rTMS on sleep parameters related to mood failed to find any significant effect on visual analog rating of mood in 13 men, although an increase in REM latency following left frontal rTMS was found that was thought to be consistent with potential antidepressant action. The parameters in this study were 120% of MT, 20 Hz, 160 trains, five stimuli per train, and an intertrain interval [ITI] of 8 seconds). A larger study by Nedjat and colleagues (1998) reported that 3 of 50 normal women receiving a single session of rTMS to the left DLPFC experienced a transient period of hypomania. Mood returned to baseline within 3 hours. While the occurrence of hypomanic symptoms suggests that rTMS may possess active mood-altering effects, the group as a whole showed no significant mood effect on visual analog ratings. Stimulation parameters in this study were 80% of MT, 20 trains, an ITI of 60 seconds, and either 10 Hz for 5 seconds or 20 Hz for 2 seconds, respectively.

Although the reports of mood effects in normal volunteers are controversial and conflicting, they nonetheless stimulated fruitful research into the use of this technique in the treatment of mood disorders, as reviewed below.

TMS as a Probe of Motor Circuit Excitability in Depression

The most traditional use of TMS has been to study the central motor pathways in healthy subjects and in patients with neurological disorders. New findings of motor system abnormalities in neuropsychiatric disorders and greater insights into the mechanisms of action of various TMS techniques invite the systematic exploration of TMS for the study of the pathophysiology of psychiatric disorders and the assessment of treatment outcomes. Nowadays neurophysiological investigations using TMS represent a growing area of psychiatric research.

As prefrontal cortex excitability can be studied only indirectly through its effects on motor cortex excitability, presumably by mediation of cortico-cortical and cortico-subcortical-motor cortex connections, several studies have explored the motor cortex excitability as a potential biological correlate of illness and recovery from depression. Several groups have described a decrease in the postexercise facilitation of motor evoked potentials (MEPs). Samii and colleagues (1996) studied postexercise MEP facilitation and suppression in 12 patients with chronic fatigue syndrome, 10 patients with unipolar or bipolar depression, and 18 healthy control subjects. All the patients were medication free. The authors found that postexercise facilitation, but not suppression, was significantly lower in patients with chronic fatigue syndrome and depression than in controls. Shajahan and colleagues (1999a) examined postexercise facilitation and suppression in 10 patients with major depressive disorder (MDD) (unipolar and bipolar) who were taking medication (various ones) and 10 healthy control subjects. Initial facilitation was observed in both groups. In the patients, however, the facilitation returned to baseline level of MEP responses significantly faster than in the control subjects. These authors followed up on their study by examining depressed patients who recovered from depression (Shajahan et al. 1999b). They compared 10 depressed patients, 10 patients (five of whom were included in the depressed group) who had recovered with medication within the previous 6 months, and 10 healthy control subjects. All the patients were taking medication. The currently depressed patients showed reduced mean postexercise facilitation compared with the other two groups, whereas the recovered patients and control subjects had no significant difference in facilitation. No significant difference in psychomotor performance was found between the depressed group and the recovered group. The authors suggested that postexercise MEP facilitation may be even more sensitive than clinical measurements. Finally, Reid and colleagues (2002) found that postexercise facilitation expressed as a percentage of baseline was 510% in 13 control subjects, 110% in 10 patients with a major depressive episode, and 190% in 11 patients with schizophrenia, with significant differences between the psychiatric groups and the control subjects.

Steele and colleagues (2000) found some evidence to suggest that there is increased motor cortical inhibition in depression. They measured the cortical silent period in 16 patients with DSM-IV depression and 19 matched control subjects and found that the silent period was significantly increased in the patient group. No correlation was found between silent period and depression score.

In a different study where medication-free patients with treatment-refractory major depressive disorder were compared with healthy control subjects, cortical excitability was found to be asymmetric, with the left hemisphere having lesser and the right hemisphere having greater excitability than in control subjects (Maeda et al. 2000a). The paired-pulse study revealed that the left primary motor cortex had significantly lower intracortical excitability at a 6-msec interstimulus interval, which is presumed to be affected by both inhibitory and facilitatory interneuronal circuits, presumably related to a change in the balance between γ-aminobutyric acid (GABA)–ergic and glutamatergic influences. There was no significant asymmetry in the control subjects. Fitzgerald and colleagues (2004) replicated the finding of a decreased left hemispherical excitability in a sample of patients with major depression who were taking medication. In line with previous studies, Bajbouj and colleagues (2006) were able to find laterality in MT with a lower excitability of the left hemisphere as compared with the right hemisphere. The silent period and intracortical inhibition were reduced in depressed patients—a finding consistent with a reduced GABAergic tone. Moreover, patients showed a significant hemispheric asymmetry in MT.

Maeda and colleagues (2000b) conducted another study to examine intracortical excitability before and after high-frequency (10-Hz) rTMS to the left dorsolateral prefrontal area. The patients' baseline excitability (i.e., the lower the left and the higher the right relative to their contralateral motor cortex) was associated with treatment outcome. In addition, responders showed "normalization" (i.e., their paired-pulse curve was no longer significantly different), whereas nonresponders had greater "asymmetry" than before pretreatment. Using TMS as a motor neurophysiological tool, Triggs and colleagues (1999), in a study of 10 depressed patients who underwent high-frequency (20-Hz) rTMS treatment to the left prefrontal area for 2 weeks, found treatment to be associated with a decrease in the MT of the ipsilateral hemisphere (i.e., increase in cortical excitability). There was a significant decrease in MT after each rTMS session compared with before the session and during the second week of rTMS treatment compared with the first. The authors, however, did not report on the possible correlation of this change in MT to their severity of the depression. They suggested, on the basis of these results, that rTMS to the prefrontal area alters brain activity at sites remote from the stimulation—a hypothesis consistent with functional imaging data (Peschina et al. 2001; Teneback et al. 1999), spectral electroencephalographic analysis (Tormos et al. 1998), and work on motor excitability (Rollnik et al. 2000). In fact, Rollnick and colleagues (2000) reported that 5-Hz stimulations to the left DLPFC exert an inhibitory effect on motor cortex function (i.e., decreased MEP amplitude). Another study found a significant increase in the ratio of MEP to M-wave amplitude, accompanied by a shortening of the silent period duration, in patients who showed marked clinical improvement (reduction in Hamilton Rating Scale for Depression score by 50% or more) following left rTMS and regardless of stimulation frequency (3 Hz vs. 10 Hz) (Chistyakov et al. 2005).

Ogawa and colleagues (2004) examined the changes in high-frequency oscillations of somatosensory evoked potentials (SEPs) before and after slow rTMS over the right primary somatosensory cortex (0.5 Hz, 50 pulses, 80% of MT intensity). The high-frequency oscillations, which represent a localized activity of intracortical inhibitory interneurons, were significantly increased after slow rTMS, whereas the SEPs were not changed. On the basis of these results, the authors suggested that slow rTMS affects cortical excitability by modulating the activity of the intracortical inhibitory interneurons beyond the time of the stimulation and that rTMS may have therapeutic effects on such disorders. Gerschlager and colleagues (2001) performed slow (1-Hz) rTMS to several frontal areas, finding that only stimulations of the premotor cortex affected the MEP responses of motor cortex. Taken together, these studies suggest that rTMS to the prefrontal areas alters brain activity remote from the site of stimulation. In addition, the findings from these studies are consistent with the literature on left-hemispheric hypoactivity in depressed patients and normalization with successful antidepressant treatment.

On the other hand, Grunhaus and colleagues (2003a) compared the MT and the MEP amplitude generated by TMS in 19 patients with major depression and 13 matched control subjects. MT was found to be similar in the two groups, and the MEP amplitude response was significantly increased by rTMS (1 session consisted of twenty 6-second trains, with a 30-second ITI at 10 Hz and 90% of MT) in both patients and control subjects. Dolberg and colleagues (2002) treated 46 depressed patients with 10-Hz rTMS to the left DLPFC for 20 sessions and found no significant effects of treatment on MT. They also found no significant difference when they compared MT baseline measures in normal control subjects with those in the group of depressed patients as a whole and those in major depressive disorder subgroups (psychotic vs. nonpsychotic, responders vs. nonresponders). Their working hypothesis that motor cortex excitability, as represented by either the MT or the averaged MEP amplitude, would differentiate between major depression patients and healthy control subjects or would correlate with changes in depression ratings following an rTMS treatment was not confirmed.

As in the traditional neurophysiological studies, limitations in the interpretation of these data arise from small sample sizes, inconsistent patient populations (based on diagnosis, medication), differences in methodology between groups, and possible lack of sensitivity and specificity. The TMS studies conducted on measures of cortical excitability have predominantly employed electromyography (hence the motor system) as an output measure. This approach is the logical consequence of the history of TMS and the ease of MEP induction with TMS. For the purpose of applying TMS to the study of the pathophysiology of major depression, however, the motor system is not the primary cortical projection of interest. Indeed, the evaluation of cortical excitability in prefrontal cortex and other multimodal association cortices would be more desirable. Even in the current form of measuring motor effects, several findings illustrate the potential of TMS to become a valuable tool in the study of the underlying pathophysiology of depression, particularly for those types involving a known motor dysfunction.

METHODOLOGICAL ISSUES IN CLINICAL TRIALS WITH TMS IN DEPRESSION

Blinding

Maintaining the blind in a randomized trial is essential to determining the ultimate clinical efficacy of TMS. Before the manufacturing of new sham coils—designed to look, act, and sound like an active coil, but without any power of effective cortical stimulation—truly blind studies were not possible, because the TMS was administered by an individual unblinded to the treatment condition. Well-designed studies using the traditional coil minimized this problem by keeping the clinical raters blinded to the treatment condition and creating a separation between the clinical team and the TMS treating physician.

Sham Control

Placebo-controlled trials represent the gold standard for establishing the efficacy of an intervention. An adequate placebo should be plausible, inactive, and simulate as closely as possible the ancillary effects of the treatment. Most controlled trials with TMS have used *sham TMS* as a placebo. Sham is typically applied by angling the coil off the head so that the magnetic field stimulates scalp muscles but does not enter the brain (Figure 5–1). This maneuver replicates the acoustic artifact and scalp muscle contraction of active TMS; however, the assumption of no brain effects has not been rigorously tested. Wassermann and colleagues (1997) found that sham TMS did not significantly effect cerebral glucose metabolism, but further studies in larger numbers with a variety of sham manipulations would help to clarify this issue. Work by Lisanby and colleagues (2001b) in rhesus monkeys suggests that certain sham manipulations may indeed induce substantial voltage in the brain. Moreover, there is evidence that some types of sham manipulations used in clinical trials actually do exert some effects on the brain (Lisanby et al. 2001a; Loo et al. 2000). The fact that most studies do not report the specifications of the sham manipulation makes comparisons across studies difficult and perhaps in part explains the large variability in sham response rates across groups. New sham coils have been designed to look and sound like an active coil by incorporating a mu-metal shield that diverts the majority of the magnetic flux generated by the internal coil such that a minimal (less than 3%) magnetic field is delivered to the cortex. However, these sham coils do not feel like active TMS, which generates a tapping sensation on the scalp. This problem of the different feel of active and sham TMS has been addressed from two directions: 1) to make active TMS feel more like sham, and 2) to make sham feel more like active. The former has been attempted through the development of an "e-shield," which is an attachment to the face of the coil that reduces the strength of the magnetic field generated at the surface of the scalp without appreciably decreasing the amount of stimulation reaching the brain (Figure 5–2). The intent is to reduce the scalp stimulation with active TMS. The second approach has been to attach electrodes to the scalp to deliver electrical stimulation during sham TMS in order to simulate the scalp sensation of active TMS. The "active" sham (Figure 5–3) is provided by a system that takes the TMS signal, determines whether the subject is receiving sham or real stimulation, and then triggers a generator to give a somatosensory "tickle" (or not),

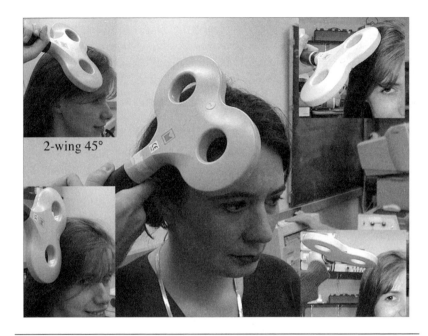

Figure 5-1.   Coil positioning for active transcranial magnetic stimulation (TMS) *(center)* as well as for several commonly used sham techniques *(insets).*

Active TMS is performed with the figure-eight coil tangential to the scalp, with the intersection of the figure eight in direct contact with the scalp. All of these sham manipulations consist of angling the coil slightly off the head such that the superficial scalp muscles are activated to simulate the sensation and acoustic artifact of repetitive TMS. This may be accomplished by tilting the coil such that two wings of the figure-eight coil touch the scalp (two-wing sham, *upper and lower left insets*) or such that only one wing of the figure eight touches (one-wing sham, *upper and lower right insets*). The degree of angulation from the plane tangential to the scalp is typically 45 or 90 degrees.

and there is auditory masking (not shown in Figure 5–3) of both the subject and the administrator. The plausibility of these two sham systems has not been systematically evaluated, but such approaches will likely afford better blinding for clinical trials than earlier approaches.

Concomitant Medications

Because TMS was first tested in a mostly medication-resistant population, most of the patients in the initial trials were taking a variety of antidepressant medications

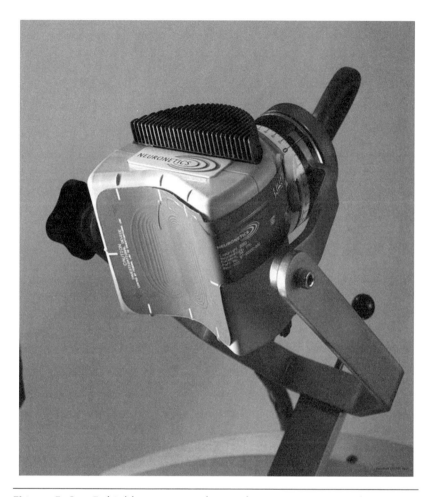

Figure 5-2. E-shield system used to make active transcranial magnetic stimulation (TMS) feel like sham TMS.

The e-shield system makes active TMS feel like sham by reducing the strength of the magnetic field generated at the surface of the scalp without appreciably decreasing the amount of stimulation reaching the brain.

as maintenance treatment. In most instances the antidepressant medications were ineffective, and patients had been taking stable doses prior to study enrollment. However, recent work reviewed below suggests that many drugs alter corticospinal excitability and parameters of intracortical inhibition (ICI) and intracortical facilitation (ICF) after either acute or chronic administration.

Temporary but significant increases in MT, MEPs, silent period, and ICI were observed 2.5 hours after 30 mg of citalopram administration, indicating a suppres-

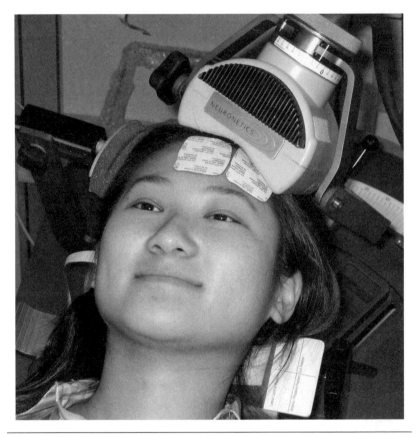

Figure 5-3. "Active" sham system that makes sham transcranial magnetic stimulation (TMS) feel like active.

The "active" sham system makes sham TMS feel like active TMS by delivering electrical stimulation during sham TMS via electrodes to the scalp to simulate the scalp sensation of active TMS.

sion of motor cortex excitability in normal subjects (Robol et al. 2004). A single intravenous dose of clomipramine exerted a significant but transitory suppression of motor cortex excitability in depressed patients by increasing MT and ICI and decreasing ICF 4 hours after drug administration (Manganotti et al. 2001). In another study, 100 mg of sertraline resulted in a steeper MEP intensity curve and a depressed paired-pulse facilitation (Ilic et al. 2002). In contrast to serotonergic drugs, MEP amplitude and ICF were increased after oral intake of 8 mg and 4 mg of reboxetine (Plewnia et al. 2002).

Experiments testing the effects of benzodiazepines on cortical excitability showed that 2.5 mg of lorazepam did not modify resting and active MTs and the amplitude of the MEP, but the duration of the silent period was prolonged with a maximum effect 5 hours after drug intake. The ICI showed a tendency toward more inhibition, whereas the ICF was almost completely suppressed. Moreover, transcallosal inhibition showed an inconsistent trend to less inhibition. In parallel to the pharmacokinetics of lorazepam, all effects peaked at 2 hours and 5 hours and were (partially) reversible after 24 hours (Ziemann et al. 1996b). Long-term use of diazepam in patients with anxiety disorders was associated with a significant increase in MT (Palmieri et al. 1999). Using a single magnetic stimulus, Di Lazzaro and colleagues (2000) found that lorazepam decreased the amplitude of the later I-waves in the descending volley; this effect was accompanied by a decrease in the amplitude of the evoked EMG response. Using the ICI paradigm, the authors also found that lorazepam increased the ICI, particularly at 4- and 5-msec ISIs. All these findings constitute direct evidence that benzodiazepines increase inhibitory circuits in the human motor cortex.

A significant dose-dependent increase of ICI was noticed after administration of 200 mg of topiramate (Reis et al. 2002). Carbamazepine, gabapentin, and lamotrigine, but not placebo, were found to abolish the normal TMS-induced facilitation of MEPs (Inghilleri et al. 2004), and 800 mg of gabapentin deepened the ICI and suppressed the ICF (Rizzo et al. 2001). Antiepileptic drugs that support the action of the inhibitory neurotransmitter GABA in the neocortex (vigabatrin, baclofen) reduced intracortical excitability but had no effect on MT. Gabapentin, whose mechanism of action has not yet been unequivocally identified, showed a similar profile. By contrast, sodium and calcium channel blockers without considerable neurotransmitter properties (carbamazepine, lamotrigine, losigamone) elevated MT but did not change intracortical excitability. The silent period was lengthened by gabapentin and carbamazepine (Ziemann et al. 1996a). In conclusion, some anticonvulsant drugs effect changes in intracortical excitability by GABA-controlled interneuronal circuits in the motor cortex, whereas others change MT by interfering with ion channel conductivity and membrane excitability.

Finally, the typical antipsychotic haloperidol was associated with an increase in corticospinal excitability, which was found to occur 4–5 weeks after medication was begun. In contrast, the atypical antipsychotic risperidone was associated with a decrease in corticospinal excitability, occurring 3–4 weeks after initiation of pharmacotherapy (Puri et al. 2003). An increase in ICI by bromocriptine, and, conversely, a decrease in ICI and an increase in ICF by haloperidol, were found by Ziemann and colleagues (1997). Because of the verified interference of different classes of drugs in cortical excitability, with specific concern about the possibility of an increased risk of seizures when these drugs are combined with high-frequency TMS, and because of the lack of significant benefit when TMS is used as an add-on treatment (Garcia-Toro et al. 2001a; Hausmann et al. 2004; Mosimann et al. 2004), it is now becoming common practice to "wash out" medication (through tapered withdrawal) before the therapeutic application of TMS and then reintroduce the medication after the treatment, in order to stabilize the clinical benefit (Schule et al. 2003). (For further discussion of washout, see pp. 137–138 below, under "Repetitive TMS," subsection "Blinded, Sham-Controlled Trials.")

CRITICAL REVIEW OF CLINICAL TRIALS WITH TMS IN DEPRESSION

Single-Pulse TMS: Open and Controlled Trials

Much of the recent work on TMS in depression has focused on repetitive TMS; however, the early single-pulse studies are of interest considering the greater safety profile of single-pulse TMS. The single-pulse TMS (<0.3 Hz) was usually administered with a large round coil centered on the vertex. In this position, the round coil stimulates broad regions of the bilateral frontal and parietal cortices. A small collection of open studies found single-pulse TMS to reduce depressive symptoms in MDD (Geller et al. 1997; Grisaru et al. 1995; Hoflich et al. 1993; Kolbinger et al. 1995; see Table 5–2). An open randomized trial found that 2 weeks of single-pulse TMS augmented speed of response to antidepressant medication in 12 patients, compared with 12 patients who received only antidepressant medications and no TMS (Conca et al. 1996). Besides the stimulation with a large, non-focal, round coil, many of these studies involved different positioning of TMS applications over the vertex, choosing multiple sites in the same patient, so speculation about activation of selective mood circuits is difficult.

The most recent report by Menkes and colleagues (1999) tested the hypothesis that single-pulse TMS to the right frontal cortex would be effective in treating depressed patients but would have minimal effect on control subjects. Eight sessions of 100 right frontal lobe TMS stimuli were given at MT and 0.5 Hz over a 6-week period. A significant antidepressant effect was noted in depressed patients on the Beck Depression Inventory (BDI) and Hamilton Rating Scale for Depression (Ham-D), whereas no change on either scale was noted in the control subjects. In a different study patients were given 10 stimuli over the frontal area of both sides for a total of 20 stimuli in a session. The subjects had daily TMS session for 5 days as an add-on therapy. In addition, six patients had their quantitative single-photon emission computed tomography (SPECT) images measured before and after TMS treatment. Compared with the value 2 days before the start of TMS therapy, the average Ham-D score dropped significantly on the day after completion of such therapy. The SPECT results showed that the regional cerebral blood flow of the bilateral frontal region had increased in four of six patients compared with pre-treatment values. These results suggest that although rTMS is steadily becoming the mainstay technique today, single-pulse TMS also possesses sufficient antidepressive effects (Fujita and Koga 2005). Further blinded trials with single-pulse

TMS comparing coil size and stimulation site will be needed to clarify if this form of stimulation will be clinically useful, even if the application of the repetitive form of TMS seems nowadays the most promising treatment.

Repetitive TMS

Open Studies

Open studies with rTMS in depression have been compelling, but the possibility of placebo response must be kept in mind in interpreting these results, given that smaller effect sizes have generally been observed in controlled, blinded trials (see next subsection). Several open studies have suggested that high frequency rTMS (in the range of 10 to 20 Hz) delivered to the left DLPFC improves symptoms in patients with MDD (see Table 5–2). In the first of these studies, George and colleagues (1995) treated six medication-resistant depressed patients with five daily rTMS sessions delivered to the left DLPFC at 20 Hz, 80% of MT, 2-second trains, 20 trains per day. Ham-D scores dropped by 26%, and two of the six patients were substantially improved. Catalá and colleagues (1996) found that daily rTMS applied to the left DLPFC improved symptoms of depression in seven medication-resistant patients with psychotic depression, whereas daily rTMS applied to the right DLPFC had no effect. In a much larger sample, Figiel and colleagues (1998) found 42% of 56 patients responded to five daily rTMS sessions, but the response rate was possibly lower in those over age 65. For each rTMS treatment, the system output was set to 110% of relaxed MT and a repetition rate of 10 Hz. Stimulation was delivered in 10 trains of 5 seconds each, with trains 30 seconds apart.

In a 2-week open trial of left prefrontal rTMS off antidepressant medications that extended the treatment to 10 days and increased the number of pulses per day (2,000 pulses per day at 20 Hz, 80% of MT, 2-second trains, 50 trains per day), the Ham-D and BDI scores decreased by 41% and 40%, respectively. After pre-rTMS antidepressant medication was resumed, improvement in mood was still significant at 1 and 3 months later. A clinical response rate and no adverse effects on neuropsychological performance were then reported in medication-resistant unipolar depressed patients (Triggs et al. 1999).

A group in Australia now has clinical experience using rTMS openly for the past 18 months in more than 85 patients with medication-resistant depression, many of whom are concurrently taking a variety of antidepressant medications, neuroleptics, and mood stabilizers (Pridmore et al. 1998). The average number of sessions has been 12, with onset of improvement typically appearing at the end of the first week. Such work demonstrates the feasibility of integrating rTMS into a clinical setting, but controlled trials are needed to establish the efficacy of this intervention. This group of investigators advocated extending the period of treatment to 3 or 4 weeks, as in their open study of 22 patients with melancholic depression referred

Table 5–2. Mood studies in normal volunteers

Study	N	Mean age	Design	Sham	Site	TMS type	Coil	Frequency (Hz)	Intensity	Train duration (sec)	ITI (sec)	Trains	Total pulses	Response
George et al. 1996	10	35	CO	None	Right/left/mid DLPFC occipital, cerebellum	rTMS	14 cm, figure 8	5	120% MT	10	120	10	500	—[a]
Pascual-Leone et al. 1996a	10	22–27	CO	None	Right/left/mid DLPFC	rTMS	14 cm, figure 8	10	110% MT	5	25	10	500	—[a]
Dearing et al. 1996	9	—[a]	CO	1-wing, 45°	Right/left DLPFC	rTMS	figure 8 and teardrop	20	80% MT	2	58	20	800	—[a]
Nedjat et al. 1998	50	—[a]	P	None	Left DLPFC	rTMS	—[a]	10 20	80% MT 80% MT	5 2	60	20	1,000 800	Mania in three cases
Mosimann et al. 2000	25	20–25	CO	1-wing, 90°	Left lateral frontal cortex	rTMS	14 cm, figure 8	20	100% MT	2	28	40	1600	No mood effect
Grisaru et al. 2001	18	26–64	CO	1-wing, 90°	Right/left DLPFC	rTMS	9 cm, figure 8	1	110% MT	500	0	1	500	—[a]
Schutter et al. 2001	12	—[a]	—[a]	2-wings, 90°	Right DLPFC	—[a]	—[a]	1	—[a]	1,200	—[a]	—[a]	1,200	↓ anxiety, ↑ left hemisphere alpha activity
Jenkins et al. 2002	19	19–38	CO	None	Right/left DLPFC	rTMS	70 mm, figure 8	1	100% MT	60	15	17	1,000	No mood effect
van Honk et al. 2003	8	20–28	CO	1-wing, 90°	Right parietal cortex	rTMS	—[a]	2	90% MT	1,200	0	1	2,400	—[a]
Barrett et al. 2004	10	20–26	CO	None	Right/left frontal cortex	rTMS	9 cm, circular	1 10	100% MT 100% MT	150 15	—[a] 10	3 45	450 675	—[a]

Note. CO=crossover; DLPFC=dorsolateral prefrontal cortex; ITI=intertrain interval; MT=motor threshold; P=parallel; rTMS=repetitive transcranial magnetic stimulation.
[a]Not reported.

for ECT in whom rTMS treatment with 1,250 pulses per day (10 Hz, 90%–100% of MT, 5-second trains, 25 trains per day) to the left DLPFC resulted in remission in 88% of cases (Pridmore et al. 1999). Although placebo response may have contributed to this effect, it may be that longer treatment is more effective and/or that patients with a melancholic subtype are more responsive to TMS.

Most of the open work with rTMS has focused on high-frequency stimulation. However, frequencies ≤1 Hz have a better safety profile and should be explored for their potentially unique therapeutic role. On this point, Feinsod and colleagues (1998) reported that 10 sessions of 1-Hz rTMS delivered with a 9-cm round coil to the right prefrontal cortex improved depression scores in 7 of 14 depressed patients. Two blinded controlled trials have now lent support to this uncontrolled observation (see discussion in next subsection).

Blinded, Sham-Controlled Trials

A series of sham-controlled trials examining the efficacy of TMS in depression have reported that high-frequency rTMS applied to the left DLPFC improves symptoms in MDD. The first controlled trial, by Pascual-Leone et al. (1996b), is still the only published trial to have compared the antidepressant efficacy of high-frequency rTMS applied to different cortical regions. Using a multiple crossover design, Pascual-Leone and colleagues reported that 5 days of high-frequency rTMS delivered to the left DLPFC (10 Hz, 90% of MT, 10-second trains, 20 trains per day) exerted marked antidepressant effects in 11 of 17 medication-resistant inpatients with psychotic depression, whereas stimulation of the right DLPFC and other areas produced no change. Only active stimulation of the left DLPFC resulted in improvement. This study is striking for its large effect size in extremely treatment-resistant patients, but most of the following studies could not replicate the same magnitude or speed of response when using similar parameters and length of stimulation.

George and colleagues (1997) found daily rTMS applied to the left DLPFC had only modest but statistically significant antidepressant activity compared with sham in a study of 12 outpatients with MDD. Each weekday the subjects received twenty 2-second, 20-Hz stimulations over 20 minutes (800 pulses per session, 10 sessions per treatment phase, total of 20 sessions overall per subject). However, Loo and colleagues (1999) failed to replicate these findings. They did not find a difference between 2 weeks of sham and active rTMS (10 Hz, 110% of MT, 5 seconds, 30 trains) in 18 medication-resistant depressed patients over 10 daily sessions. Given that both groups in Loo et al.'s study improved, the question has been raised as to whether the sham employed (45-degree coil tilt) may have been somewhat active (Lisanby et al. 2001a; Loo et al. 2000).

Berman and colleagues (2000) were able to detect a difference between sham and active TMS (20 Hz, 80% of MT, 2 seconds, 20 trains) in 20 medication-resistant depressed patients when they used a 45-degree coil tilt as sham coil. This coil was enclosed in a thick casing (used for water cooling of the coil) that elevated the coil windings about 0.5 cm off the scalp. The clinical response was significant but modest in magnitude (14-point drop in Ham-D scores with active and 0 drop with sham). Herwig and colleagues (2003) reported similar findings with real stimulation that improved depression on test measures (Ham-D and Montgomery-Åsberg Depression Rating Scale [MADRS]) moderately but significantly better compared with sham. In the real condition, 4 of 13 patients responded, with a mean improvement in Ham-D and/or MADRS scores of at least 50%, whereas none responded to sham. More recently, patients with medication-resistant depression were randomly assigned to receive 15 sessions of active or sham rTMS delivered to the left DLPFC. The response rate for the TMS group was 30.6%, significantly greater than the 6.1% rate in the sham group. The remission rate for the TMS group was 20%, which is significantly greater than the 3% rate in the sham group. The authors concluded that although all the patients in this study had medication resistance and over half the sample met DSM-IV criteria for chronic depression, rTMS could still produce clinically significant antidepressant effects (Avery et al. 2006).

Two parallel-group studies of rTMS in the elderly have been negative. Manes and colleagues (2001) found response rates of 30% with sham and 30% with active rTMS (20 Hz, 80% of MT, five daily treatments) in 20 elderly depressed patients. Using a higher intensity of MT (100%) and 2 weeks of treatment, Mosimann and colleagues (2004) failed to find a difference between active and sham rTMS in 25 elderly patients. These controlled observations confirm open data from Figiel and colleagues (1998), who reported that only 23% of patients over age 65 responded to rTMS, compared with 56% of younger patients. It has been suggested that lower response rates in the elderly may result from inadequate dosing (Kozel et al. 2000). Alternatively, cerebral atrophy would increase the distance from the coil to the brain, thereby decreasing the strength of the induced electric current. Dosing relative to MT may not adequately compensate for this increase in distance, since cortical atrophy is not necessarily symmetrical in all brain regions.

Several groups have examined the utility of TMS as an add-on to pharmacotherapy in the treatment of depression. While an open study by Conca and colleagues (1996) suggested that single-pulse TMS to multiple scalp locations in addition to various medications was more effective than medications alone, a sham-controlled trial by Garcia-Toro and colleagues (2001b) failed to find a benefit with left-DLPFC 20-Hz rTMS augmentation of sertraline therapy. In a study by Lisanby and colleagues (2001b), 36 patients began taking sertraline and were randomly assigned to receive 10 daily sessions of sham, 1-Hz rTMS to the right DLPFC, or 10-Hz rTMS to the left DLPFC. The therapeutic results were disappointing, with effect sizes of only 0.24 for 20-Hz and 0.20 for 1-Hz TMS. Patients who were classified as not medication resistant at baseline showed substantial improvement regardless of TMS condition, whereas medication-resistant patients showed little change. Medication-resistant patients showed a small but statistically significant benefit in the high-frequency rTMS condition. In a double-blind, controlled trial of 46 outpatients meeting DSM-IV criteria for nonpsychotic depressive episode (Rumi et al. 2005), rTMS at 5 Hz definitively accelerated the onset of action and augmented the response to amitriptyline. There was a significant decrease in Ham-D scores after just the first week of treatment. The decrease in Ham-D scores in the rTMS group was significantly greater compared with the sham group throughout the 4 weeks of the study. In another double-blind, randomized, sham-controlled study, Rossini and colleagues (2005) recruited 99 inpatients with a major depressive episode and randomly assigned them to receive venlafaxine, sertraline, or escitalopram in combination with a 2-week period of sham or active 15-Hz rTMS delivered to the left DLPFC. The active rTMS group showed a significantly faster reduction in Ham-D scores compared with the sham group—a finding that supports the efficacy of rTMS in hastening the response to antidepressant drugs in patients with MDD.

Although there is still not convincing evidence that TMS can speed onset of action, better effects might be seen with TMS as an add-on to ongoing pharmacotherapy to augment response. Indeed, most studies of TMS in depression have allowed patients to continue taking stable doses of antidepressant medications during the TMS trial. Garcia-Toro and colleagues (2001a) randomly assigned depressed patients taking stable doses of antidepressant medications for 6 weeks to receive sham or active rTMS (20 Hz). The authors found a modest clinical benefit to active rTMS (drop in depression scores of 7 points with active and 2 points with sham; response rates of 25% with active and 5% with sham). In contrast, in a double-blind, controlled study (Poulet et al. 2004), active rTMS and sham resulted in similar antidepressant effects in combination with paroxetine. A similar delay in improvement in scale scores was seen in both groups, so rTMS seemed not to be efficient as an add-on treatment to pharmacological medication in patients with nonresistant major depression. A study by Hausmann and colleagues (2004) suggested that rTMS used as an "add-on" strategy, and applied in a unilateral and a bilateral stimulation paradigm, does not exert an additional antidepressant effect.

Given the lack of a clear and significant benefit for TMS when used as an add-on, it is now becoming common practice to wash out patients during the therapeutic application of TMS and to reintroduce the medication after the treatment in order to stabilize the clinical benefit. Koerselman and colleagues (2004) found that over a subsequent 12-week follow-up without resumption of medication, the active rTMS group (20 Hz, 20 trains of 2 seconds, 30 seconds between trains, and 80% of MT) continued to improve significantly compared with the placebo group; the authors concluded that depressive symptoms may continue to decrease in severity after the cessation of rTMS stimulation. On the other hand, Schule and colleagues (2003) examined whether antidepressant pharmacotherapy can stabilize clinical improvement after rTMS monotherapy. Twenty-six drug-free patients with a major depressive episode participated in an open rTMS trial over 2 weeks (10–13 sessions, 10 Hz, left prefrontal stimulation at 100% of MT intensity). The patients were then followed up during standardized antidepressant pharmacotherapy with mirtazapine for a further 4 weeks. After 2 weeks of rTMS monotherapy, 39% of the patients had responded to rTMS by at least 50% reduction in their Ham-D scores. Treatment interruption after rTMS (an interval of 1–5 days between the last rTMS treatment and the first administration of mirtazapine) resulted in a significant increase in the Ham-D score of rTMS responders. The degree of the deterioration was dependent on the length of interval without treatment. However, this deterioration was reversed and the further clinical course stabilized by subsequent mirtazapine treatment. The overall response rate after rTMS and mirtazapine treatment (alone or in combination) was 77%. These results suggest that antidepressant pharmacotherapy is able to further improve the clinical response to rTMS and that responders to rTMS monotherapy should receive subsequent psychopharmalogical treatment without interruption in order to avoid a deterioration of symptoms.

TMS shows promise as a novel antidepressant treatment. Systematic and large-scale studies are needed to identify patient populations most likely to benefit and treatment parameters most likely to produce success. Most data support an antidepressant effect of high-frequency rTMS administered to the left prefrontal cortex. The absence of psychosis, younger age, and certain brain physiological markers might predict treatment success. Technical parameters possibly affecting treatment success include intensity and duration of treatment, but these suggestions require systematic testing (Gershon et al. 2003). A double-blind, sham-controlled multicenter study on the efficacy of high-frequency rTMS applied to the left DLPFC for 6 weeks has tested in 301 patients whether more pulses per day (3,000 pulses/day) and longer periods of stimulation are more effective to evoke clinical response in a controlled setting (results unpublished as of fall 2006).

Anyway, it is still an open question whether the antidepressant effects of rTMS are region- or frequency-dependent. Other groups have examined the efficacy of lower frequencies, which have the benefit of a better safety profile compared with high-frequency rTMS. Two groups have found that 1-Hz rTMS of the right DLPFC appears to exert antidepressant effects of comparable magnitude to 10-Hz left DLPFC rTMS (Klein et al. 1999; Tormos et al. 1999). Klein and colleagues (1999) demonstrated, in a double-blind, sham-controlled trial (N=71), that 1-Hz rTMS administered with a round coil positioned on the right DLPFC for 10 daily sessions was more effective than sham; 17 of 36 patients (47%) had a ≤50% drop in Ham-D, compared with 6 of 35 (17%) in the sham group. This work confirmed open trial findings by the same group (Feinsod et al. 1998). A much smaller double-blind study replicated these results, with the active group showing a better clinical response compared with the sham group (Kauffmann et al. 2004). Response was achieved in 4 of 7 patients (57%) in the active group and 2 of 5 patients (40%) in the sham group. Furthermore, 2 of the 5 patients crossed over to active from sham and had an average decrease of 45% in Ham-D scores. On follow-up, most patients in the treatment group experienced relapse after 2–3 months, whereas patients in the sham group who had improved relapsed in 2 weeks. The authors concluded that if rTMS in the low-frequency range of 1 Hz in the treatment of medication-resistant depression as an adjunct to antidepressants has beneficial effects, further studies should be done to explore maintenance treatment strategies.

In the first direct comparison of 1-Hz and 10-Hz rTMS laterality effects, Tormos and colleagues (1999) randomly assigned patients with MDD ($N=45$) to one of four groups (10 Hz left, 1 Hz left, 1 Hz right, or sham DLPFC rTMS). Both 1 Hz to the right and 10 Hz to the left DLPFC significantly reduced depressive symptoms. These findings fit with the hypothesis that rTMS reduces depressive symptoms by inhibiting right DLPFC (1 Hz) or by exciting left DLPFC (10–20 Hz), in line with models for lateralization in prefrontal systems. While the findings of inhibitory and excitatory effects of 1-Hz and 10-Hz rTMS over motor cortex are supportive of this hypothesis (e.g., Chen et al. 1997; Pascual-Leone et al. 1994), direct examination of the neurophysiological action of these rTMS stimulation parameters is clearly needed to substantiate this hypothesized mechanism.

The role of frequency has been challenged in recent studies in which patients were randomly assigned to different frequency groups in parallel study designs. In a study by Padberg and colleagues (1998), 18 patients with medication-resistant depression were randomly assigned to receive 5 days of single-pulse TMS, 10-Hz rTMS, or sham delivered to the left DLPFC. Each group received a total of 250 pulses per day. Both the single-pulse TMS and the rTMS groups showed modest improvement (drop in Ham-D scores by 5 points and 3 points, respectively, compared with increase of 1.5 points in the sham group). Only the single-pulse group differed significantly from sham, and there was no significant difference between the single-pulse TMS and the 10-Hz TMS groups. George and colleagues (George et al. 2000; Nahas et al. 1998) completed a larger study of 30 patients with depression who were randomly assigned to receive 5-Hz, 20-Hz, or sham rTMS to the left prefrontal cortex. Both active conditions yielded a modest improvement after 2 weeks of stimulation, and there was no significant difference between the 5-Hz and 20-Hz groups. Although the sample may have been too small to detect a small difference between these two frequencies, the potential that lower frequencies that are safer may be effective has major implications for future clinical practice.

More recently, Hoppner and colleagues (2003) applied a placebo-controlled condition designed to investigate the influence of the two different stimulation procedures. High-frequency rTMS (20 Hz) delivered to the left DLPFC, low-frequency rTMS (1 Hz) delivered to the right DLPFC, or sham stimulations (10 patients in each group) as add-on treatment at 10 days within 2 weeks. Differences between the rTMS procedures regarding depressive symptoms could not be found. Motor abnormalities, however, significantly improved exclusively after real stimulation procedures. Patients with less severe deficits in psychomotor speed and concentration responded more intensively than patients with severe deficits. Fitzgerald and colleagues (2003) demonstrated that both left-DLPFC high-frequency rTMS and right-DLPFC low-frequency rTMS have benefits in patients with medication-resistant major depression. Twenty 5-second left-DLPFC high-frequency rTMS trains at 10 Hz and five 60-second right-DLPFC low-frequency trains at 1 Hz were applied daily. The authors concluded that treatment for at least 4 weeks is necessary for clinically meaningful benefits to be achieved. rTMS given at low frequency over the right frontal cortex appeared to be as effective a treatment of refractory depression as high-frequency treatment over the left frontal cortex (Isenberg et al. 2005). A significant reduction in Ham-D, BDI, and Clinical Global Impression scores was found at the end of treatment for both groups (left-DLPFC high-frequency and right-DLPFC low-frequency). The treatment response rate found (32%) was typical of other response rates reported in the literature. Considering there are suggestions that lower frequencies may even fare better (Kimbrell et al. 1999), the utility of low-frequency TMS in clinical treatment deserves exploration.

Although left-DLPFC high-frequency rTMS and right-DLPFC low-frequency rTMS have both been shown to have antidepressant effects, doubts remain about the magnitude of previously demonstrated treatment effects. Fitzgerald and colleagues (2006) evaluated sequentially combined left-DLPFC high-frequency rTMS and right-DLPFC low-frequency rTMS for treatment-resistant depression in a 6-week double-blind, randomized, sham-controlled trial. Three trains of right-DLPFC low-frequency rTMS of 140-second duration at 1 Hz were applied daily, followed immediately by 15 trains of 5-second duration of left-DLPFC high-frequency rTMS at 10 Hz. There was a significantly greater response to active than to sham stimulation at 2 weeks and across the full duration of the study. A significant proportion of the study group receiving active treatment met response (44%) or remission (36%) criteria by study end compared with the sham stimulation group (8% and 0%, respectively). The authors concluded that the sequential application of both left-DLPFC high-frequency rTMS and right-DLPFC low-frequency rTMS has a substantial treatment efficacy with a clinically significant response over 4–6 weeks of active treatment.

It bears remembering that the optimal stimulation site for antidepressant effects may not have been identified yet. For example, all of the studies to date have stimulated left or right prefrontal cortex, while other sites of stimulation are entirely unexamined (Schutter and van Honk 2005). As noted earlier, van Honk and colleagues (2003) found mood effects in healthy volunteers with parietal stimulation, but this site has not been tested in depression. Further work using controlled designs is needed to determine whether the antidepressant effects of rTMS are region-, frequency-, or intensity-dependent, and to test the efficacy of more robust parameters in a sample large enough to provide adequate statistical power. Multicenter trials sponsored both by industry and by the National Institute of Mental Health are presently under way to address some of these questions.

rTMS Versus ECT

There has been great interest in determining whether rTMS could offer an alternative to ECT for severe or treatment-resistant depression, particularly since the adverse-effect profile of rTMS is relatively benign. Although rTMS is frequently referred to as a potential replacement for ECT, only four studies to date have rigorously compared the efficacy of these two treatments in a parallel design. In an open study of 40 patients, Grunhaus and colleagues (2000) found that, overall, ECT was superior to rTMS. However, while ECT was superior to rTMS in patients with delusional depression, rTMS and ECT had equal efficacy in nonpsychotic patients. The same group (Grunhaus et al. 2003b) reported on a controlled, randomized comparison of ECT and rTMS in 40 patients with nonpsychotic MDD referred for ECT. ECT was performed according to established protocols. Thirteen patients were treated unilaterally, and 7 patients were treated bilaterally. Repetitive TMS was performed over the left DLPFC at 90% of MT. Patients were treated with 20 sessions (five times per week for 4 weeks) of 10-Hz treatments (1,200 pulses per treatment day) at 90% of MT. The overall response rate was 58% (23 of 40 patients responded to treatment). In the ECT group, 12 (60%) responded and 8 (40%) did not; in the rTMS group, 11 (55%) responded and 9 (45%) did not. Thus, patients responded as well to either ECT or rTMS. Using bilateral ECT, Janicak and colleagues (2002) completed a similar randomized study involving 25 patients with major depression (unipolar or bipolar) who were deemed clinically appropriate for ECT. The patients were randomly assigned to rTMS (10–20 treatments, 10 Hz, 110% of MT applied to the left DLPFC for a total of 10,000–20,000 stimulations) or a course of bitemporal ECT (4–12 treatments). As in the study by Grunhaus et al. (2003b), no difference in efficacy between ECT and TMS was found (ECT, 64%; rTMS, 55%) (Janicak et al. 2002). Finally, Dannon and colleagues (2002) demonstrated that patients treated with rTMS or ECT showed the same percentage of clinical stabilization at 3 and 6 months of follow-up.

Of all the studies comparing ECT and rTMS with regard to clinical efficacy in the treatment of depression, there is only one in which both the clinical and neurocognitive effects of unilateral ECT and rTMS were compared (Schulze-Rauschenbach et al. 2005). Thirty patients with treatment-refractory nonpsychotic major depression received an average of 10 treatments with either unilateral

ECT or left-DLPFC rTMS and were assessed for objective and subjective cognitive impairments before and about a week after treatment. Treatment response was comparable (46% of the ECT group and 44% of the rTMS group showed a reduction in Ham-D scores of 50% or more). In patients treated with rTMS, cognitive performance remained constant or improved and memory complaints alleviated, whereas in the ECT group memory recall deficits emerged and memory complaints remained. The investigators concluded that rTMS has the same efficacy as unilateral ECT and, unlike the latter, no adverse memory effects.

Yet another approach has been to combine rTMS with ECT. Pridmore and colleagues (2000) randomly assigned 32 patients to receive TMS or right unilateral ECT. The number of treatments was not predetermined but was selected by the patient's treating psychiatrist. The response rate based on change in Ham-D score was identical in the two groups (66%), but ECT was superior on self-report measures. The same group of investigators compared the efficacy of six ECT treatments with two ECT treatments in combination with eight TMS sessions (Pridmore et al. 2000). While they found no difference between ECT and ECT plus TMS, it is important to note that administration of only six unilateral ECT treatments is not optimal treatment. As in TMS augmentation of antidepressant medications, the theory behind such trial designs is that TMS may augment response to a standard treatment such as ECT. This approach may theoretically have the benefit of allowing a decrease in the frequency or total number of ECT treatments. Maintenance treatment with rTMS following a course of ECT has not yet been reported but is an example of future directions for this work.

All of these studies have the limitation that the patients were not blinded to the form of treatment, and some have questioned whether the ECT comparison group represented optimal ECT practice. Nevertheless, it would be impossible to blind the patient to the treatment modality in this case (since sham ECT would not be considered ethically acceptable), and all studies have found rTMS to have a more favorable side-effect profile.

CONCLUSION

The body of literature on the use of TMS in depression is rapidly growing, and many of the findings have been encouraging. Several meta-analyses have examined the antidepressant efficacy of rTMS (Holtzheimer et al. 2001; Martin et al. 2001, 2003) and found evidence for statistical benefit of rTMS. However, the effect size could be described as moderate and in some cases of limited clinical significance. For example, Burt and colleagues (2002) found the average percentage of improvement with active TMS was 28.94% (SD=23.19) and with sham, 6.63% (SD=25.56). Relatively few patients met standard criteria for response or remission. It is also true, however, that the meta-analyses are heavily weighted toward the earlier studies that used what may now be considered inadequate dosages and durations of rTMS.

It is important to note several limitations in the cited studies. Perhaps most importantly, none of the key findings have been rigorously replicated. Most studies included small sample sizes making it harder to detect effects. Nearly all of the published trials were of a short trial duration compared with psychopharmacological trials, and to date there has been only a few published works on continuation or maintenance treatments. Treatment response rates across groups have varied widely, as have sham response rates.

This lack of replication and range in response rates should perhaps not be surprising, considering the large number of treatment variables that must be taken into account (e.g., stimulation parameters, treatment schedule, site of stimulation, coil shape, method of site localization, sham technique, depression subtype). Only a limited range of these myriad parameters has been explored. Despite these limitations, some conclusions may be drawn from the current studies on the use of TMS for depression. With the exception of Loo and colleagues (1998), most of the published blinded, sham-controlled studies have reported a significant effect of TMS.

The role of laterality and frequency in this antidepressant effect is far less certain. In studies that found an effect, this effect had a rapid onset within 1–2 weeks, which is faster than most medications with the exception of psychostimulants. In addition to having a fast onset, the apparent therapeutic response is also short lived when maintenance treatment is not provided. Some studies report a relapse within 1–2 weeks. If TMS will find a future clinical role in the treatment of depression, strategies to prevent relapse will be needed.

Unanswered questions regarding the utility of TMS in depression include those regarding the ideal stimulation paradigm (including parameters, coil shape, frequency of sessions), the optimal site of stimulation (including the methods for identifying it on an individual basis), predictors of response, and the mechanism of action. Ongoing research directions for TMS in the treatment of depression include studies with larger sample sizes, multicenter comparisons, maintenance strategies, and parallel designs exploring the multiple variables of TMS stimulation parameters. With the results of the past decade of research with TMS in depression, and the outcome of large multicenter trials, we are close to determining the role that TMS may ultimately have in our clinical armamentarium for the treatment of depression.

REFERENCES

Abrams R, Taylor MA: Diencephalic stimulation and the effects of ECT in endogenous depression. Br J Psychiatry 129:482–485, 1976

Avery DH, Holtzheimer PE III, Fawaz W, et al: A controlled study of repetitive transcranial magnetic stimulation in medication-resistant major depression. Biol Psychiatry 59:187–194, 2006

Bajbouj M, Lisanby SH, Lang UE, et al: Evidence for impaired cortical inhibition in patients with unipolar major depression. Biol Psychiatry 59:395–400, 2006

Barbas H: Complementary roles of prefrontal cortical regions in cognition, memory, and emotion in primates. Adv Neurol 84:87–110, 2000

Barrett J, Della-Maggiore V, Chouinard PA, et al: Mechanisms of action underlying the effect of repetitive transcranial magnetic stimulation on mood: behavioral and brain imaging studies. Neuropsychopharmacology 29:1172–1189, 2004

Berman RM, Narasimhan M, Sanacora G, et al: A randomized clinical trial of repetitive transcranial magnetic stimulation in the treatment of major depression. Biol Psychiatry 47:332–337, 2000

Bickford RG, Guidi M, Fortesque P, et al: Magnetic stimulation of human peripheral nerve and brain: response enhancement by combined magnetoelectrical technique. Neurosurgery 20:110–116, 1987

Burt T, Lisanby SH, Sackeim HA: Neuropsychiatric applications of transcranial magnetic stimulation: a meta analysis. Int J Neuropsychopharmacol 5:73–103, 2002

Catalá MD, Rubio B, Pascual-Leone A: Lateralized effect of rapid-rate transcranial magnetic stimulation of dorsolateral prefrontal cortex on depression (abstract). Neurology 46:A327, 1996

Chen R, Classen J, Gerloff C, et al: Depression of motor cortex excitability by low-frequency transcranial magnetic stimulation. Neurology 48:1398–1403, 1997

Chistyakov AV, Kaplan B, Rubichek O, et al: Antidepressant effects of different schedules of repetitive transcranial magnetic stimulation vs clomipramine in patients with major depression: relationship to changes in cortical excitability. Int J Neuropsychopharmacol 8:223–233, 2005

Conca A, Koppi S, König P, et al: Transcranial magnetic stimulation: a novel antidepressive strategy? Neuropsychobiology 34:204–207, 1996

Dannon PN, Dolberg OT, Schreiber S, et al: Three- and six-month outcome following courses of either ECT or rTMS in a population of severely depressed individuals: preliminary report. Biol Psychiatry 51:687–690, 2002

Davidson RJ, Pizzagalli D, Nitschke JB, et al: Depression: perspectives from affective neuroscience. Annu Rev Psychol 53:545–574, 2002

Dearing JE, George MS, Greenberg BD, et al: Effects of prefrontal repetitive transcranial magnetic stimulation (rTMS) on mood and anxiety in healthy volunteers: a replication study (NR182), in 1996 New Research Program and Abstracts, American Psychiatric Association 149rd Annual Meeting, New York, May 4–9, 1996. Washington, DC, American Psychiatric Association, 1996

Devanand DP, Lisanby SH, Lo E, et al: Effects of electroconvulsive therapy on plasma vasopressin and oxytocin. Biol Psychiatry 44:610–616, 1998

Di Lazzaro V, Oliviero A, Meglio M, et al: Direct demonstration of the effect of lorazepam on the excitability of the human motor cortex. Clin Neurophysiol 111:794–799, 2000

Dolberg OT, Dannon PN, Schreiber S, et al: Magnetic motor threshold and response to TMS in major depressive disorder. Acta Psychiatr Scand 106:220–223, 2002

Drevets WC: Functional anatomical abnormalities in limbic and prefrontal cortical structures in major depression. Prog Brain Res 126:413–431, 2000

Epstein CM, Figiel GS, McDonald WM, et al: Rapid rate transcranial magnetic stimulation in young and middle-aged refractory depressed patients. Psychiatric Annals 28:36–39, 1998

Feinsod M, Kreinin B, Chistyakov A, et al: Preliminary evidence for a beneficial effect of low-frequency, repetitive transcranial magnetic stimulation in patients with major depression and schizophrenia. Depress Anxiety 7(2):65–68, 1998

Figiel GS, Epstein C, McDonald WM, et al: The use of rapid-rate transcranial magnetic stimulation (rTMS) in refractory depressed patients. J Neuropsychiatry Clin Neurosci 10:20–25, 1998

Fink M, Ottosson J-O: A theory of convulsive therapy in endogenous depression: significance of hypothalamic functions. Psychiatry Res 2:49–61, 1980

Fink M, Kahn RL, Green MA: Experimental studies of the electroshock process. Dis Nerv Syst 19:113–118, 1958

Fitzgerald PB, Brown TL, Marston NA, et al: Transcranial magnetic stimulation in the treatment of depression: a double-blind, placebo-controlled trial. Arch Gen Psychiatry 60:1002–1008, 2003

Fitzgerald PB, Brown TL, Marston NA, et al: Motor cortical excitability and clinical response to rTMS in depression. J Affect Disord 82:71–6, 2004

Fitzgerald PB, Benitez J, de Castella A, et al: A randomized, controlled trial of sequential bilateral repetitive transcranial magnetic stimulation for treatment-resistant depression. Am J Psychiatry 163:88–94, 2006

Fox P, Ingham R, George MS, et al: Imaging human intra-cerebral connectivity by PET during TMS. Neuroreport 8:2787–2791, 1997

Fujita K, Koga Y: Clinical application of single-pulse transcranial magnetic stimulation for the treatment of depression. Psychiatry Clin Neurosci 59:425–432, 2005

Garcia-Toro M, Mayol A, Arnillas H, et al: Modest adjunctive benefit with transcranial magnetic stimulation in medication-resistant depression. J Affect Disord 64:271–275, 2001a

Garcia-Toro M, Pascual-Leone A, Romera M, et al: Prefrontal repetitive transcranial magnetic stimulation as add on treatment in depression. J Neurol Neurosurg Psychiatry 71:546–548, 2001b

Geller V, Grisaru N, Abarbanel JM, et al: Slow magnetic stimulation of prefrontal cortex in depression and schizophrenia. Progr Neuropsychopharmacol Biol Psychiatry 21:105–110, 1997

George MS, Wassermann EM, Williams WA, et al: Daily repetitive transcranial magnetic stimulation (rTMS) improves mood in depression. Neuroreport 6:1853–1856, 1995

George MS, Wassermann EM, Williams WA, et al: Changes in mood and hormone levels after rapid-rate transcranial magnetic stimulation (rTMS) of the prefrontal cortex. J Neuropsychiatry Clin Neurosci 8:172–180, 1996

George MS, Wassermann EM, Kimbrell TA, et al: Mood improvement following daily left prefrontal repetitive transcranial magnetic stimulation in patients with depression: a placebo-controlled crossover trial. Am J Psychiatry 154:1752–1756, 1997

George MS, Lisanby SH, Sackeim HA: Transcranial magnetic stimulation: applications in neuropsychiatry. Arch Gen Psychiatry 56:300–311, 1999

George MS, Nahas Z, Molloy M, et al: A controlled trial of daily left prefrontal cortex TMS for treating depression. Biol Psychiatry 48:962–970, 2000

Gerschlager W, Siebner HR, Rothwell JC: Decreased corticospinal excitability after subthreshold 1 Hz rTMS over lateral premotor cortex. Neurology 57:449–455, 2001

Gershon AA, Dannon PN, Grunhaus L: Transcranial magnetic stimulation in the treatment of depression. Am J Psychiatry 160:835–845, 2003

Grisaru N, Abarbanel J, Belmaker RH: Slow magnetic stimulation of motor cortex and frontal lobe in depression and schizophrenia. Acta Neuropsychiatr 7(suppl):10–12, 1995

Grisaru N, Bruno R, Pridmore S: Effect on the emotions of healthy individuals of slow repetitive transcranial magnetic stimulation applied to the prefrontal cortex. J ECT 17:184–189, 2001

Grunhaus L, Dannon P, Schrieber S: Effects of transcranial magnetic stimulation on severe depression: similarities with ECT (abstract). Biol Psychiatry 43(suppl):76S-#254, 1998

Grunhaus L, Dannon PN, Schreiber S, et al: Repetitive transcranial magnetic stimulation is as effective as electroconvulsive therapy in the treatment of nondelusional major depressive disorder: an open study. Biol Psychiatry 47:314–324, 2000

Grunhaus L, Polak D, Amiaz R, et al: Motor-evoked potential amplitudes elicited by transcranial magnetic stimulation do not differentiate between patients and normal controls. Int J Neuropsychopharmacol 6:371–378, 2003a

Grunhaus L, Schreiber S, Dolberg OT, et al: A randomized controlled comparison of electroconvulsive therapy and repetitive transcranial magnetic stimulation in severe and resistant nonpsychotic major depression. Biol Psychiatry 53:324–331, 2003b

Hajak G, Cohrs S, Tergau F, et al: Sleep and rTMS: investigating the link between transcranial magnetic stimulation, sleep and depression. Electroencephalogr Clin Neurophysiol Suppl 51:315–321, 1999

Hausmann A, Kemmler G, Walpoth M, et al: No benefit derived from repetitive transcranial magnetic stimulation in depression: a prospective, single centre, randomised, double blind, sham controlled "add on" trial. J Neurol Neurosurg Psychiatry 75:320–322, 2004

Herwig U, Lampe Y, Juengling FD, et al: Add-on rTMS for treatment of depression: a pilot study using stereotaxic coil-navigation according to PET data. J Psychiatr Res 37:267–275, 2003

Hoflich G, Kasper S, Hufnagel A, et al: Application of transcranial magnetic stimulation in treatment of drug-resistant major depression: a report of two cases. Hum Psychopharmacol 8:361–365, 1993

Holtzheimer PE 3rd, Russo J, Avery DH: A meta-analysis of repetitive transcranial magnetic stimulation in the treatment of depression. Psychopharmacol Bull 35:149–169, 2001

Hoppner J, Schulz M, Irmisch G, et al: Antidepressant efficacy of two different rTMS procedures: high frequency over left versus low frequency over right prefrontal cortex compared with sham stimulation. Eur Arch Psychiatry Clin Neurosci 253:103–109, 2003

Ilic TV, Korchounov A, Ziemann U: Complex modulation of human motor cortex excitability by the specific serotonin reuptake inhibitor sertraline. Neurosci Lett 319:116–120, 2002

Inghilleri M, Conte A, Frasca V, et al: Antiepileptic drugs and cortical excitability: a study with repetitive transcranial stimulation. Exp Brain Res 154:488–493, 2004

Isenberg K, Downs D, Pierce K, et al: Low frequency rTMS stimulation of the right frontal cortex is as effective as high frequency rTMS stimulation of the left frontal cortex for antidepressant-free, treatment-resistant depressed patients. Ann Clin Psychiatry 17:153–159, 2005

Janicak PG, Dowd SM, Martis B, et al: Repetitive transcranial magnetic stimulation versus electroconvulsive therapy for major depression: preliminary results of a randomized trial. Biol Psychiatry 51:659–667, 2002

Jenkins J, Shajahan PM, Lappin JM, et al: Right and left prefrontal transcranial magnetic stimulation at 1 Hz does not affect mood in healthy volunteers. BMC Psychiatry 2 (January 9):1, 2002 (Epub)

Kauffmann CD, Cheema MA, Miller BE: Slow right prefrontal transcranial magnetic stimulation as a treatment for medication-resistant depression: a double-blind, placebo-controlled study. Depress Anxiety 19:59–62, 2004

Kennedy SH, Evans KR, Kruger S, et al: Changes in regional brain glucose metabolism measured with positron emission tomography after paroxetine treatment of major depression. Am J Psychiatry 158:899–905, 2001

Kimbrell TA, Little JT, Dunn RT, et al: Frequency dependence of antidepressant response to left prefrontal repetitive transcranial magnetic stimulation (rTMS) as a function of baseline cerebral glucose metabolism. Biol Psychiatry 46:1603–1613, 1999

Klein E, Kreinin I, Chistyakov A, et al: Therapeutic efficacy of right prefrontal slow repetitive transcranial magnetic stimulation in major depression: a double-blind controlled study. Arch Gen Psychiatry 56:315–320, 1999

Koerselman F, Laman DM, van Duijn H, et al: A 3-month, follow-up, randomized, placebo-controlled study of repetitive transcranial magnetic stimulation in depression. J Clin Psychiatry 65:1323–1328, 2004

Kolbinger H, Höflich G, Hufnagel A, et al: Transcranial magnetic stimulation (TMS) in the treatment of major depression: a pilot study. Hum Psychopharmacol 10:305–310, 1995

Kozel FA, Nahas Z, deBrux C, et al: How coil-cortex distance relates to age, motor threshold and possibly the antidepressant response to repetitive transcranial magnetic stimulation (rTMS). J Neuropsychiatry Clin Neurosci 12:376–384, 2000

Lisanby SH, Devanand DP, Prudic J, et al: Prolactin response to ECT: effects of electrode placement and stimulus dosage. Biol Psychiatry 43:146–155, 1998

Lisanby SH, Gutman D, Luber B, et al: Sham TMS: intracerebral measurement of the induced electrical field and the induction of motor-evoked potentials. Biol Psychiatry 49:460–463, 2001a

Lisanby SH, Luber B, Finck AD, et al: Deliberate seizure induction with repetitive transcranial stimulation in nonhuman primates. Arch Gen Psychiatry 58:199–200, 2001b

Lisanby SH, Pascual-Leone A, Sampson SM, et al: Augmentation of sertraline antidepressant treatment with transcranial magnetic stimulation (abstract). Biol Psychiatry 49(suppl):81S, 2001c

Loo C, Mitchell P, Sachdev P, et al: rTMS: a sham-controlled trial in medication-resistant depression (abstract). Biol Psychiatry 43(suppl):95s-#317, 1998

Loo C, Mitchell P, Sachdev P, et al: Double-blind controlled investigation of transcranial magnetic stimulation for the treatment of resistant major depression. Am J Psychiatry 156:946–948, 1999

Loo CK, Taylor JL, Gandevia SC, et al: Transcranial magnetic stimulation (TMS) in controlled treatment studies: are some "sham" forms active? Biol Psychiatry 47:325–331, 2000

Maeda F, Keenan J, Freund S, et al: Transcranial magnetic stimulation studies of cortical excitability in depression (abstract). Biol Psychiatry 46(suppl):169S, 2000a

Maeda F, Keenan JP, Pascual-Leone A: Interhemispheric asymmetry of motor cortical excitability in major depression as measured by transcranial magnetic stimulation. Br J Psychiatry 177:169–173, 2000b

Manes F, Jorge R, Morcuende M, et al: A controlled study of repetitive transcranial magnetic stimulation as a treatment of depression in the elderly. Int Psychogeriatr 13:225–231, 2001

Manganotti P, Bortolomasi M, Zanette G, et al: Intravenous clomipramine decreases excitability of human motor cortex: a study with paired magnetic stimulation. J Neurol Sci 184:27–32, 2001

Martin JLR, Barbanoj MJ, Schlaepfer TE, et al: Transcranial magnetic stimulation for treating depression. Cochrane Database of Systematic Reviews, Issue 4, Article No CD003493; DOI: 10.1002/14651858.CD003493, 2001

Martin JL, Barbanoj MJ, Schlaepfer TE, et al: Repetitive transcranial magnetic stimulation for the treatment of depression: systematic review and meta-analysis. Br J Psychiatry 182:480–491, 2003

Mayberg HS: Positron emission tomography imaging in depression: a neural systems perspective. Neuroimaging Clin N Am 13:805–815, 2003

Menkes DL, Bodnar P, Ballesteros RA: Slow-rate transcortical magnetic stimulation (sTMS)—a non-invasive and effective treatment for major depression (abstract). Neurology 50:A318, 1998

Menkes DL, Bodnar P, Ballesteros RA, et al: Right frontal lobe slow frequency repetitive transcranial magnetic stimulation (SF r-TMS) is an effective treatment for depression: a case-control pilot study of safety and efficacy. J Neurol Neurosurg Psychiatry 67:113–115, 1999

Michelucci R, Valznia F, Passarelli D, et al: Rapid-rate transcranial magnetic stimulation and hemispheric language dominance: usefulness and safety in epilepsy. Neurology 44:1697–1700, 1994

Mosimann UP, Rihs TA, Engeler J, et al: Mood effects of repetitive transcranial magnetic stimulation of left prefrontal cortex in healthy volunteers. Psychiatry Res 94:251–256, 2000

Mosimann UP, Schmitt W, Greenberg BD, et al: Repetitive transcranial magnetic stimulation: a putative add-on treatment for major depression in elderly patients. Psychiatry Res 126:123–133, 2004

Mottaghy FM, Keller CE, Gangitano M, et al: Correlation of cerebral blood flow and treatment effects of repetitive transcranial magnetic stimulation in depressed patients. Psychiatry Res 115:1–14, 2002

Nahas Z, Speer AM, Molloy M, et al: Preliminary results concerning the roles of frequency and intensity in the antidepressant effect of daily left prefrontal rTMS (abstract). Biol Psychiatry 43(suppl):94s-#315, 1998

Nedjat S, Folkerts HW, Michael ND, et al: Evaluation of side effects after rapid-rate transcranial magnetic stimulation over the left prefrontal cortex in normal volunteers (abstract). Electroencephalogr Clin Neurophysiol 107:96P, 1998

Nobler MS, Oquendo MA, Kegeles LS, et al: Decreased regional brain metabolism after ECT. Am J Psychiatry 158:305–308, 2001

Ogawa A, Ukai S, Shinosaki K, et al: Slow repetitive transcranial magnetic stimulation increases somatosensory high-frequency oscillations in humans. Neurosci Lett 358:193–196, 2004

Padberg F, Zwanzger P, Thoma H, et al: TMS in major depression: impact of frequency and intensity on the therapeutic effect in pharmacotherapy-refractory patients (abstract). Electroencephalogr Clin Neurophysiol 107:96P, 1998

Palmieri MG, Iani C, Scalise A, et al: The effect of benzodiazepines and flumazenil on motor cortical excitability in the human brain. Brain Res 815:192–199, 1999

Pascual-Leone A, Gates JR, Dhuna A: Induction of speech arrest and counting errors with rapid-rate transcranial magnetic stimulation. Neurology 41:697–702, 1991

Pascual-Leone A, Valls-Sole J, Wassermann EM, et al: Responses to rapid-rate transcranial magnetic stimulation of the human motor cortex. Brain 117:847–858, 1994

Pascual-Leone A, Catalá MD, Pascual AP: Lateralized effect of rapid-rate transcranial magnetic stimulation of the prefrontal cortex on mood. Neurology 46:499–502, 1996a

Pascual-Leone A, Rubio B, Pallardo F, et al: Rapid-rate transcranial magnetic stimulation of left dorsolateral prefrontal cortex in drug-resistant depression. Lancet 348:233–237, 1996b

Paus T, Jech R, Thompson CJ, et al: Transcranial magnetic stimulation during positron emission tomography: a new method for studying connectivity of the human cerebral cortex. J Neurosci 17:3178–3184, 1997

Paus T, Castro-Alamancos MA, Petrides M: Cortico-cortical connectivity of the human mid-dorsolateral frontal cortex and its modulation by repetitive transcranial magnetic stimulation. Eur J Neurosci 14:1405–1411, 2001

Peschina W, Conca A, Konig P, et al: Low frequency rTMS as an add-on antidepressive strategy: heterogeneous impact on 99m Tc-HMPAO and 18 F-FDG uptake as measured simultaneously with the double isotope SPECT technique: pilot study. Nucl Med Commun 22:867–873, 2001

Petrides M, Pandya DN: Dorsolateral prefrontal cortex: comparative cytoarchitectonic analysis in the human and the macaque brain and corticocortical connection patterns. Eur J Neurosci 11:1011–1136, 1999

Plewnia C, Hoppe J, Hiemke C, et al: Enhancement of human cortico-motoneuronal excitability by the selective norepinephrine reuptake inhibitor reboxetine. Neurosci Lett 330:231–234, 2002

Post RM, Kimbrell TA, McCann UD, et al: Repetitive transcranial magnetic stimulation as a neuropsychiatric tool: present status and future potential. J ECT 15:39–59, 1999

Poulet E, Brunelin J, Boeuve C, et al: Repetitive transcranial magnetic stimulation does not potentiate antidepressant treatment. Eur Psychiatry 19:382–383, 2004

Pridmore S, Katsikitis M, van Roof M: rTMS versus ECT in severe major depressive episode (abstract). Electroencephalogr Clin Neurophysiol 107:96P–97P, 1998

Pridmore S, Rybak M, Turnier-Shea P, et al: A naturalistic study of response in melancholia to transcranial magnetic stimulation (TMS). German Journal of Psychiatry 2:13–21, 1999

Pridmore S, Bruno R, Turnier-Shea Y, et al: Comparison of unlimited numbers of rapid transcranial magnetic stimulation (rTMS) and ECT treatment sessions in major depressive episode. Int J Neuropsychopharmacol 3:129–134, 2000

Puri BK, Davey NJ, Zaman R: Excitability of the motor cortex in schizophrenia following typical and atypical antipsychotics: two serial case reports. Int J Clin Pract 57:831–833, 2003

Reid PD, Daniels B, Rybak M, et al: Cortical excitability of psychiatric disorders: reduced post-exercise facilitation in depression compared to schizophrenia and controls. Aust N Z J Psychiatry 36:669–673, 2002

Reis J, Tergau F, Hamer HM, et al: Topiramate selectively decreases intracortical excitability in human motor cortex. Epilepsia 43:1149–1156, 2002

Rizzo V, Quartarone A, Bagnato S, et al: Modification of cortical excitability induced by gabapentin: a study by transcranial magnetic stimulation. Neurol Sci 22:229–232, 2001

Robol E, Fiaschi A, Manganotti P: Effects of citalopram on the excitability of the human motor cortex: a paired magnetic stimulation study. J Neurol Sci 221:41–46, 2004

Rollnik JD, Schubert M, Dengler R: Subthreshold prefrontal repetitive transcranial magnetic stimulation reduces motor cortex excitability. Muscle Nerve 23:112–114, 2000

Rossini D, Magri L, Lucca A, et al: Does rTMS hasten the response to escitalopram, sertraline, or venlafaxine in patients with major depressive disorder? A double-blind, randomized, sham-controlled trial. J Clin Psychiatry 66:1569–1575, 2005

Rumi DO, Gattaz WF, Rigonatti SP, et al: Transcranial magnetic stimulation accelerates the antidepressant effect of amitriptyline in severe depression: a double-blind placebo-controlled study. Biol Psychiatry 57:162–166, 2005

Sackeim HA, Prudic J, Devanand DP, et al: Effects of stimulus intensity and electrode placement on the efficacy and cognitive effects of electroconvulsive therapy. N Engl J Med 328:839–846, 1993

Samii A, Wassermann EM, Ikoma K, et al: Decreased postexercise facilitation of motor evoked potentials in patients with chronic fatigue syndrome or depression. Neurology 47:1410–1414, 1996

Schule C, Zwanzger P, Baghai T, et al: Effects of antidepressant pharmacotherapy after repetitive transcranial magnetic stimulation in major depression: an open follow-up study. J Psychiatr Res 37:145–153, 2003

Schulze-Rauschenbach SC, Harms U, Schlaepfer TE, et al: Distinctive neurocognitive effects of repetitive transcranial magnetic stimulation and electroconvulsive therapy in major depression. Br J Psychiatry 186:410–416, 2005

Schutter DJ, van Honk J: A framework for targeting alternative brain regions with repetitive transcranial magnetic stimulation in the treatment of depression. J Psychiatry Neurosci 30:91–97, 2005

Schutter DJ, van Honk J, d'Alfonso AA, et al: Effects of slow rTMS at the right dorsolateral prefrontal cortex on EEG asymmetry and mood. Neuroreport 12:445–447, 2001

Shajahan PM, Glabus MF, Gooding PA, et al: Reduced cortical excitability in depression. Impaired post-exercise motor facilitation with transcranial magnetic stimulation. Br J Psychiatry 174:449–454, 1999a

Shajahan PM, Glabus MF, Jenkins JA, et al: Postexercise motor evoked potentials in depressed patients, recovered depressed patients, and controls. Neurology 53:644–646, 1999b

Soares JC, Mann JJ: The functional neuroanatomy of mood disorders. J Psychiatr Res 31:393–432, 1997

Steele JD, Glabus MF, Shajahan PM, et al: Increased cortical inhibition in depression: a prolonged silent period with transcranial magnetic stimulation (TMS). Psychol Med 30:565–570, 2000

Teneback CC, Nahas Z, Speer AM, et al: Changes in prefrontal cortex and paralimbic activity in depression following two weeks of daily left prefrontal TMS. J Neuropsychiatry Clin Neurosci 11:426–435, 1999

Tormos JM, Catala MD, Juan C, et al: Effects of repetitive transcranial magnetic stimulation on EEG. Neurology 50:A317–A318, 1998

Tormos JM, Catala MD, Pascual-Leone A: Transcranial magnetic stimulation. Rev Neurol 29:165–171, 1999

Triggs WJ, McCoy KJ, Greer R, et al: Effects of left frontal transcranial magnetic stimulation on depressed mood, cognition, and corticomotor threshold. Biol Psychiatry 45:1440–1446, 1999

van Honk J, Schutter DJ, Putman P, et al: Reductions in phenomenological, physiological and attentional indices of depressive mood after 2 Hz rTMS over the right parietal cortex in healthy human subjects. Psychiatry Res 120:95–101, 2003

Wassermann EM, Kimbrell TA, George MS, et al: Local and distant changes in cerebral glucose metabolism during repetitive transcranial magnetic stimulation (abstract). Neurology 48:A107, 1997

Ziemann U, Lonnecker S, Steinhoff BJ, et al: Effects of antiepileptic drugs on motor cortex excitability in humans: a transcranial magnetic stimulation study. Ann Neurol 40:367–378, 1996a

Ziemann U, Lonnecker S, Steinhoff BJ, et al: The effect of lorazepam on the motor cortical excitability in man. Exp Brain Res 109:127–135, 1996b

Ziemann U, Tergau F, Bruns D, et al: Changes in human motor cortex excitability induced by dopaminergic and anti-dopaminergic drugs. Electroencephalogr Clin Neurophysiol 105:430–437, 1997

6

TRANSCRANIAL MAGNETIC STIMULATION IN MANIA

Nimrod Grisaru, M.D.

Bella Chudakov, M.D.

Alex Kaptsan, M.D.

Alona Shaldubina, Ph.D.

Julia Applebaum, M.D.

R. H. Belmaker, M.D.

Mania is a severe psychiatric disorder that often results in hospitalization and severe disruption of work and family relationships. Although many new pharmacological treatments are available (Belmaker 2004), all seem to require a time course of 2–3 weeks for clinical results. During this period the patient with mania often requires physical restraint, as well as sedation with benzodiazepines that presents a risk of falls, aspiration, or disinhibited behavior. Clinicians often feel that electroconvulsive therapy (ECT) has more rapid onset of action than pharmacological treatment in mania, but it is difficult to obtain consent and cooperation for ECT in manic patients. Thus, new, rapidly acting treatments for mania are worthy of pursuit.

TMS AS ADD-ON TREATMENT

Comparison of TMS Delivered to the Left Versus Right Prefrontal Cortex

ECT is effective in mania as well as in depression (Black et al. 1987; Sikdar et al. 1994; Small et al. 1988, 1991). Since transcranial magnetic stimulation (TMS) may have ECT-like properties (Belmaker and Fleischmann 1995), we decided to study TMS to determine if it has efficacy in mania (Grisaru et al. 1998). Because the studies in depressed patients and healthy control subjects suggested a laterality of TMS effects, we decided to compare left and right prefrontal TMS in patients with mania.

The difficulties of drug-free studies of mania are well known (Licht et al. 1997), and we designed our study on the basis of previous work in mania by our group (Biederman et al. 1979; Klein et al. 1999) as an add-on study of left versus right prefrontal TMS to ongoing unrestricted drug treatment. On the basis of rapid response of mania to ECT, we hypothesized that the effect of TMS would be apparent early enough and strongly enough to be measurable even against the background of ongoing pharmacotherapy.

A patient admitted to the Beersheva Mental Health Center could enter the study if he or she met DSM-IV criteria for mania. No changes in clinical pharmacotherapy were made because of study participation. Patients with a history of epilepsy, neurosurgery, brain trauma, cardiac pacemaker implant, or drug abuse were excluded. The study was approved by our Helsinki Committee (Institutional Review Board), and all patients gave written informed consent. Patients were hospitalized for a mean of 8.6 days (range 1–38 days) before entering the study. Eighteen patients were enrolled. Two dropped out—one after four TMS treatments because of severe worsening and a positive urine for drugs, and the other before any TMS treatment because of change in diagnosis. Of the 16 patients with mania who completed the study, 12 did not have psychosis and 4 had psychosis. Seven were male and 9 were female; the average age was 36 years (range 20–52 years).

Of the 9 patients receiving left prefrontal TMS, 6 patients were receiving lithium; 1 patient, carbamazepine; 1 patient, valproate; and 1 patient, no mood stabilizer. Eight patients of this group were also receiving neuroleptics (in chlorpromazine equivalents, mean total daily dose=340 mg; range 150–600 mg). Of the 7 patients receiving right prefrontal TMS, 5 were receiving lithium; 2, carbamazepine; and 1, no mood stabilizer. Four patients of this group were also receiving neuroleptics (in chlorpromazine equivalents, mean total daily dose= 240 mg; range 75–600 mg).

Patients were assessed at four time points: 24 hours before the first TMS treatment (baseline), 3 and 7 days after the first treatment, and at the end of the study (day 14). Day 14 was usually four days after the final TMS. The following instruments were used: Clinical Global Impression scale (CGI; Guy 1976), Young Mania Rating Scale (YMRS; Young et al. 1978), and Brief Psychiatric Rating Scale (BPRS; Overall and Gorham 1962).

A Cadwell high-speed magnetic stimulator with a 9-cm diameter circular coil was used. Each patient was assessed for magnetic motor threshold (MT) (Hallett and Cohen 1989) before the first treatment, and 80% of individual patient MT was then administered for all treatment days (George et al. 1995). Mean patient MT was 67% for the left treatment group (range 50%–80%) and 72% for the right treatment group (range 55%–85%).

Patients were given 10 daily consecutive sessions, with 20 trains per session. Frequency was 20 Hz for 2 seconds per train, and the intertrain interval (ITI) was 1 minute. Each of the participants was given the stimuli over the right prefrontal cortex or the left prefrontal cortex, as randomly assigned.

The BPRS improvement score at day 14 was significantly different for left versus right-treated patients (Figure 6–1). For total BPRS, two-way repeated measures analysis of variance (ANOVA) with covariance for baseline showed a significant effect of time (F=3.9, df=2,28, P=0.03) and a significant interaction of time and side of transcranial magnetic stimulation (F=3.4, df=1.2, 17.2, P<0.08, Greenhouse-Geiser corrected). Post hoc Scheffé test showed a significant effect of side of TMS on day 14 (P=0.01).

These results suggest that TMS stimulation in mania of the right prefrontal cortex has therapeutic effects. The right side is the opposite from the lobe reported to have antidepressant effects. Interestingly, right unilateral ECT was not found to be effective in mania in a small group of patients (Milstein et al. 1987). The effects of TMS in psychiatry may be complex, since certain stimulation patterns enhance neuronal activity and cause (e.g., a motor movement; Hallett and Cohen 1989); whereas other stimulation parameters can disrupt neuronal outflow and cause (e.g., speech arrest; Pascual-Leone et al. 1991). Thus, further studies of frequency, intensity, and location of the magnetic stimulus will be necessary before the contrast with ECT is proven.

Comparison of TMS Delivered to the Right Prefrontal Cortex and Sham TMS

The results of Grisaru and colleagues (1998) discussed in the previous section could have been due to worsening of mania by left TMS, as happens with monoamine reuptake inhibitor antidepressants (Wielosz 1983). Thus, we designed a trial to compare TMS delivered to the right prefrontal cortex and sham TMS in the treatment of mania (Kaptsan et al. 2003).

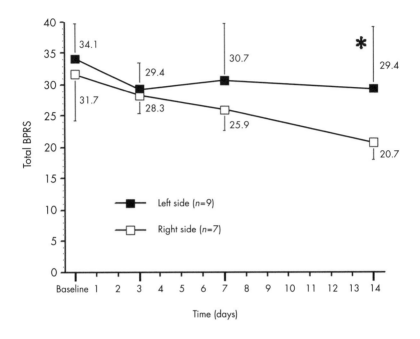

Figure 6–1. Antimanic effect of transcranial magnetic stimulation (TMS) delivered to the right versus left prefrontal cortex, as assessed by total Brief Psychiatric Rating Scale (BPRS) score (mean±SD).

Two-way analysis of variance (with repeated measures) with covariance for baseline showed significant effect of time ($P=0.03$) and significant interaction of time and side of TMS delivery ($P=0.05$).

*Post hoc Scheffé test, $P=0.013$ (day 14).

A patient admitted to the Beer Sheva Mental Health Center in Israel could enter the study if he or she met DSM-IV criteria for mania by consensus of two psychiatrists after clinical interview. No changes in clinical pharmacotherapy were made because of study participation. Patients with a history of epilepsy, neurosurgery, brain trauma, cardiac pacemaker implant, or drug abuse were excluded. The study was approved by our Helsinki Committee, and all patients gave written informed consent.

Twenty-five hospitalized patients were enrolled in the study, and none was a subject in a previous TMS study. Patients were hospitalized for a mean of 14.6 days (range 2–64 days) before entering the study, except for one patient with 82 days of hospitalization (the patient had had several phases in his hospitalization, and thus number of days before TMS was not a meaningful measure). The reason for the long pre-TMS hospitalization was the severity of the psychotic-manic state of most of the patients. In this period they were not able to sign informed consent or to cooperate with the study requirements.

Six of the patients dropped out: 3 after one right active TMS treatment because of manic uncooperativness unrelated to TMS treatment; 1 after three right active treatments because of physical illness not due to TMS therapy; 1 during detection of threshold, reporting headache and unpleasant feelings; and 1 after five sessions of sham treatment because of severe worsening of mania and a positive urine test for drugs. Of the 19 patients who completed the study, 16 had psychotic mania and 3 had nonpsychotic mania. Nine were men (5 in the right TMS group) and 10 were women (6 in the right TMS group). The patients' mean age was 41.6 years (range 19–65 years); the mean age of the patients given right TMS was 43.8 years, and that of the patients given sham TMS was 39.6 years. Patients were randomly assigned by one of the authors (R.H.B.) unrelated to patient treatment, according to a prearranged random order.

Among the 11 patients receiving right active TMS, concomitant drug therapy consisted of valproate acid (mean dosage = 800 mg/day) for 6 patients, lithium (mean dosage = 1,425 mg/day) for 4 patients, and no mood stabilizer for 1 patient. Ten of these patients also received neuroleptics (mean total daily dose = 490 mg in chlorpromazine equivalents, range 200–1,100 mg), and 1 patient received olanzapine (15 mg/day).

Among the 8 patients receiving sham TMS, 4 were receiving lithium, 2 were receiving valproate, 1 was receiving lithium plus valproate, and 1 was receiving lithium and carbamazepine. All of them were also receiving neuroleptics (mean total daily dose = 445 mg in chlorpromazine equivalents, range 50 mg–750 mg).

Patients were assessed at four time points: 24 hours before the first TMS treatment (baseline), 3 and 7 days after the first treatment, and at the end of the study (day 14). The CGI, YMRS, and BPRS were used in the assessment. Rating scales were evaluated by a senior psychiatrist located normally on another clinical unit who was blind to the treatment and not involved in the TMS treatment and the clinical treatment of the patients. The ward staff was not involved in the study design, and the TMS treatment was done in the human TMS laboratory, located away from the wards. Patients were blind to the hypothesis of the study.

A Cadwell high-speed magnetic stimulator with a 9-cm diameter circular coil was used. Each patient was assessed for MT only before the first treatment. MT was defined as the lowest stimulation intensity over the motor cortex capable of inducing a finger movement at least 5 times out of 10 . Eighty percent of the individual patient MT was then administered on all treatment days. Mean patient MT was 63% for the right TMS group (range 52%–75%) and 65% for the sham group (range 40%–100%). Mean patient MT was 63.6% (range 60%–67%) for the anticonvulsant treatment active subgroup and 62.4% (range 52%–75%) for the non–anticonvulsant treatment active subgroup.

Patients were given 10 daily consecutive sessions with 20 trains per session.

Frequency was 20 Hz for 2 seconds per train; the ITI was 1 minute. Each of the participants was given the stimuli over the right prefrontal cortex or sham position (vertical position of the coil, angled 90 degrees relative to the head but slightly off the scalp), randomly assigned by one of us (R.H.B.). The right prefrontal cortex was F3 on a rubber shower-cap with marked electroencephalography points. There was no beneficial effect of TMS delivered to the right prefrontal cortex compared with sham TMS (Kaptsan et al. 2003).

These results do not support a therapeutic effect of TMS delivered to the right prefrontal cortex in the treatment of mania. The combined results of the two studies discussed in detail in this chapter (Grisaru et al. 1998; Kaptsan et al. 2003) could be interpreted to mean that TMS delivered to the left prefrontal cortex may have blocked the effect of concomitant antimanic medication. Several factors should be noted, however: 16 of the 19 patients in Kaptsan et al.'s (2003) study had psychotic mania. This group had done more poorly in the previous study of TMS in mania (Grisaru et al. 1998), as well as in studies of psychotic depression versus nonpsychotic depression with TMS (Grunhaus et al. 2000). The mean total daily dose in chlorpromazine equivalents was 490 mg in the Kaptsan et al. study for the right TMS group and 445 mg for the sham TMS group, whereas in Grisaru et al.'s study it was 240 mg for right TMS and 340 mg for left TMS. The MT was 72 for right TMS and 67 for left TMS for the Grisaru et al. study and 63 for right TMS and 65 for sham TMS in the Kaptsan et al. study. Thus, lower TMS doses were given in the Kaptsan et al. study (comparing TMS with sham), and this may have reduced TMS efficacy. Mean days of hospitalization before TMS were 8.6 in the left versus right TMS study and 14.6 in the TMS versus sham study, suggesting inclusion of patients with more resistant mania in Kaptsan et al.'s study.

Some TMS researchers have expressed concern about the nature of sham TMS, and the possibility exists that the sham in Kaptsan et al. (2003) study was active enough to obscure differences between the two treatment groups. It is also possible that a longer treatment period, a higher treatment intensity, or different parameters of location and frequency might be more therapeutic in mania. Testing a new treatment as an add-on to an effective treatment is a severe test. Most antidepressants in controlled studies do not show additive effects to another effective antidepressant (Nemets et al. 2001). Thus, it will be important in the future to study TMS as monotherapy in mild cases of mania whenever ethically and practically possible.

Michael and Erfurth (2004) gave five sessions during weeks 1 and 2 and three sessions during weeks 3 and 4 to manic patients in an open design. Nine bipolar inpatients diagnosed with mania were treated with right prefrontal rapid TMS in an open and prospective study. Eight of nine patients received TMS as add-on treatment to an insufficient or only partially effective drug therapy. During the 4 weeks of TMS treatment, there was a sustained reduction of manic symptoms, as measured by the Bech-Rafaelsen Mania Scale (BRMAS), in all patients. Because of the open and add-on design of the study, a clear causal relationship between TMS treatment and reduction of manic symptoms could not be established. However, the data are consistent with the concept that TMS delivered to the right prefrontal cortex is safe and efficacious as an add-on in the treatment of bipolar mania, showing laterality opposed to the proposed effect of rapid TMS in the treatment of depression.

EFFECTS OF REPETITIVE TMS IN ANIMAL MODELS OF MANIA

To explore the effects of repetitive TMS in an animal model of mania, we used the amphetamine-induced hyperactivity model (Shaldubina et al. 2001). Amphetamine-induced hyperactivity is a well investigated model of mania that includes reasonable face validity (increased activity, increase in secondary reinforcement value, increased aggression) and predictive validity, because the effects are usually inhibited by lithium treatment (Gessa et al. 1995; Lyon 1991, 1990; Robbins and Sahakian 1980; Robbins et al. 1983) and were also reported to be reduced by carbamazepine (Maj et al. 1985) and valproate (Maitre et al. 1984).

Methods

Three experiments were performed to evaluate the effects of subacute (two sessions, 24 hours apart), daily chronic (7 days), and twice-daily chronic (7 days) rTMS treatment in the amphetamine-induced hyperactivity model. Male Sprague-Dawley rats (Harlan, Jerusalem; $n=20$ for experiment 1; $n=40$ for experiment 2; $n=20$ for experiment 3), weighing 200–250 grams at the beginning of experiment, were housed in an "in-lab, rat only" colony room with 12-hour light-dark cycle, constant temperature (22°C) and free access to food (standard rat chow) and water. Rats were given a 1-week habituation period prior to the beginning of the experiment during which they were handled by the experimenter for 1 minute every day. All experimental procedures were executed during the light phase of the light/dark cycle.

rTMS treatment was delivered with a Cadwell high-speed magnetic stimulator and a 5-cm round coil. Each treatment session lasted 2 seconds and used 25-Hz frequency at maximal machine capacity. During treatment, rats were held firmly, attached to a table, by one experimenter while another one applied rTMS or a sham audible control. As described elsewhere (Fleischmann et al. 1995), the coil was held immediately above but not touching the rat's head, with the pointer of the coil above the vertex of the skull and the handle of the coil parallel to the rat's vertebral column (see Fleischmann et al. 1995 for illustration). Control animals were held in a manner identical to TMS-treated animals, with a coil held above their head, and they were exposed to the audible artifact of TMS given about 10 cm away.

For experiment 1, rats were exposed to 2 treatment sessions, with the first delivered approximately 24 hours prior to amphetamine injection and the second delivered immediately after amphetamine injection, prior to placement in the automated activity monitors. For experiment 2, rats received 7 daily rTMS sessions and were tested for amphetamine-induced hyperactivity approximately 24 hours after the last session. For experiment 3, rats received 7 days of twice-daily (morning and afternoon, approximately 9 hours apart) rTMS treatments (totaling 14 sessions). The last session was administered immediately after amphetamine injection and prior to placement in the automated activity monitors. Control rats for each experiment were handled the same as the treatment group only the rTMS apparatus was not activated and was replaced by sham audible artifact. The 2- and 7-session schedules were chosen because they had been demonstrated to be effective in a rat model of depression (Fleischmann et al. 1995). The twice-daily schedule was added because a similar schedule of electroconvulsive shock had been reported to enhance amphetamine hyperactivity (Evans et al. 1976).

Immediately after amphetamine injection (for experiment 2) or immediately after the last rTMS session that followed the amphetamine injection (for experiments 1 and 3), rats were placed in automated activity monitors (Elvicom, Herzelia, Israel) measuring $38 \times 38 \times 35.5$ cm and left there for 30 minutes. Amount of locomotor activity, both horizontal and vertical, was recorded for each 10 minutes session and for the entire 30 minutes.

Results

Subacute rTMS treatment produced a significant decrease in horizontal amphetamine-induced activity (ANOVA, treatment effect: $F_1 = 6.62$, $P < 0.02$). Daily rTMS treatment for 7 days significantly decreased amphetamine-induced horizontal hyperactivity (ANOVA, treatment effect: $F_1 = 5.46$, $P < 0.03$). The effect of twice-daily treatment with rTMS was opposite to the effects of the previous treatment schedules. Twice-daily rTMS treatment augmented horizontal amphetamine-induced hyperactivity (ANOVA, treatment effect: $F_1 = 5.36$, $P < 0.04$) (see Table 6–1).

The results of Shaldubina and colleagues (2001) did not reveal a clear picture of TMS effects on amphetamine-induced hyperactivity. We had hypothesized that TMS might reduce amphetamine-induced hyperactivity, as does lithium (Robbins and Sahakian 1980), and this effect was indeed apparent after 2 or after 7 daily TMS treatments. However, TMS administered twice daily *enhanced* amphetamine-induced hyperactivity. The last effect may be similar to ECT effects, because chronic twice-daily electroconvulsive shock in rats has been demonstrated to

Table 6–1. Rat horizontal activity after acute amphetamine administration, after various schedules of repetitive transcranial magnetic stimulation (rTMS)

Schedule	Counts (mean ± SEM)		*P*
	rTMS	Sham	
Subacute TMS (two TMS treatments 24 hours apart)	1,680 ± 60	1,830 ± 40	< 0.05
Daily TMS for 7 days	1,708 ± 64	1,875 ± 40	< 0.05
Twice-daily TMS for 14 days	2,780 ± 160	3,200 ± 190	< 0.05

increase amphetamine-induced hyperactivity (Evans et al. 1976), apparently in a manner similar to its enhancement of apomorphine-induced hyperactivity (Lerer and Belmaker 1982; Modigh et al. 1984).

In humans, TMS stimulation of the brain may have effects depending on the area stimulated (George et al. 1996). Reports suggest that left prefrontal cortex rapid stimulation is antidepressant and right prefrontal cortex stimulation is anti-manic (George et al. 1997; Grisaru et al. 1998), although slow stimulation of the right prefrontal cortex may have antidepressant activity (Klein et al. 1999). In rats, available coils stimulate the whole brain, although a small region-specific coil in rats may be available in the future. Since localized stimulation is not available at present, it is not yet possible to use the rat model to further examine the lateralization question. Further clinical trials of rTMS delivered to the right prefrontal cortex in nonpsychotic patients with mania are warranted.

REFERENCES

Belmaker RH: Invited review: Bipolar disorder. N Engl J Med 351:476–486, 2004

Belmaker RH, Fleischmann A: Transcranial magnetic stimulation: a potential new frontier in psychiatry. Biol Psychiatry 38:419–421, 1995

Biederman J, Lerner Y, Belmaker RH: Combination of lithium carbonate and haloperidol in schizoaffective disorder: a controlled study. Arch Gen Psychiatry 36:327–333, 1979

Black DW, Winokur G, Nasrallah A: Treatment of mania: a naturalistic study of electroconvulsive therapy versus lithium in 438 patients. J Clin Psychiatry 48:132–139, 1987

Evans JP, Grahame-Smith DG, Green AR, et al: Electroconvulsive shock increases the behavioural responses of rats to brain 5-hydroxytryptamine accumulation and central nervous system stimulant drugs. Br J Pharmacol 56:193–199, 1976

Fleischmann A, Prolov K, Abarbanel J, et al: The effect of transcranial magnetic stimulation of rat brain on behavioral models of depression. Brain Res 699:130–132, 1995

George MS, Wassermann EM, Williams WA, et al: Daily repetitive transcranial magnetic stimulation (rTMS) improves mood in depression. Neuroreport 6:1853–1856, 1995

George MS, Wassermann EM, Williams WA, et al: Changes in mood and hormone levels after rapid-rate transcranial magnetic stimulation (rTMS) of the prefrontal cortex. J Neuropsychiatry Clin Neurosci 8:172–180, 1996

George MS, Wassermann EM, Kimbrell TA, et al: Mood improvement following daily left prefrontal repetitive transcranial magnetic stimulation in patients with depression: a placebo-controlled crossover trial. Am J Psychiatry 154:1752–1756, 1997

Gessa GL, Pani L, Serra G, et al: Animal models of mania, in Depression and Mania: From Neurobiology to Treatment. Edited by Gessa GL, Fratta W, Pani L et al. New York, Raven, 1995, pp 43–66

Grisaru N, Chudakov B, Yaroslavsky Y, et al: Transcranial magnetic stimulation in mania: a controlled study. Am J Psychiatry 155:1608–1610, 1998

Grunhaus L, Dannon PN, Schreiber S, et al: Repetitive transcranial magnetic stimulation is as effective as electroconvulsive therapy in the treatment of nondelusional major depressive disorder: an open study. Biol Psychiatry 47:314–324, 2000

Guy W: ECDEU Assessment Manual for Psychopharmacology—Revised (DHEW Publ No ADM 76-338). Rockville, MD, U.S. Department of Health, Education, and Welfare, Public Health Service, Alcohol, Drug Abuse, and Mental Health Administration, NIMH Psychopharmacology Research Branch, Division of Extramural Research Programs, 1976, pp 218–222

Hallett M, Cohen LG. Magnetism: a new method for stimulation of nerve and brain. JAMA 262:538–541, 1989

Kaptsan A, Yaroslavsky Y, Applebaum J, et al: Right prefrontal TMS versus sham treatment of mania: a controlled study. Bipolar Disord 5:36–39, 2003

Klein E, Kreinin I, Chistyakov A, et al: Therapeutic efficacy of right prefrontal slow repetitive transcranial magnetic stimulation in major depression: a double-blind controlled study. Arch Gen Psychiatry 56:315–320, 1999

Lerer B, Belmaker RH: Receptors and the mechanism of action of ECT. Biol Psychiatry 17:497–511, 1982

Licht RW, Gouliaev G, Vestergaard P, et al: Generalisability of results from randomised drug trials: a trial on antimanic treatment. Br J Psychiatry 170:264–267, 1997

Lyon M: Animal models of mania and schizophrenia, in Behavioral Models in Psychopharmacology. Edited by Willner P. Cambridge, UK, Cambridge University Press, 1990, pp 253–310

Lyon M: Animal models for the symptoms of mania, in Animal Models in Psychiatry, I. Neuromethods 18. Edited by Boulton AA, Baker GB, Martin-Iverson MD. Clifton, NJ, Humana Press, 1991, pp 197–244

Maitre L, Baltzer V, Mondadoni C, et al: Psychopharmacological and behavioral effects of anti-epileptic drugs in animals, in Anticonvulsants in Affective Disorders. Edited by Emrich HM, Okuna T, Miller AA. Amsterdam, Elsevier, 1984, pp 3–13

Maj J, Chojnacka-Wojcik E, Lewandowska A, et al: The central action of carbamazepine as a potential antidepressant drug. Pol J Pharmacol Pharm 37:47–56, 1985

Michael N, Erfurth A: Treatment of bipolar mania with right prefrontal rapid transcranial magnetic stimulation. J Affect Disord 78:253–257, 2004

Milstein V, Small JG, Klapper MH, et al: Uni- versus bilateral ECT in the treatment of mania. Convuls Ther 3:1–9, 1987

Modigh K, Balldin J, Eriksson E, et al: Increased responsiveness of dopamine receptors after ECS: a review of experimental and clinical evidence, in ECT: Basic Mechanisms. Edited by Lerer B, Weiner RD, Belmaker RH. London, John Libbey, 1984, pp 18–27

Nemets B, Fux M, Levine J, et al: Combination of antidepressant drugs: the case of inositol. Hum Psychopharmacol 16:37–43, 2001

Overall JE, Gorham DR: The Brief Psychiatric Rating Scale. Psychol Rep 10:799–812, 1962

Pascual-Leone A, Gates JR, Dhuna A: Induction of speech arrest and counting errors with rapid-rate transcranial magnetic stimulation. Neurology 41:697–702, 1991

Robbins TW, Sahakian BJ: Animal models of mania, in Mania: An Evolving Concept. Edited by Belmaker RH, van Praag HM. Lancaster, UK, MTP Press, 1980, pp 143–216

Robbins TW, Watson BA, Gaskin M, et al: Contrasting interactions of pipradrol, *d*-amphetamine, cocaine, cocaine analogues, apomorphine and other drugs with conditioned reinforcement. Psychopharmacology (Berl) 80:113–119, 1983

Shaldubina A, Kaptsan A, Belmaker RH, et al: Transcranial magnetic stimulation in an amphetamine hyperactivity model of mania. Bipolar Disord 3:30–34, 2001

Sikdar S, Kulhara P, Avasthi A, et al: Combined chlorpromazine and electroconvulsive therapy in mania. Br J Psychiatry 164:806–810, 1994

Small JG, Klapper MH, Kellams JJ, et al: Electroconvulsive treatment compared with lithium in the management of manic states. Arch Gen Psychiatry 45:727–732, 1988

Small JG, Milstein V, Small IF: Electroconvulsive therapy for mania. Psychiatr Clin North Am 14:887–903, 1991

Wielosz M: Effects of electroconvulsive shock on monoaminergic systems in the rat brain. Pol J Pharmacol Pharm 35:127–130, 1983

Young RC, Biggs JT, Ziegler VE, et al: A rating scale for mania: reliability, validity and sensitivity. Br J Psychiatry 133:429–435, 1978

7

TRANSCRANIAL MAGNETIC STIMULATION IN ANXIETY DISORDERS

Benjamin D. Greenberg, M.D., Ph.D.

Transcranial magnetic stimulation (TMS) has grown increasingly familiar to clinical psychiatrists over the last decade. The different TMS techniques include single-pulse TMS, paired-pulse TMS, and repetitive TMS (rTMS). As is noted elsewhere in this volume, these TMS techniques may be combined with a variety of neuroimaging, cognitive, or pharmacological tools (see, e.g., Chapter 2, "Methods of Administering Transcranial Magnetic Stimulation"; Chapter 3, "Basic Neurophysiological Studies With Transcranial Magnetic Stimulation"; and Chapter 9, "Transcranial Magnetic Stimulation and Brain Imaging," in this volume; see also Pascual-Leone et al. 1997; Ziemann et al. 1996). Only cortical structures are themselves accessible to TMS using current technology. However, TMS appears capable of affecting activity in deeper brain structures that are functionally linked to cortical brain regions (see Chapter 9, this volume).

While progress in research using TMS generally has further exemplified its potential, direct applications to anxiety disorders have been infrequent, with the great majority of TMS work in psychiatry focusing on depression. The potential of TMS in research in anxiety disorders, as in other disorders, includes pathophysiology and delineation of physiological endophenotypes of relevance to involvement of genetic factors and of particular neuroanatomical networks in anxiety disorders. Its potential clinical usefulness remains of great interest but has only be-gun to be explored. Only a few exploratory studies of TMS as a treatment have been reported. Some early studies have been viewed as treatment trials (e.g., Greenberg et al. 1997), when they were really intended to explore the use of TMS as a neuroanatomical probe of structures and circuits potentially involved in clin-ical phenomena. Because of the limited work available, a review of TMS in anxiety disorders must focus on its potential in research on mechanisms of illness, treat-ment response, and clinical treatment.

TMS IN OBSESSIVE-COMPULSIVE DISORDER: PROBING PATHOPHYSIOLOGICAL MODELS

Obsessive-compulsive disorder (OCD) is characterized by recurrent intrusive thoughts, images, or feelings that lead to repetitive behaviors. The intrusions (ob-sessions) persist against the patient's attempts to eradicate them and are accompa-nied by marked and often overwhelming anxiety. The symptoms are associated with significant, and often dramatic, impairment in the abilities of affected indi-viduals to carry out their occupational and social roles.

Neuroanatomical Models of OCD Pathophysiology

Neuroanatomical models of OCD pathophysiology have been developed over the last two decades, primarily on the basis of evidence from functional neuroimaging (see next subsection, "Neuroimaging and Neurosurgical Evidence in OCD"). These models attempt to explain both how intrusive thoughts might arise and how performance of a compulsion could temporarily reduce obsessions and the associ-ated anxiety. The models share certain functionally linked brain areas, principally prefrontal cortex (including orbital and medial prefrontal cortex), "paralimbic" structures (anterior cingulate gyrus and anterior temporal, parahippocampal, and insular cortices), basal ganglia (including caudate nucleus, putamen, and globus pallidus), and thalamus (e.g., Modell et al. 1989; Rapoport 1991). These areas are associated with aspects of cognition and emotion likely to be important in OCD symptoms. These aspects of cognition and emotion include 1) response inhibi-tion, planning, verifying of operations/error detection, and mood regulation (pre-frontal cortex); 2) assigning of importance to external stimuli via integration with emotional states, and modulation of arousal and intense emotion (paralimbic cor-tex); 3) automatic filtering of stimuli and mediation of stereotyped, rule-guided behaviors, outside of consciousness and motivation (basal ganglia); and 4) trans-mission of processed information, through excitatory input, back to the cortex (thalamus).

OCD models emphasize abnormal activity in cortico-striato-pallido-thalamic (CSPT) circuits. In these models, activity of any component element can influence overall activity in the circuit and the likelihood of symptom occurrence. Dysfunction in any of a number of these areas might therefore give rise to OCD symptoms. Furthermore, stimulation that modulated activity within these neuronal loops would allow tests of hypotheses regarding whether and how particular kinds of information processing in these functionally related networks was associated with OCD symptoms. Various research measures, including neuroimaging, cognitive measures, and electrophysiological tests assessing both local and distributed effects of stimulation could make important contributions as this research advances.

Neuroimaging and Neurosurgical Evidence in OCD

Although dysfunction at any one of several places along neuroanatomical circuits potentially involved in OCD could, in theory, account for its symptoms, more regionally specific proposals have been made. For example, one hypothesis is that a primary locus of abnormality is within the orbitofrontal cortex (Insel 1992), the region most consistently implicated in OCD by imaging studies. Although orbitofrontal cortex is not as easily accessible to TMS as more dorsal regions that have been the focus of most TMS research in psychiatry, effects consistent with effects of TMS on orbitofrontal cortex have been reported (van Honk et al. 2002b).

Another, and widely held, working hypothesis is that OCD symptoms arise as a response to defective filtering of cortical input by the basal ganglia. One result of this abnormal processing would be dysregulated, and increased excitatory thalamic output to the cerebral cortex (termed *defective thalamic gating*), leading to excessive, aberrantly modulated activity in the cortex and subsequently in other components of CSPT circuits. TMS studies, including those with the paired-pulse TMS, may provide converging evidence relevant to the hypothesis of abnormal striatal function in OCD, as discussed below.

There have been a number of recent reviews of the neuroimaging evidence implicating the aforementioned circuitry in OCD (Rauch 2003; Saxena et al. 2001), and only a few relevant issues will be dealt with here. Structural neuroimaging studies, using several different techniques, have found basal ganglia abnormalities in OCD that are consistent with the hypothesis that striatal dysfunction contributes to symptomatology. It is worth noting that abnormalities in regional brain volumes may not be consistent across OCD patients. As noted earlier, abnormalities in a number of functionally related areas might predispose individuals to the development of OCD. Not only might the disorder have a heterogeneous etiology, increasing the likelihood of failure to find an actual difference in a small study sample (a type 2 statistical error), it also might be that different OCD symptom subtypes are associated with abnormalities in different functional networks (Mataix-Cols et al. 2004). Of course, structural abnormalities, even if present, may be apparent on some measures but not others (e.g., Bartha et al. 1998; Russell et al. 2002).

Functional neuroimaging work has been generally more consistent in OCD, implicating prefrontal mechanisms and related structures, including striatum, thalamus, anterior cingulate, and temporal paralimbic areas, in OCD symptomatology across a fairly large number of studies (for a review, see Hoehn-Saric and Greenberg 1997). For example, there are well-replicated findings that OCD patients who are not taking medication have prefrontal (usually orbitofrontal) cortex hypermetabolism or increased perfusion, both in the resting state (Baxter et al. 1992; Schwartz et al. 1996) and after symptom provocation (e.g., Rauch et al. 1994). Successful pharmacological treatment of OCD with serotonin reuptake inhibitor antidepressants is associated with normalization of this "hyperfrontality" (Baxter et al. 1992; Hoehn-Saric et al. 2001), as is successful treatment with behavior therapy (Baxter et al. 1992; Schwartz et al. 1996). Symptom provocation and resting state studies also demonstrate increased activity in basal ganglia, thalamus, and anterior cingulate gyrus.

Other evidence supporting overactive prefrontal-subcortical function in OCD comes from neurosurgical treatment of a patient subgroup. In cases of disabling OCD that prove extremely refractory to all proven pharmacological and behavioral treatments, focal sterotactic neurosurgery—mainly anterior cingulotomy and anterior capsulotomy in the United States, which target neurocircuitry implicated in OCD by neuroimaging work (Rauch 2003)—has led to significant symptom improvement (Greenberg et al. 2003). A new development, application of deep brain stimulation, which is now standard therapy for movement disorders (Greenberg and Rezai 2003), has provided initial results suggesting that directly changing activity in CSPT circuits can improve symptoms of otherwise intractable OCD. Interestingly, symptom improvements after chronic stimulation of the thalamo-prefrontal fibers and adjacent ventral striatum have been associated with reduction in prefrontal cortex metabolism on positron emission tomography (PET) after chronic treatment (Nuttin et al. 2003).

Thus, the evidence consistent with neuroanatomical models of OCD, first presented in the 1980s, continues to accumulate. Studies combining TMS with neuroimaging and using structural and functional imaging could help assess, in more detail, the relation of activity in components of CSPT circuits to OCD symptoms. For example, one modification of the CSPT dysregulation hypothesis of OCD notes a distinction between a more ventral or "direct" CSPT circuit and the parallel but more dorsal "indirect" pathway and suggests that the balance of activity in the two divisions may be important in modulating OCD symptoms (Saxena et al. 2001). The hypothesis predicts that increased activity in the direct pathway from prefrontal cortex to striatum–globus pallidus–thalamus and back to prefrontal cortex would increase obsessional doubt and compulsive checking, while, in contrast, increased activity in the parallel indirect pathway might decrease symptoms. According to this view, either decreasing activity in the direct pathway or increasing activity in the indirect pathway would be beneficial in OCD. While altering the direct/indirect pathway balance might be accomplished pharmacologically, it could also, in theory, be produced by rTMS at particular cortical sites if cortical input were relatively segregated to the dorsal or ventral pathways (see Mega and Cummings 1994). It remains to be determined whether such an anatomically selective effect of cortical TMS on activity in subcortical regions receiving cortical input is possible. Studies combining TMS and functional neuroimaging may represent the most powerful approach to this question. Conversely, combined TMS and neuroimaging or neurophysiological studies could, in theory, also help test recent proposals that different OCD symptom subtypes may be mediated by different neuroanatomical networks (Mataix-Cols et al. 2004).

rTMS as an Anatomical Probe in OCD

As discussed in the previous subsection, functional neuroimaging, neuroanatomical, and neurosurgical data suggest that rTMS, by directly altering prefrontal activity, might affect OCD symptoms. In a preliminary controlled study of rTMS as an anatomical probe in OCD (Greenberg et al. 1997), we administered single sessions of high-frequency stimulation to left and right dorsolateral prefrontal cortex and to a parieto-occipital control site, in a randomized design. The prefrontal locations were defined as the site 5 cm anterior and 2 cm inferior to the hand area of primary motor cortex on each side. The 12 OCD patients studied had, on average, moderately severe symptoms (a mean baseline Yale-Brown Obsessive Compulsive Scale [Y-BOCS] score of about 20), even though 8 of them were treated with antiobsessional serotonin reuptake inhibitors. Each site was stimulated, 2 days apart, with 20-Hz trains of 2 seconds each, once per minute for 20 minutes (800 pulses total per session) with an figure-eight focal coil attached to a Cadwell high-speed magnetic stimulator. rTMS intensity was 80% of abductor pollicis brevis twitch threshold.

We observed that right lateral prefrontal rTMS was followed by a significant reduction in compulsive urges, lasting at least 8 hours, in this group of OCD patients who were mainly moderately affected but included two severely ill individuals (Greenberg et al. 1997). This effect was not seen after left prefrontal or parieto-occipital stimulation. These OCD patients, who were not clinically depressed at baseline as a group, also reported significant mood elevation for 30 minutes after right prefrontal stimulation. The finding of a laterally specific effect on symptoms was unexpected but interesting, given studies finding 1) correlations between symptom provocation and orbitofrontal perfusion were opposite in the right and left hemispheres (Rauch et al. 1994), 2) disruption of abnormally correlated metabolic activity in brain regions in the right hemisphere was associated with symptom improvement (Schwartz et al. 1996), and 3) the location of anterior capsulotomy lesions in the right, but not the left, hemisphere appeared to be a key determinant of neurosurgical efficacy in OCD (Lippitz et al. 1999).

Our initial observations (Greenberg et al. 1997) suggested that a single rTMS session might have reduced compulsive urges by changing neuronal activity well beyond the period of acute stimulation. However, despite its controlled design, the study had a number of limitations, including the possibility of placebo effects, relatively crude anatomical localization, and, importantly, lack of independent measures of cortical or subcortical function. Nevertheless, the findings raise the intriguing possibility that right prefrontal rTMS directly interrupted ongoing cortical activity related to compulsive urges. Alternatively, stimulation may have indirectly enhanced activity in subcortical regions, which might have suppressed compulsions. These possibilities await testing in further studies combining rTMS with measures of regional brain activity in OCD, including functional neuroimaging, cognitive tests, and electrophysiological methods.

Paired-Pulse TMS as a Physiological Probe in OCD

Paired-pulse TMS is well established as a probe of inhibitory and excitatory modulation in the primary motor cortex. The method is based on observations that TMS pulses too weak to produce motor evoked potentials (MEPs) themselves modulate the responses to stronger pulses, above the threshold to produce MEPs, when the weak pulses are presented milliseconds before the suprathreshold stimuli. Interest has focused on several phenomena, including the threshold excitability (the lowest energy that produces MEPs) and intracortical inhibition (ICI) (the reduction in MEP amplitude when the weak and test pulses are separated by 2–5 milliseconds). Pharmacological studies in nonpatient volunteers suggest that ICI is likely to be mediated by activation of γ-aminobutyric acid (GABA)–ergic cortical interneurons (Ziemann et al. 1996). Abnormal ICI has been demonstrated in a number of neuropsychiatric disorders thought to involve abnormal basal ganglia function (Ridding et al. 1995). In patients with Tourette's syndrome or focal dystonias, illnesses both thought to involve basal ganglia pathology that are related to OCD, paired-pulse inhibition was reduced compared with the inhibition in nonpatients (Ziemann et al. 1997).

Intrigued by these reports, we performed similar experiments in OCD patients and also detected reduced inhibitory modulation with paired-pulse TMS (Greenberg et al. 1998, 2000). Reduced ICI was similar to that seen in Tourette's syndrome (Ziemann et al. 1997). Although the reduction in ICI was greatest in patients with comorbid OCD and tics, reduced ICI was observed even in OCD patients without tics. However, we also observed that both resting and active motor thresholds (MTs) were reduced in OCD patients compared with control subjects, suggesting either an increased excitability intrinsic to motor cortex or an increased excitatory drive from thalamocortical projections. Both phenomena might relate to the consistent findings of increased cortical activity in OCD discussed earlier. It is of significant interest that the two abnormalities observed—reduced ICI and enhanced cortical excitability—could both be due to an abnormality in basal ganglia function, consistent with theories of OCD and Tourette's syndrome pathogenesis (Baxter et al. 1996; Peterson et al. 1998). These findings from studies using paired-pulse TMS provide additional evidence that OCD and Tourette's syndrome, related to each other by phenomenology and heritability, may also have overlapping pathophysiological features. Further studies will be necessary to determine whether this phenomenon is preferentially observed in neuropsychiatric illnesses proposed to be related to OCD and Tourette's syndrome. Likewise, additional work will be necessary to determine whether paired TMS measures can help suggest new pharmacological treatment approaches in OCD or help monitor therapeutic effects of agents that may act to decrease excitatory drive via reducing glutaminergic excitatory drive (Coric et al. 2003) or enhancing inhibitory mechanisms. However, with regard to the latter hypothesis, the clinical utility of benzodiazepines and anticonvulsants in OCD has been mixed at best (Hollander et al. 2003). In contrast, there is some empirical support for the idea that changes in glutaminergic function might be relevant to effects of successful pharmacological treatment of OCD (Rosenberg et al. 2000).

rTMS as an OCD Treatment?

Interest in TMS as a possible therapeutic modality in OCD has several sources. There is increasing recognition that OCD burdens a significant proportion of the population with functional impairment, being among the top 10 causes of disability in developed societies (Murray and Lopez 1997). In addition, it is also clear that available medication and behavioral treatments, while extremely beneficial for many patients, have limited efficacy or limited acceptance (true of both behavioral and medication approaches) in many others. Unfortunately, despite some promising leads (Hollander et al. 2002), development of fundamentally new and effective medication treatment modalities has been largely lacking in recent years.

Despite this need for more effective treatments, very few studies have explored the potential utility of rTMS as a treatment in anxiety disorders in general, or specifically in OCD. A recent Cochrane systematic review (Martin et al. 2003) could find only three published rTMS studies in OCD, of which only two, with very different designs, were designed to explore therapeutic effects of rTMS. Martin and colleagues (2003) could conclude, in that review, only that the data were insufficient to judge the clinical utility of rTMS in OCD. That result, unsurprising as it was given the fact that so few studies had been published, perhaps best serves to underscore the continuing interest in the clinical use of TMS for OCD, and by extension in other conditions in which anxiety is a core clinical feature.

In one of the two available treatment studies (both of which were small pilot trials), 12 patients with resistant OCD were randomly assigned to receive rTMS delivered to either the right or left prefrontal cortex daily for 2 weeks and were assessed by an independent rater at 1 and 2 weeks and 1 month later (Sachdev et al. 2001). There were significant improvements in obsessions, compulsions, and total scores on the Y-BOCS after 2 weeks and at 1-month follow-up. The improvement remained significant for obsessions and tended toward significance for total Y-BOCS scores after correction for changes in depression scores—a finding of interest given the relationships between the severity of OCD and depression, which very often occur comorbidly. There were no significant differences between right- and left-sided delivery of TMS. Two subjects (33%) in each group showed a clinically significant improvement that persisted at I month, but with relapse later in 1 subject. The authors (Sachdev et al. 2001) rightly noted that without a sham treatment group in this study, the possibility that this was a placebo response could not be ruled out. The authors concluded that rTMS warrants further investigation to better establish its efficacy and examine the best parameters for response in OCD.

The only other published study to explore rTMS as a potential OCD treatment—the only published controlled rTMS trial in OCD—used a very different technique (Alonso et al. 2001). Patients were randomly assigned to 18 sessions of real or sham rTMS. The total sample was small ($N=18$), with only 10 patients receiving active stimulation. In contrast to the Sachdev et al. (2001) study discussed earlier and the study by our group finding that focal right prefrontal stimulation had an effect on compulsive urges (Greenberg et al. 1997), Alonso and colleagues used a much slower train (1 Hz), which led to a significantly lower number of total pulses being delivered over the course of the trial. This detail is of interest because the total number of pulses delivered might relate to the therapeutic response. In addition, the investigators used a TMS coil that induced less focal stimulation over the prefrontal cortex than was induced in prior work. Intensity was 110% of MT for real rTMS and 20% of MT for sham stimulation. No significant changes were detected in either group after treatment. Two of 10 patients who received real rTMS, with checking compulsions, and 1 of 8 patients receiving sham treatment, with sexual/religious obsessions, were considered responders. The authors' conclusion that low-frequency rTMS of the right prefrontal cortex failed to produce significant improvement of OCD is of interest in light of another report that short-term TMS (2 days) at 1 Hz failed to affect either obsessions, compulsions, or tics in patients with Tourette's syndrome in a sham-controlled, crossover study (Munchau et al. 2002). The conclusion remains that further studies are indicated to assess the efficacy and to clarify the optimal stimulation characteristics of rTMS in OCD.

TMS IN POSTTRAUMATIC STRESS DISORDER

There is some preliminary research on therapeutic effects of TMS in posttraumatic stress disorder (PTSD). Cardinal symptoms of the illness are reexperiencing of the traumatic event(s) (such as visual flashbacks), avoidant behavior, and hyperarousal accompanied by marked anxiety. These symptoms, which by definition evolve after an extremely dangerous and frightening experience, cause significant interference in occupational and social functioning.

Recent theories of PTSD pathogenesis suggest that mechanisms involved in normal threat assessment become dysregulated so that fear responses associated with the original traumatic situation become overgeneralized and fail to extinguish (Rauch et al. 1997). This model makes the commonsense proposal that brain regions associated with fear conditioning and extinction are important in PTSD. These areas include the amygdala, involved in threat assessment, in reallocation of resources in response to threat, and in fear conditioning itself; the hippocampus, thought to encode and access contextual information; and the medial prefrontal cortex, particularly the affective division of the anterior cingulate gyrus, believed to promote fear extinction via its descending influence on the amygdala. Dysfunction in any of these regions might therefore contribute to PTSD symptomatology. Accumulating neuroimaging evidence that has provided support for this emerging conception of the neural circuitry mediating the symptoms of PTSD has been reviewed elsewhere (Pitman et al. 2001). For the purposes of this review, it is most important to note that limbic and paralimbic activation appears associated with traumatic memory–related anxiety, and prefrontal input could modulate PTSD-related subcortical activity.

The possibility that prefrontal cortex stimulation might affect regional brain activity associated with PTSD symptoms was the focus of a small pilot study in which two PTSD patients had repeated low-frequency rTMS (1 Hz, 80% of MT), delivered openly to right dorsolateral prefrontal cortex via a focal coil (McCann et al. 1998). One patient, who received 17 daily sessions of 1,200 pulses each over a 1-month period, reported selective improvement in PTSD symptoms without a change in global anxiety; the second patient, who had 1-Hz rTMS over the same region 30 times during a 6-week period, also reported significant symptom improvement. In each case the apparent beneficial effect of TMS persisted for less than 1 month after rTMS was discontinued. After rTMS, fluorodeoxyglucose-PET scans displayed a reduction in metabolism from pre-rTMS levels, which were higher than those in a reference healthy population, preferentially on the right (with the important caveat that the baseline scans were obtained months before rTMS administration in both cases). This open pilot study in PTSD patients did not exclude placebo effects, or changes in severity due to the natural course of the illness, as explanations for the observed changes in clinical state.

Another preliminary study of TMS in PTSD used a single session of even lower-frequency stimulation. Ten PTSD patients had a single session of 0.3-Hz stimulation at the maximum output of a Magstim single-pulse stimulator. A total of 30 pulses were applied bilaterally over motor cortex with a nonfocal coil (Grisaru et al. 1998). Both self and observer ratings of PTSD symptoms improved transiently, generally 1–7 days after the procedure. Low-frequency rTMS was well tolerated in this PTSD patient group. However, although there was some evidence of a therapeutic effect on PTSD symptoms, the effect was transient.

A later study by a different group (Rosenberg et al. 2002) treated 12 patients with comorbid PTSD and depression openly with rTMS over left frontal cortex as an adjunct to antidepressant medications. rTMS parameters were 90% of MT, 1 Hz or 5 Hz, 6,000 stimuli over 10 days. Whereas an antidepressant response was found in 75% of the patients (sustained 2 months later in 50% of the patients), with improvement in anxiety, hostility, and insomnia, core PTSD symptoms only improved minimally.

In a recent controlled trial (Cohen et al. 2004), 24 patients with PTSD were randomly assigned to low-frequency (1 Hz), high-frequency (10 Hz), or sham rTMS in a double-blind design. Patients had 10 daily sessions over 2 weeks. Ten daily treatments of 10-Hz rTMS (at 80% of MT) applied over the right dorsolateral prefrontal cortex had notable therapeutic effects on the core PTSD symptoms of reexperiencing and avoidance. Anxiety was also reduced after a course of rTMS applied over the right dorsolateral prefrontal cortex. These effects, obtained under controlled conditions, suggest that additional work is warranted.

CONCLUSION

This review has illustrated how TMS studies in anxiety disorders might make several specific contributions. Studies with TMS promise to improve our understanding of physiological abnormalities and neuroanatomical networks, which could mediate symptoms of this group of illnesses. Such findings may elucidate pathogenesis and provide impetus for pharmacological studies, including investigations of, for instance, possible therapeutic effects of agents that might normalize an excessive cortical excitability in OCD observed with TMS as a physiological probe.

Other kinds of TMS research might contribute to our understanding of physiological or regional correlates of factors predisposing to development of anxiety disorders. For example, using the paired-pulse TMS technique, our group measured the threshold and amplitude of MEPs to single and paired TMS in 46 healthy volunteers (23 women, 23 men) who were given the NEO Personality Inventory—Revised (NEO PI-R; Costa and McCrae 1992), a widely used measure of the five-factor model of personality. The ratio of paired-pulse conditioned to unconditioned MEP amplitude, a measure of intracortical inhibitory processing, was found to correlate with Neuroticism (N), a stable measure of trait-level anxiety and other negative emotions (Wassermann et al. 2001). This finding reflected a factor that contributed to both personality and cortical regulation. This relationship was not statistically significant in women, probably because of confounding hormonal influences on excitability that vary over the menstrual cycle (Smith et al. 1999). Decreased ICI may be related more to trait anxiety and depression, which are high in a number of neuropsychiatric disorders, including OCD. Interestingly, the MEP threshold (significantly lowered in OCD, as discussed earlier) was unrelated to Neuroticism.

Another intriguing use of TMS is to investigate brain mechanisms underlying specific emotions, including those elicited in a situationally specific manner, which is a common feature of anxiety disorders. For instance, rTMS research in healthy subjects suggests that the emotions anger and anxiety are lateralized in the prefrontal cortex. In an intriguing placebo-controlled study, 1-Hz rTMS at 130% of the individual MT applied over the right prefrontal cortex reduced the vigilant emotional response to fearful faces in eight healthy subjects. These data provide further support for the lateralization of social anxiety in the prefrontal cortex (van Honk et al. 2002a). Such approaches, used in multidisciplinary studies with complementary measures of behavior, emotional traits, and cerebral activity, promise to further advance our understanding of relationships between clinically relevant behaviors and activity in specific neural networks.

As emphasized earlier in this chapter, investigation of possible therapeutic effects of rTMS in OCD or in any anxiety disorder remains at a preliminary stage, although there have been promising initial observations in OCD. These provocative findings require systematic testing in controlled studies. Other research in progress might help guide trials of rTMS as a treatment. For example, a new development, deep brain stimulation (DBS), which targets subcortical sites for severe and extremely treatment-refractory (so-called intractable) OCD (Greenberg and Rezai 2003), may, in combination with functional neuroimaging, be particularly powerful in elucidating the relationship between activity within these networks and symptoms of illness. Moreover, it is possible that combined DBS-imaging studies could point to involvement of dorsal cortical regions that are accessible to high-frequency TMS, in contrast to orbital and medial prefrontal cortex, which for anatomical reasons will require higher TMS intensities and therefore lower frequencies to ensure that the treatment remains within safety guidelines for nonconvulsive TMS. Investigation of all of these stimulation targets in treatment trials is to be encouraged.

REFERENCES

Alonso P, Pujol J, Cardoner N, et al: Right prefrontal repetitive transcranial magnetic stimulation in obsessive-compulsive disorder: a double-blind, placebo-controlled study. Am J Psychiatry 158:1143–1145, 2001

Bartha R, Stein MB, Williamson PC, et al: A short echo 1H spectroscopy and volumetric MRI study of the corpus striatum in patients with obsessive-compulsive disorder and comparison subjects. Am J Psychiatry 155:1584–1591, 1998

Baxter LR Jr, Schwartz JM, Bergman KS, et al: Caudate glucose metabolic rate changes with both drug and behavior therapy for obsessive-compulsive disorder. Arch Gen Psychiatry 49:681–689, 1992

Baxter LR Jr, Saxena S, Brody AL, et al: Brain mediation of obsessive-compulsive disorder symptoms: evidence from functional brain imaging studies in the human and nonhuman primate. Semin Clin Neuropsychiatry 1:32–47, 1996

Cohen HZ, Kaplan Z, Kotler M, et al: Repetitive transcranial magnetic stimulation of the right dorsolateral prefrontal cortex in posttraumatic stress disorder: a double-blind, placebo-controlled study. Am J Psychiatry 161:515–524, 2004

Coric V, Milanovic S, Wasylink S, et al: Beneficial effects of the antiglutamatergic agent riluzole in a patient diagnosed with obsessive-compulsive disorder and major depressive disorder. Psychopharmacology (Berl) 167:219–220, 2003

Costa PT, McCrae RR: NEO Personality Inventory—Revised. Lutz, FL, Psychological Assessment Resources, 1992

Greenberg BD, Rezai AR: Mechanisms and state of the art of deep brain stimulation in neuropsychiatry. CNS Spectr 8:522–526, 2003

Greenberg BD, George MS, Martin JD, et al: Effect of prefrontal repetitive transcranial magnetic stimulation in obsessive-compulsive disorder: a preliminary study. Am J Psychiatry 154:867–869, 1997

Greenberg BD, Ziemann U, Harmon A, et al: Decreased neuronal inhibition in cerebral cortex in obsessive-compulsive disorder on transcranial magnetic stimulation. Lancet 352:881–882, 1998

Greenberg BD, Ziemann U, Cora-Locatelli G, et al: Altered cortical excitability in obsessive-compulsive disorder. Neurology 54:142–147, 2000

Greenberg BD, Price LH, Rauch SL, et al: Neurosurgery for intractable obsessive-compulsive disorder and depression: critical issues. Neurosurg Clin North Am 14:199–212, 2003

Grisaru N, Amir M, Cohen H, et al: Effect of transcranial magnetic stimulation in posttraumatic stress disorder: a preliminary study. Biol Psychiatry 44:52–55, 1998

Hoehn-Saric R, Greenberg BD: Psychobiology of obsessive-compulsive disorder: anatomical and physiological considerations. International Review of Psychiatry 9:15–30, 1997

Hoehn-Saric R, Schlaepfer TE, Greenberg BD, et al: Cerebral blood flow in obsessive-compulsive patients with major depression: effect of treatment with sertraline or desipramine on treatment responders and non-responders. Psychiatry Res 108:89–100, 2001

Hollander E, Bienstock CA, Koran LM, et al: Refractory obsessive-compulsive disorder: state-of-the-art treatment. J Clin Psychiatry 63 (suppl 6):20–29, 2002

Hollander E, Kaplan A, Stahl SM: A double-blind, placebo-controlled trial of clonazepam in obsessive-compulsive disorder. World J Biol Psychiatry 4:30–34, 2003

Insel TR: Toward a neuroanatomy of obsessive-compulsive disorder. Arch Gen Psychiatry 49:734–744, 1992

Lippitz BE, Mindus P, Meyerson BA, et al: Lesion topography and outcome after thermocapsulotomy or gamma knife capsulotomy for obsessive-compulsive disorder: relevance of the right hemisphere. Neurosurgery 44:452–458; discussion, 458–460, 1999

Martin JLR, Barbanoj MJ, Pérez V, et al: Transcranial magnetic stimulation for the treatment of obsessive-compulsive disorder. Cochrane Database of Systematic Reviews, Issue 2, Article No: CD003387; DOI: 10.1002/14651858.CD003387, 2003

Mataix-Cols D, Wooderson S, Lawrence N, et al: Distinct neural correlates of washing, checking, and hoarding symptom dimensions in obsessive-compulsive disorder. Arch Gen Psychiatry 61:564–576, 2004

Mega MS, Cummings JL: Frontal-subcortical circuits and neuropsychiatric disorders. J Neuropsychiatry Clin Neurosci 6:358–370, 1994

McCann UD, Kimbrell TA, Morgan CM, et al: Repetitive transcranial magnetic stimulation for posttraumatic stress disorder. Arch Gen Psychiatry 55:276–279, 1998

Modell JG, Mountz JM, Curtis GC, et al: Neurophysiologic dysfunction in basal ganglia/ limbic striatal and thalamocortical circuits as a pathogenetic mechanism of obsessive-compulsive disorder. J Neuropsychiatry Clin Neurosci 1:340–341, 1989

Munchau A, Bloem BR, Thilo KV, et al: Repetitive transcranial magnetic stimulation for Tourette syndrome. Neurology 59:1789–1791, 2002

Murray CJ, Lopez AD: Global mortality, disability, and the contribution of risk factors: Global Burden of Disease Study. Lancet 349(9063):1436–1442, 1997

Nuttin BJ, Gabriels LA, Cosyns PR, et al: Long-term electrical capsular stimulation in patients with obsessive-compulsive disorder. Neurosurgery 52:1263–1272; discussion 1272–1274, 2003

Pascual-Leone A, Grafman J, Cohen LG, et al: Transcranial magnetic stimulation: a new tool for the study of higher cognitive functions in humans, in Handbook of Neuropsychology, Vol 11. Edited by Grafman J, Boller F. Amsterdam, Elsevier, 1997, pp 267–292

Peterson BS, Skudlarski P, Anderson AW, et al: A functional magnetic resonance imaging study of tic suppression in Tourette syndrome. Arch Gen Psychiatry 55:326–333, 1998

Pitman RK, Shin LM, Rauch SL: Investigating the pathogenesis of posttraumatic stress disorder with neuroimaging. J Clin Psychiatry 62 (suppl 17):47–54, 2001

Rapoport JL: Recent advances in obsessive-compulsive disorder. Neuropsychopharmacology 5:1–10, 1991

Rauch SL: Neuroimaging and neurocircuitry models pertaining to the neurosurgical treatment of psychiatric disorders. Neurosurg Clin N Am 14:213–223, vii-viii, 2003

Rauch SL, Jenike MA, Alpert NM, et al: Regional cerebral blood flow measured during symptom provocation in obsessive-compulsive disorder using oxygen-15–labeled carbon dioxide and positron emission tomography. Arch Gen Psychiatry 51:62–70, 1994

Rauch SL, Savage CR, Alpert NM, et al: The functional neuroanatomy of anxiety: a study of three disorders using positron emission tomography and symptom provocation. Biol Psychiatry 42:446–452, 1997

Ridding MC, Sheean G, Rothwell JC, et al: Changes in the balance between motor cortical excitation and inhibition in focal, task specific dystonia. J Neurol Neurosurg Psychiatry 59:493–498, 1995

Rosenberg DR, MacMaster FP, Keshavan MS, et al: Decrease in caudate glutamatergic concentrations in pediatric obsessive-compulsive disorder patients taking paroxetine. J Am Acad Child Adolesc Psychiatry 39:1096–1103, 2000

Rosenberg PB, Mehndiratta RB, Mehndiratta YP, et al: Repetitive transcranial magnetic stimulation treatment of comorbid posttraumatic stress disorder and major depression. J Neuropsychiatry Clin Neurosci 14:270–276, 2002

Russell A, Cortese B, Lorch E, et al: Localized functional neurochemical marker abnormalities in dorsolateral prefrontal cortex in pediatric obsessive-compulsive disorder. J Child Adolesc Psychopharmacol 13 (suppl 1):S31–S38, 2002

Sachdev PS, McBride R, Loo CK, et al: Right versus left prefrontal transcranial magnetic stimulation for obsessive-compulsive disorder: a preliminary investigation. J Clin Psychiatry 62:981–984, 2001

Saxena S, Bota RG, Brody AL: Brain-behavior relationships in obsessive-compulsive disorder. Semin Clin Neuropsychiatry 6:82–101, 2001

Schwartz JM, Stoessel PW, Baxter LR Jr, et al: Systematic changes in cerebral glucose metabolic rate after successful behavior modification treatment of obsessive-compulsive disorder. Arch Gen Psychiatry 53:109–113, 1996

Smith MJ, Keel JC, Greenberg BD, et al: Menstrual cycle effects on cortical excitability. Neurology 53:2069–2072, 1999

van Honk J, Hermans EJ, d'Alfonso AA, et al: A left-prefrontal lateralized, sympathetic mechanism directs attention towards social threat in humans: evidence from repetitive transcranial magnetic stimulation. Neurosci Lett 319:99–102, 2002a

van Honk J, Schutter DJ, d'Alfonso AA, et al: One Hz rTMS over the right prefrontal cortex reduces vigilant attention to unmasked but not to masked fearful faces. Biol Psychiatry 52:312–317, 2002b

Wassermann EM, Greenberg BD, Nguyen MB, et al: Motor cortex excitability correlates with an anxiety-related personality trait. Biol Psychiatry 50:377–382, 2001

Ziemann U, Lonnecker S, Steinhoff BJ, et al: Effects of antiepileptic drugs on motor cortex excitability in humans: a transcranial magnetic stimulation study. Ann Neurol 40:367–378, 1996

Ziemann U, Paulus W, Rothenberger A: Decreased motor inhibition in Tourette's disorder: evidence from transcranial magnetic stimulation. Am J Psychiatry 154:1277–1284, 1997

8

Transcranial Magnetic Stimulation Studies of Schizophrenia

Ralph E. Hoffman, M.D.

Transcranial magnetic stimulation (TMS) offers new tools for selectively probing and altering brain function. This chapter provides a review of TMS studies involving patients with schizophrenia. These studies can be divided roughly into two classes: those that use single- or paired-pulse TMS to assess cortical inhibition, and those that explore effects of extended trains of repetitive TMS in altering symptoms.

Studies of pathophysiological mechanisms of schizophrenia have often considered cortical excitability and inhibition. This conceptual orientation is motivated by the fact

Studies described in this chapter were generously supported by the following: two Independent Investigator Awards from the National Alliance for Research on Schizophrenia and Depression; National Institute of Mental Health Grants R21 MH63326 and 1-R01 MH06707; grants from the Donaghue Medical Foundation and the Dana Foundation to Dr. Hoffman; and Program Grant RR00125 from the National Institutes of Health/National Center for Research Resources/General Clinical Research Centers.

179

that characteristic symptoms of schizophrenia such as auditory hallucinations and delusions can be viewed as "activation" or "breakthrough" symptoms—behaviors, thoughts, or perceptions that are inappropriate, intrusive, or out of place. Supporting this view are functional magnetic resonance imaging (fMRI) data showing that auditory hallucinations are accompanied by activation of a distributed network of cortical and subcortical regions involving Broca's area and bitemporal cortex (Shergill et al. 2000) and a single-photon emission computed tomography (SPECT) neuroimaging study linking excessive activation of the left temporal cortex to delusions (Puri et al. 2001). Studies of early stages of sensory processing using prepulse inhibition and evoked potentials suggest that the cerebral cortex is less able to suppress responses to inputs in patients with schizophrenia (Alder et al. 1982; Swerdlow and Koob 1987), which again suggests alterations of cortical excitability and/or inhibition.

The origin of disturbed cortical dynamics in schizophrenia remains unclear. Preliminary SPECT evidence has been reported suggesting that in vivo benzodiazepine receptor binding negatively correlates with positive symptoms in schizophrenia (Busatto et al. 1997). To the extent that these receptors correspond to a subunit of the inhibitory γ-aminobutyric acid (GABA) type A receptor (GABA$_A$) complex, these data suggest an impairment in inhibitory systems. At a microanatomic level, postmortem analysis has demonstrated reduced GABAergic chandelier axons in the cerebral cortex of patients with schizophrenia relative to normal control subjects and patients with depression (Volk et al. 2002). Because chandelier neurons comprise a major class of inhibitory interneurons, these data support the view that schizophrenia is characterized by impairments in cortical inhibition.

TMS offers a method for assessing cortical excitability and inhibition directly in the living human brain. Technical limitations at this time restrict such studies to the motor cortex. However, functional alterations of cortical dynamics in schizophrenia responsible for characteristic symptoms such as hallucinations and delusions may generalize to the motor cortex. If so, these TMS methods could prove to be very useful in characterizing underlying pathophysiological disturbances.

ASSESSMENT OF CORTICAL EXCITABILITY AND INHIBITION

Motor Threshold and Latency

The most straightforward TMS-based method for assessing cortical excitability is to determine threshold for eliciting motor activity through electromyographic recordings of peripheral muscles (referred to as *motor evoked potentials,* or MEPs) while administering single-pulse TMS to the motor cortex. Lower motor threshold (MT) can be interpreted as higher cortical excitability. Abarbanel and colleagues (1996) compared

MT and size of MEPs elicited by single-pulse TMS in 10 patients with depression, 10 patients with schizophrenia, and 10 normal subjects. For the schizophrenia group, MT was reduced, with increased amplitude of MEP following similar levels of cortical stimulation. The authors speculated that group differences may have been a medication effect, however. Time from TMS stimulation to onset of MEP was not different for the three groups. A study by Puri and colleagues (1996) found that although MTs themselves were not different in patients with schizophrenia compared with normal subjects, latency of MEPs in response to TMS was significantly shorter in the patients with schizophrenia, thus suggesting some curtailment of inhibitory mechanisms. It is worth noting that drug effects were unlikely to account for group differences in this study, since seven of nine of the patients with schizophrenia were drug-naive. A third study, by Pascual-Leone and colleagues (2002), challenged these findings. MEP response threshold and latency of seven unmedicated patients with schizophrenia were not significantly different than that of seven normal control subjects. The authors suggested that a reason for shorter latencies in the schizophrenia group reported by Puri et al. is that in their study subjects voluntarily activated target muscles, whereas in the Pascual-Leone et al. study target muscles were examined in a nonactivated state. Pascual-Leone et al. (2002) also reported abnormalities in laterality of MT in patients with schizophrenia. They found that in normal subjects there was nearly a 10% higher MT for the left hemisphere compared with the right hemisphere. However, the opposite was found to be true for both medicated and nonmedicated patients with schizophrenia. These findings were consistent with that of Daskalakis and colleagues (2002), who showed that resting MT (RMT) was significantly reduced for nonmedicated patients ($N=15$) relative to normal control subjects ($N=15$) on the left side but not on the right.

These methods may also be helpful in characterizing effects of antipsychotic medication. In the Pascual-Leone et al. (2002) study, MT of medicated patients with schizophrenia was found to be increased about 5% compared with that of unmedicated patients with this disorder. These differences were replicated by Daskalakis et al. (2002). However, another study found no differences between medicated and unmedicated patients with schizophrenia in terms of RMT (Davey et al. 1997). There were differences in methodology in this study compared with the Pascual-Leone et al. (2002) and Daskalakis et al. (2002) studies that may account for differing results. In the Davey et al. (1997) study, the stimulation coil was not positioned at the motor cortical site of maximum MEP but instead was placed on the top of the head. Second, MT in the Davey et al. study was determined during voluntary contraction of muscles.

Induced Cortical Silent Period

One approach used to characterize motor cortical inhibitory dynamics specifically entails administering TMS pulses while the subject maintains weak, voluntary tonic contractions of the target muscle. TMS produces a subsequent "silent period" whereby the corresponding MEP drops transiently to baseline levels. Reduced duration of the TMS-induced silent period is an indicator of reduced cortical inhibition. Fitzgerald and colleagues (2002b) compared duration of silent period induced by single-pulse TMS in 22 medicated patients with schizophrenia and 21 normal control subjects and found that this measure was, as predicted, reduced in the former group. This finding was replicated in a study by Daskalakis and colleagues (2002) of 15 unmedicated patients and 15 normal control subjects (Figure 8–1). Silent period duration was found to be normal in a group of medicated patients with schizophrenia in this same study (Figure 8–1), suggesting that antipsychotic drugs partially normalize abnormal cortical inhibitory processes. Along these lines, Davey and colleagues (1997) reported weaker suppression of electromyographic response in the medicated patients with schizophrenia compared with medicated patients during the early component of the silent period.

Paired-Pulse Inhibition

Paired-pulse TMS paradigms can be used to study inhibitory as well as facilitative cortical processes. In this method, an initial, conditioning subthreshold TMS pulse is followed shortly thereafter by a second suprathreshold test TMS pulse. Amplitude of MEP changes produced by the conditioning pulse can be mapped relative to the interpulse interval, which ranges from 1 to 20 milliseconds. Shorter interpulse intervals (i.e., 1–6 msec) generally produce reductions in the MEP response to the test pulse, whereas longer interpulse intervals (i.e., 10–20 msec) amplify MEP responses to the test pulse.

Applying these methods to medicated patients with schizophrenia, a reduction in paired-pulse inhibition was detected when these patients were compared with normal control subjects (Fitzgerald et al. 2002b)—a finding that was replicated by Pascual-Leone and colleagues (2002). Daskalakis and colleagues (2002) found that paired-pulse inhibition was lower in unmedicated patients relative to normal control subjects. The results from the medicated patients in their study were intermediate between and not statistically different from those of normal subjects and nonmedicated patients. When the two groups of patients were combined, total Positive and Negative Syndrome Scale scores correlated negatively with inhibition induced by paired-pulse methods (Figure 8–2). These data suggest a possible causal or permissive role of curtailed inhibitory processes in the genesis of symptoms of schizophrenia. Pascual-Leone and colleagues (2002) also reported enhanced cortical facilitation in medicated patients relative to nonmedicated patients and normal control subjects when paired-pulse effects were studied at 12 msec and 20 msec. In contrast, no group differences for facilitation were reported by Daskalakis and colleagues (2002).

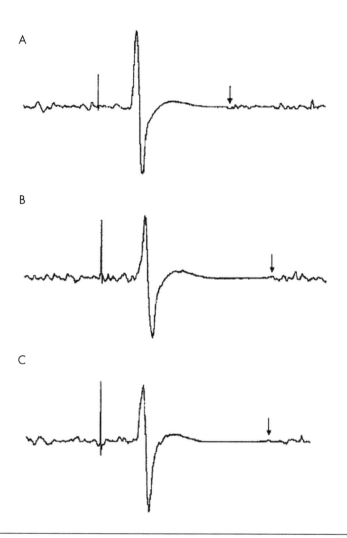

Figure 8-1. Electromyographic recordings from the tonically active first dorsal interosseus muscle following 40% suprathreshold transcranial magnetic stimulation.

(A) reflects patient with schizophrenia who is not receiving medication. (B) reflects a patient with schizophrenia who is receiving medication; and (C) reflects healthy control subjects. Each waveform represents the average of 15 trials. The silent period starts at the onset of the motor evoked potential and ends with the return of motor activity marked by the arrow.

Source. Reprinted from Daskalakis ZJ, Christensen BK, Chen R, et al.: "Evidence for Impaired Cortical Inhibition in Schizophrenia Using Transcranial Magnetic Stimulation." *Archives of General Psychiatry* 59:347–354, 2002, p. 351. Copyright 2002, American Medical Association. All rights reserved. Used with permission.

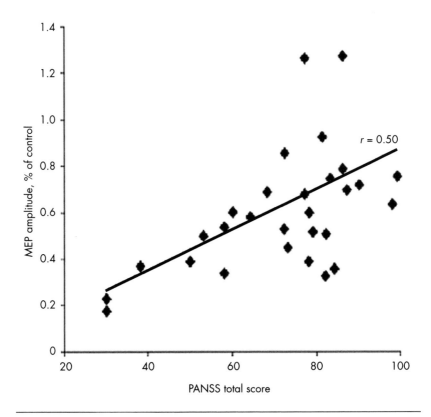

Figure 8–2. Relationship between between Positive and Negative Syndrome Scale (PANSS) total score and cortical inhibition in 30 patients with schizophrenia.

MEP = motor evoked potential elicited by test pulses using the paired-pulse paradigm.

Source. Reprinted from Daskalakis ZJ, Christensen BK, Chen R, et al.: "Evidence for Impaired Cortical Inhibition in Schizophrenia Using Transcranial Magnetic Stimulation." *Archives of General Psychiatry* 59:347–354, 2002, p. 351. Copyright 2002, American Medical Association. All rights reserved. Used with permission.

Transcallosal Inhibition

Finally, inhibitory effects mediated by cross-callosal projections can also be studied via TMS. Along these lines, TMS of the motor cortex has been shown to inhibit tonic electromyographic activity in ipsilateral muscle groups—presumably via momentary inhibition of the contralateral motor cortex. Boroojerdi and colleagues (1999) reported the first use of this approach in patients with schizophrenia. The delay between transcallosal stimulation and inhibition of electromyographic response was significantly longer in 10 medicated patients with schizophrenia compared with 10 age- and gender-matched normal control subjects. Moreover, the duration of inhibition produced by transcallosal TMS was *increased* in the former group. The latter finding is of special interest insofar as the direction of the abnormality is opposite to the silent period effects of TMS effects observed in patients with schizophrenia cited above. A later study of transcallosal inhibition by Fitzgerald and colleagues (2002a) included a larger number of subjects (25 medicated patients with schizophrenia and 20 control subjects). The patient group again demonstrated longer transcallosal suppression of motor contractions compared with normal subjects, although no change in the latency of effect was observed. Obviously medication effects need to be considered in understanding these group differences. Along those lines, the Fitzgerald et al. (2002a) study reported relatively a robust positive correlation ($r=0.64$) between dose of olanzapine given and duration of transcallosal inhibition.

Another approach to studying transcallosal cortical inhibition used a dual-pulse method in which TMS pulses are administered to both motor cortices. In this approach, subthreshold TMS given as a conditioning pulse to motor cortex inhibits the MEP of a second suprathreshold TMS pulse administered to the opposite hemisphere. Using this approach, Fitzgerald and colleagues (2000a) compared a normal control group ($n=16$) and a group of patients with schizophrenia (medicated, $n=23$) and found that the latter demonstrated reduced effects of the TMS conditioning pulse—a finding consistent with studies using same-side dual-pulse methods in schizophrenia. Also using the dual-pulse method, Daskalakis and colleagues (2002) found reduced transcallosal inhibition in unmedicated patients compared with control subjects—a finding that was absent for their group of medicated patients.

Summary

In summary, these studies suggest that schizophrenia is associated with reduced cortical inhibition in the motor cortex, although findings are not always replicated clearly across studies. Motor threshold appears to demonstrate enhanced cortical excitability in schizophrenia, especially on the left side. Studies demonstrating a reduced silent period in patients with schizophrenia suggest reduced cortical inhibition may be reversible by antipsychotic drugs. However, drug effects may be complex, since one study found that antipsychotic medication produced less early inhibition of MEPs (Davey et al. 1997), and another study (Fitzgerald et al. 2000a) suggested that antipsychotic drugs extend the duration of transcallosal inhibition induced by TMS. Perhaps a better way to conceptualize the effects of antipsychotic drugs per these paradigms is that intrinsic cortical inhibition is rendered more diffuse or less focused. In terms of paired-pulse methods, the Daskalakis et al. (2002) study is the most revealing, since the subject groups in that study were relatively large and both medicated and nonmedicated patients were studied. Daskalakis et al.'s data again suggest that schizophrenia is associated with reduced cortical inhibition that is reversed in part by antipsychotic drugs.

All of the studies reviewed above examined effects of TMS delivered to the motor cortex. The excitatory and inhibitory dynamics of motor cortex in response to TMS may, however, be distinct from those of other cortical areas. It is possible, however, that future TMS studies using measures other than MEPs will be able to accurately assess facilitative and inhibitory processes in non-motor cortical areas. Along these lines, Bohning and colleagues (1999) have demonstrated the capacity to interleave 1-Hz rTMS with data acquisition time intervals during fMRI scanning. Nahas and colleagues (2001) applied this methodology to the study of rTMS effects in prefrontal cortex in normal subjects. They reported dose-related responses to rTMS both directly underneath the coil and in the contralateral prefrontal region. It should be possible to use paired-pulse methods in combination with functional neuroimaging to study, for instance, prefrontal inhibitory and excitability dynamics in patients with schizophrenia relative to other subject groups.

STUDIES USING REPETITIVE TRAINS OF TMS IN SCHIZOPHRENIA

In the remainder of this chapter, studies are considered that use repetitive TMS (rTMS) in attempts to alter cortical dynamics in patients with schizophrenia. The first such study was reported by Geller and colleagues (1997). Ten patients with schizophrenia and 10 patients with depression were studied to determine if mood changes could be induced and whether different effects could be obtained in different patient groups. Very-low-frequency (once per 30 seconds) rTMS was administered on each side of the brain, 15 pulses each. Two of 10 patients with schizophrenia appeared to improve, at least transiently. Feinsod and colleagues (1998) reported a nonblind study in which 7 of 10 patients with schizophrenia experienced decreased anxiety and restlessness in response to low-frequency frontal rTMS. On the other hand, a later double-blind study examining the effects of low-frequency rTMS delivered to right prefrontal cortex did not find any improvement following active stimulation relative to sham stimulation (Klein et al. 1999a). This study was prompted by an earlier study demonstrating antidepressant effects using low-frequency rTMS delivered to right prefrontal cortex in patients with major depression (Klein et al. 1999b).

The first study examining effects of higher-frequency rTMS delivered to prefrontal cortex in patients with schizophrenia was reported by Cohen and colleagues (1999). rTMS at 20 Hz was given daily to patients in open-label fashion to left prefrontal cortex in 2-second trains once per minute for 20 minutes for 10 days. Patients had chronic schizophrenia with predominantly negative symptoms. Five of six patients had hypofrontality as determined by a SPECT scan. The results after rTMS indicated no change in hypofrontality. However, negative symptoms showed a general decrease ($P<0.02$). A trend toward improvement in neuropsychological test performance was also noted, although only performance in a delayed visual memory task achieved statistical significance ($P<0.05$).

Rollnik and colleagues (2000) examined, in a double-blind, crossover design, the effects of higher-frequency rTMS delivered to left prefrontal cortex in 12 schizophrenia patients with negative symptoms. This approach was motivated by studies suggesting that higher-frequency rTMS has an activating influence on cortical function (Post et al. 1997), and other studies demonstrating hypofrontality in schizophrenia (Schroder et al. 1996; Weinberger and Berman 1996; Wolkin et al. 1992). In Rollnik et al.'s study, rTMS was delivered to left dorsolateral prefrontal cortex each day for 2 weeks. Each stimulation session consisted of twenty 2-second pulse trains at 20 Hz and 80% of MT. The Brief Psychiatric Rating Scale score decreased following active rTMS ($P<0.05$) compared with sham stimulation, whereas depressive and anxiety symptoms did not change significantly. Interestingly, symptom changes detected in this trial did not appear to reflect predominantly negative symptoms.

Another study investigated effects of 10-Hz rTMS administered to left prefrontal cortex (Yu et al. 2002). The main goal was to determine effects on P300 abnormalities and elevated prolactin levels induced by antipsychotic drugs. Partially normalization of each of these abnormalities was detected, although only five patients were studied. Given that elevated prolactin levels were likely due to dopamine blockade, partial normalization of prolactin suggests that a mechanism of action of prefrontal rTMS in the higher-frequency range is enhanced dopaminergic function. This view is consistent with another recent TMS study in healthy humans in which high-frequency rTMS delivered to prefrontal cortex was shown to increase dopamine release as detected with 11C-labeled raclopride positron-emission tomography (PET) (Strafella et al. 2001). It has been argued that reductions in dopamine delivered to prefrontal areas may be the cause of negative symptoms (Weinberger 1987).

In addition, our group has used rTMS to as an investigational intervention for auditory hallucinations. Auditory hallucinations are a common symptom in schizophrenia, occurring in 60%–70% of cases and often producing severe distress, disability, and behavioral control. In about 25% of patients, auditory hallucinations respond poorly or not at all to currently available antipsychotic medication (Shergill et al. 1999). One important feature of auditory hallucinations is that they generally are experienced as spoken speech with discernible loudness, timbre, and other "percept-like" features. These characteristics suggest direct involvement of speech perception neurocircuitry. Support for this view derived from the observation that patients with auditory hallucinations, compared with healthy control subjects, are more likely to experience perceptual illusions of words or word phrases when listening to acoustic noise (Alpert 1985; Bentall and Slade 1985). These early findings suggest excessive sensitivity or reactivity of speech perception systems.

Neuroimaging studies suggest activation of brain areas during auditory hallucinations that are ordinarily active during speech perception. For instance, an fMRI study of three patients demonstrated activation in Heschl's gyrus during auditory hallucinations (Dierks et al. 1999). Heschl's gyrus is in the anterior superior temporal cortex and comprises a primary auditory processing primary acoustic processing part of the brain. Other neuroimaging studies have detected activation in temporoparietal cortex during auditory hallucinations (Lennox et al. 2000; Silbersweig et al. 1995). This brain region is adjacent to Wernicke's area and is also active during speech perception (Benson et al. 2001).

Multiple studies have suggested that 1-Hz extended-duration (~15 minute) rTMS produces sustained reductions in activation in the brain area directly stimulated (Chen et al. 1997) as well as in other brain areas functionally connected to the former (Wassermann et al. 1997). We consequently predicted that 1-Hz rTMS delivered to areas of the brain dedicated to speech perception might reduce auditory hallucinations (Hoffman et al. 1999, 2000). We targeted left temporoparietal cortex because of the findings from the neuroimaging studies cited earlier and because this area is readily accessible to scalp stimulation (Figure 8–3). We initially reported a study of 12 right-handed schizophrenic patients with medication-resistant auditory hallucinations, in which we compared effects of 1-Hz active rTMS to sham stimulation, using a double-blind crossover design. Stimulation was administered at 80% of MT. Sham stimulation was administered to the same location with the coil tilted 45 degrees off the scalp using the "two-wing" method (i.e., with both "wings" of the coil touching the scalp). Because this was the first time that rTMS was administered in this brain area, we were very cautious regarding patient safety/tolerability. The first day the patient received 4 minutes of stimulation, and the stimulation duration was then increased by 4-minute increments to 16 minutes on the final, fourth day. Hallucination severity was rated by using a Hallucination Change Score that was anchored to the patient's own narrative description of his hallucinations at baseline. This level of severity was assigned a score of 10. Subsequent assessments in which no hallucinations occurred within the prior 24 hours were assigned a 0, and assessments in which hallucinations were twice as severe were assigned a score of 20.

When we compared endpoint data, statistically significant improvements in auditory hallucinations were detected for active rTMS relative to sham stimulation ($P<0.01$). Therapeutic effects were brief, generally lasting less than 1 week. Concomitant anticonvulsant medication was found to curtail the symptom-reducing

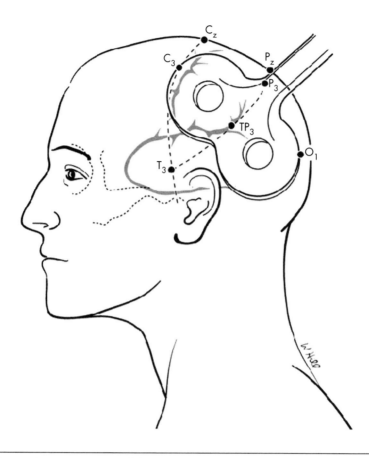

Figure 8-3. Location of the stimulation for Hoffman and colleagues' initial repetitive transcranial magnetic stimulation (rTMS) trials for auditory hallucinations.

TP_3 was defined as being midway between T_3 and P_3 according to the 10–20 International electroencephalographic electrode deployment system. This region falls near the posterior border of Wernicke's area and overlies the supramarginal gyrus in most cases. C_3 is the site used to elicit motor thresholds.

Source. Reprinted from Hoffman RE, Hawkins KA, Gueorguieva R, et al.: "Transcranial Magnetic Stimulation of Left Temporoparietal Cortex and Medication-Resistant Auditory Hallucinations." *Archives of General Psychiatry* 60:49–56, 2003, p. 51. Copyright 2003, American Medical Association. All rights reserved. Used with permission.

effects of rTMS—an effect that was highly statistically significant. Because anticonvulsant drugs limit transsynaptic propagation of cortical activation (Applegate et al. 1997), these data suggest that putative therapeutic effects of rTMS require propagation of activation. Other positive symptoms of schizophrenia were relatively unchanged by rTMS in this protocol, suggesting that rTMS effects were relatively selective and specifically related to pathophysiology producing auditory hallucinations.

We consequently sought to determine if a more extended trial of rTMS administered to left temporoparietal cortex could produce more clinically significant, sustained reductions in auditory hallucinations. A sample of 50 patients was studied (Hoffman et al. 2003, 2005). All enrolled patients met DSM-IV criteria for schizophrenia or schizoaffective disorder on the basis of the Structured Clinical Interview for DSM-IV, and reported experiencing auditory hallucinations at least five times per day. Forty-two of the patients met criteria for medication resistance, defined as daily auditory hallucinations persisting in spite of at least two adequate trials of antipsychotic medications that included at least one atypical antipsychotic medication. Ages ranged from 19 to 58 years. Exclusion criteria were the same as in our earlier protocol (Hoffman et al. 2000). Patients were randomly allocated to either active rTMS ($n = 27$) or sham stimulation ($n = 23$). There were no statistically significant differences in age, gender, number of prior hospitalizations, duration of current hallucination episode (defined as the number of months since the patient last had a remission of auditory hallucinations of 4 weeks or greater), number of patients with medication-resistant auditory hallucinations, or prior treatment with electroconvulsive therapy. Length of time of unremitting auditory hallucinations was extended, with a mean of approximately 10 years in each group. No change in dose of antipsychotic or thymoleptic medication was made for 4 weeks prior to trial entry and during the trial itself. Study participants, clinical raters, and all personnel responsible for the clinical care of the participants remained blind to allocated condition. As in our first study, 1-Hz stimulation was again administered halfway between T_3 and P_3 (referred to hereafter as TP_3) on the basis of the International 10–20 electroencephalographic (EEG) system, but with a modestly higher field strength (90% of MT vs. the 80% of MT that was used in our first study). Patients in this trial received 8 minutes of stimulation on day 1, 12 minutes of stimulation on day 2, and 16 minutes of stimulation for the next 7 days (excluding weekends), for a total of 132 minutes of stimulation, compared with 40 minutes in the first trial. Sham stimulation was administered at the same location, strength, and frequency, with the coil angled 45 degrees away from the skull in a "single-wing" tilt position. A neuropsychological battery was administered at baseline and at the end of each leg of the trial. Patients were assessed at baseline and after three active rTMS/sham stimulation sessions on the basis of the Hallucination Change Score described earlier and the Auditory Hallucinations Rating Scale (AHRS) developed by our group (Hoffman et al. 2003), which assesses seven phenomenological components: hallucination frequency, loudness, "realness," number of speaking voices, typical length of individual hallucinations, degree that the patient could ignore hallucinations, and level of distress produced. These assessments were conducted after every third stimulation session, as were the Positive and Negative Syndrome Scale (PANSS) and two neuropsychological screening tasks: the Hopkins Verbal Memory Task (Benedict et al. 1998) and the Letter-Number Working Memory task (Gold et al. 1997). The Clinical Global Impression scale (CGI) was scored after each leg of the trial. A full neuropsychological test battery was administered at baseline and after each leg of the trial.

In terms of safety and tolerability, only headache (transient and responsive to acetaminophen) and light-headedness (generally lasting less than a half hour) were expressed at a higher frequency for patients receiving active rTMS versus sham stimulation. Concentration complaints during active rTMS were no more frequent than for sham stimulation. Two patients in the open-label active group reported mild memory impairment. The research team later learned that one of these patients had just begun talking benztropine prescribed by his outpatient psychiatrist, which could account for these memory difficulties. This patient's memory complaints lasted 3–4 days and improved when the benztropine was discontinued. Memory complaints for the second case were only for 1 day. There were four dropouts. One patient from the active trial and one patient from the sham trial were removed because of drops in the Hopkins Verbal Learning Task beyond our "stop" criteria. For the patient in the active trial, retesting demonstrated a return to baseline functioning. For the sham patient, worsening neuropsychological test performance was accompanied by worsening auditory hallucinations, which may have produced these difficulties. One patient enrolled in the sham phase was removed from the study by his clinical psychiatrist because of worsening psychotic symptoms. One patient dropped out after one session of active rTMS because he complained that his "head felt weird." Changes in performance for the full neuropsychological battery did not reveal any noticeable trends toward declining function for patients following the double-masked active trial or differences in change scores comparing patients randomized to active versus sham stimulation.

In terms of clinical outcomes, the Hallucination Change Score, our primary outcome measure, was significantly lower for active compared with sham groups for the day 7 assessment ($t_{44}=2.53$, $P<0.015$) and the final (day 10) assessment ($t_{43}=2.70$, $P<0.01$). The Hallucination Change Score dependence over time was characterized by using a random-time model. The time effect ($F_{1,41.4}=39.43$, $P<0.0001$) and the interaction between treatment and time ($F_{1,41.4}=7.88$, $P<0.0076$) were significant. The active group demonstrated a significant linear decrease in the hallucination change scores over time ($t_{24.6}=-7.87$, $P<0.001$) as did sham group ($t_{22.6}=-2.13$, $P=0.0446$). Patients were classified as responders if hallucination severity was reduced by at least 50%. Using this criterion, we found that 14 of 27 patients (51.9%) achieved responder status in the active group, compared with 4 of 23 (17.4%) in the sham group ($\chi^2=6.4$, $P=0.01$). For CGI scores, the mean ($\pm$SD) of 2.84 ± 0.85 for the active group was reduced relative to the sham group (mean$\pm$SD$=3.80\pm.88$, $t_{46}=-3.80$, $P=0.0004$). Anticonvulsant drug treatment was not statistically associated with clinical outcome.

The one AHRS variable that demonstrated significant treatment effects was frequency. The change of hallucination frequency over time was modeled by a random-intercept, random-time model. There was a significant time effect ($F_{1,46.7} = 17.96$, $P = 0.0001$) and a significant interaction between time and treatment ($F_{1,46.7} = 11.47$, $P = 0.0014$; see Figure 8–4). The active group demonstrated a significant linear decrease in the frequency of hallucinations over time ($t_{25.9} = -5.09$, $P < 0.0001$, whereas the sham group did not show a significant linear decrease ($t_{20.7} = -0.64$, $P = 0.53$). A composite variable was created as the sum of the seven AHRS variables. There was a significant time effect ($F_{1,47.2} = 20.04$, $P = 0.0001$) and a borderline significant interaction between time and treatment ($F_{1,47.2} = 3.91$, $P = 0.054$). The active group demonstrated a significant linear decrease over time ($t_{25.2} = 3.81$, $P = 0.0008$), while the sham group showed a significant but smaller linear decrease over time ($t_{11.9} = 2.35$, $P = 0.020$).

Baseline AHRS phenomenological characteristics were assessed to determine if any variable appeared to be a moderator of rTMS effects as defined by Kraemer and colleagues (2002). One variable—hallucination frequency—had a significant interaction with treatment type (sham vs. active; $F_{1,41} = 7.70$, $P = 0.008$) and therefore qualifies as a candidate moderator of rTMS efficacy. Moderator effects were optimized if hallucinators were dichotomized into high- and low-frequency hallucinations on the basis of whether auditory hallucinations occurred on average greater than once every 10 minutes or not. Those patients with more frequent auditory hallucinations demonstrated a greater differential effect when compared with patients receiving sham stimulation, whereas patients with lower hallucination frequency demonstrated less robust differences between active and sham rTMS.

Other variables emerged as "nonspecific predictors," defined as variables demonstrating statistically significant correlations with endpoint auditory Hallucination Change Scores but nonsignificant statistical interactions between these variables and group allocation. These variables included the number of acoustically distinct voices heard at baseline ($r = 0.50$ between this variable and endpoint Hallucination Change Score), California Verbal Learning Test (Elwood 1995) short-term recall ($r = 0.47$) and CVLT long-term recall ($r = 0.35$). The former suggests that greater number of speaking voices comprising auditory hallucinations reflects pathophysiology that is harder to reverse by rTMS. CVLT findings are of interest given that verbal memory is known to rely on left temporoparietal cortex (Fiez et al. 1996; Ojemann 1978), thus suggesting that greater pathophysiological involvement of this cortical area produces greater resistance to rTMS.

Clinical trials using rTMS for auditory hallucinations have now been reported by other groups. d'Alfonso and colleagues (2002), using a rTMS protocol applied in a nonblind fashion, reported consistent results. Eight patients with persistent auditory hallucinations were given a trial of 1-Hz rTMS with stimulation at 80% of MT and duration at 20 minutes of stimulation per day for 10 days. Statistically

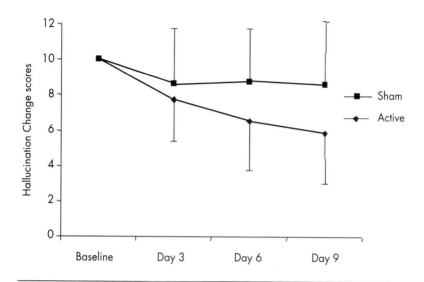

Figure 8–4. Hallucination Change scores across the four assessment periods of the double-blind phase of the study by Hoffman et al. (2005).

Error bars are standard deviations. Data at each time point reflect last observation carried forward.

Source. Reprinted from *Biological Psychiatry*, Volume 58, Hoffman et al., "Temporoparietal Transcranial Magnetic Stimulation for Auditory Hallucinations: Safety, Efficacy and Moderators in a Fifty Patient Sample," p. 100, copyright 2005, with permission from the Society of Biological Psychiatry.

significant improvements in auditory hallucinations were detected relative to baseline, but the improvements were modest. Reduced response may reflect at least three factors. First, one of the eight patients was left-handed and therefore had a 50-50 chance of being right-hemisphere dominant, which could have reduced the effects of rTMS administered to the left hemisphere. Second, another patient required a reduction in stimulation from 80% to 50% due to pain at the site of stimulation, which also may have reduced rTMS effects. Third, stimulation in this study was not administered to left temporoparietal cortex but instead to a more anterior left temporal region 2 cm above T_3 per the International 10–20 EEG electrode placement system. Given that T_3 often falls on the superior temporal gyrus (Homan et al. 1987), it is possible that a 2-cm displacement in a superior direction may have moved the stimulation coil off the temporal lobe to a sensorimotor cortex in some cases.

Poulet and colleagues (2005) described 10 dextral patients with schizophrenia and auditory hallucinations who were randomly assigned to receive 5 days of active versus sham rTMS delivered to TP_3 at 90% of MT in a crossover design. Each week of stimulation was separated by a 1-week washout period. The design was unique insofar as a total of 2,000 pulses were administered each day in two separate sessions (1,000 pulses each). Thus, the daily dose of rTMS given was roughly twice that of our later clinical trial (Hoffman et al. 2005). Improvements at least as robust as those reported in that study were observed after 5 days; mean improvement of total AHRS scores was on average 56%, with no improvement detected following the sham phase of the trial. Nonresponders were treated with medication with anticonvulsant properties, whereas responders were not—a finding that confirmed a prediction based on our earlier report (Hoffman et al. 2000). Also of interest is that this group later reported data for 14 patients receiving active rTMS and 10 patients receiving sham rTMS in a 5-day protocol of 2,000 pulses each day (Brunelin et al. 2006). Robust improvements in total AHRS scores were detected following active rTMS but not following sham rTMS. Moreover, source monitoring capacity—ability to recall the source of a list of words—was studied. This list included words previously read by the patient and words not previously seen. Source monitoring defects elicited by this task have been postulated to produce or contribute to the genesis of auditory hallucinations (Keefe et al. 1999). Source monitoring performance improved following active rTMS but not sham rTMS. Reductions in AHRS scores correlated with source monitoring improvement at a trend level ($r=0.37$, $P=0.06$).

Lee and colleagues (2005) randomly allocated 39 patients with treatment-resistant auditory hallucinations to three groups: active rTMS to the TP_3, active rTMS to the right homologous region (TP_4), and sham stimulation. Symptoms were evaluated with the AHRS, PANSS, and CGI. Active rTMS delivered both to left and to right temporoparietal sites produced greater overall symptomatic improvements per CGI scores relative to sham stimulation ($P=0.004$ and $P=0.002$, respectively). However, summed AHRS scores did not show significantly greater improvements for either active site versus sham stimulation. Right-sided rTMS did show reductions in the attentional salience subscale of the AHRS relative to sham stimulation at a trend level ($P=0.07$).

Chibbaro and colleagues (2005) studied 16 patients with schizophrenia and auditory hallucinations. rTMS at 1 Hz was administered at 90% of MT during four sessions on successive days. The duration of each stimulation session was 15 minutes. Half the patients received active rTMS, and half received sham stimulation. Both patient groups demonstrated a significant reduction in auditory hallucinations as well as in other positive symptoms at the end of the first week. However, at later time points up to and including 8 weeks following the trial, improvements in the sham group disappeared, whereas improvement was retained for patients receiving active rTMS.

There have also been two studies with negative findings for rTMS applied to the TP_3 temporoparietal site. The first, reported by McIntosh and colleagues

(2004), used the lower-dosed 4-day protocol that we previously described (Hoffman et al. 2000) and found no significant improvement in auditory hallucinations for active rTMS versus sham stimulation. Of note is that the stimulation was halted every minute for 15 seconds, which may have disrupted physiological effects of rTMS. The second study, reported by Fitzgerald et al. (2005), studied 33 patients with treatment-resistant auditory hallucinations. rTMS was applied for 10 sessions for 15 minutes at 1 Hz and 90% of MT. Active treatment did not result in a greater therapeutic effect than sham on any measure except for the loudness of hallucinations, in which there was a significant reduction in the active versus the sham group over time.

The positioning of the rTMS coil for such trials is likely to be an important parameter. Its importance is underscored by the fact that the anatomic distribution of language functions can vary considerably across individuals (Ojemann 1991). We consequently initiated an rTMS trial in which the location of magnetic stimulation was determined by topographic location of patient-specific fMRI maps of abnormally functioning cortical neurocircuitry. In the first three cases, activation maps of hallucination periods were generated by having patients depress a button during scanning for the duration of individual episodes of hallucinations. Significance maps of correlations of hallucination periods signaled by this method and voxel-specific blood oxygen level–dependent (BOLD) activation were generated, with correction for the likely hemodynamic delay of BOLD signal relative to actual brain activation. An alternative method for mapping functionally engaged neurocircuitry was developed for three additional patients whose hallucinations were constant during wakefulness. In these cases, there were no nonhallucination periods during fMRI scanning that could be used as a comparison condition to delineate hallucination-specific activation. Studies have indicated that BOLD correlation maps such as these delineate functional connectivity between cortical regions (Arfanakis et al. 2000; Cordes et al. 2000; Hampson et al. 2002; Lowe et al. 1998, 2000; Xiong et al. 1999). Our assumption is that auditory hallucinations incorporate Wernicke's region but also involve other brain regions that are functionally connected to Wernicke's region. For patients with constant hallucinations, correlation maps relative to Wernicke's area were therefore generated for BOLD signal fluctuations during scanning periods. For these six patients, a BrainLAB frameless stereotactic system (BrainLAB AG, Munich, Germany) was used to identify scalp locations corresponding to underlying regions of interest. rTMS was administered to three regions identified by fMRI maps plus a sham stimulation region based on these data. Each site received 3 days of 1-Hz stimulation of 16 minutes' duration each at 90% of MT. An additional 3 days of stimulation was given at the site, and this demonstrated the greatest reduction in hallucinations. Four of 6 patients demonstrated a clinically significantly improvement using this fMRI-guided protocol.

One other research group has attempted to position rTMS for patients with auditory hallucinations by using stereotactic methods. Brain areas showing apparent activation during inner speech based on either fMRI maps or structural MRI were targeted. Active stimulation was applied over Broca's area and over the superior temporal gyrus corresponding to the primary auditory cortex (Brodmann areas 22/42). rTMS did not lead to a significant reduction of hallucination severity for the patients overall. However, for the four patients for whom rTMS positioning was based on individualized fMRI maps, improvements following rTMS to the superior temporal site approached significance compared to sham stimulation ($P=0.06$)

In summary, although the number of studies using rTMS as a potential clinical intervention for schizophrenia is small, these studies show promise in terms of advancing our understanding of pathophysiological mechanisms. Higher-frequency rTMS studies in schizophrenia focusing on the prefrontal cortex could provide important insights regarding the pathophysiology of hypofrontality and possible linkages to subcortical dopamine dysregulation.

Low-frequency rTMS targeting speech processing areas has been studied more extensively, with many but not all studies showing greater efficacy for active rTMS compared with sham stimulation. Factors that may moderate rTMS response include concomitant anticonvulsant drug therapy, differing dosages of rTMS (i.e., stimulation strength, total number of pulses per day, and number of days of stimulation), and possibly position of the stimulation coil. These data provide evidence that speech perception neurocircuitry participates in the generation of auditory hallucinations and suggest a potential alternative clinical intervention for this syndrome. Future clinical trials are likely to benefit from strategies using individualized neuroimaging to position rTMS. Clinical utility of this intervention may be enhanced by identification of specific predictors of response that identify individuals who are especially likely to benefit.

Finally, it is worth noting that single- and paired-pulse rTMS methodologies and related methodologies for discerning cortical inhibition impairments—if they could be applied to areas other than motor cortex—could direct and refine repetitive TMS trials in clinical populations. As noted earlier, Nahas and colleagues (2001) have shown that fMRI scanning can be interleaved with rTMS so that BOLD signals can be used to map regional activation of rTMS elicited during scanning itself. It may be possible to use such methods in combination with paired-pulse methodologies, in which a subthreshold TMS pulse is followed by a second pulse that produces detectable activation on fMRI scanning. A control condition could consist of suprathreshold pulses delivered in the absence of a conditioning subthreshold pulse. By comparing conditions across trials, it may be possible to delineate reductions in BOLD signal activation due to subthreshold conditioning pulse. These methods could then be used to delineate temporal or frontal regions in patients with schizophrenia exhibiting especially egregious impairments in cortical inhibition that could then be targeted with suppressive 1-Hz rTMS. Alternatively, areas of excessively inhibited cortical regions could be challenged with activating, high-frequency rTMS. Multifaceted research of this sort has not yet been executed, but each of the steps has already been worked out conceptually and methodologically. In the mean time, TMS has already provided a range of interesting and illuminating findings in patients with schizophrenia.

REFERENCES

Abarbanel JM, Lembert T, Yaroslavski U, et al: Electrophysiological responses to transcranial magnetic stimulation in depression and schizophrenia. Biol Psychiatry 40:148–150, 1996

Alder LE, Pachtman E, Franks RD, et al: Neurophysiological evidence for a defect in neural mechanisms involved in sensory gating in schizophrenia. Biol Psychiatry 17:639–654, 1982

Alpert M: The signs and symptoms of schizophrenia. Compr Psychiatry 26:103–112, 1985

Applegate CD, Samoriski GM, Ozduman K: Effects of valproate, phenytoin, and MK-801 in a novel model of epileptogenesis. Epilepsia 38:631–636, 1997

Arfanakis K, Cordes D, Haughton VM, et al: Combining independent component analysis and correlation analysis to probe interregional connectivity in fMRI task activation datasets. Magn Reson Imaging 18:921–930, 2000

Benedict RHB, Schretlen D, Groninger L, et al: Hopkins Verbal Learning Test—Revised: normative data and analysis of inter-form and test-retest reliability. Clin Neuropsychol 12:43–55, 1998

Benson RR, Whalen DH, Richardson M, et al: Parametrically dissociating speech and non-speech perception in the brain using fMRI. Brain Language 78:364–396, 2001

Bentall RP, Slade PD: Reality testing and auditory hallucinations. Br J Clin Psychol 24:159–169, 1985

Bohning DE, Shastri A, McConnell KA, et al: A combined TMS/fMRI study of intensity-dependent TMS over motor cortex. Biol Psychiatry 45:385–394, 1999

Boroojerdi B, Topper R, Foltys H, et al: Transcallosal inhibition and motor conduction studies in patients with schizophrenia using transcranial magnetic stimulation. Br J Psychiatry 175:375–379, 1999

Brunelin J, Poulet E, Bediou B, et al: Low frequency repetitive transcranial magnetic stimulation improves source monitoring deficit in hallucinating patients with schizophrenia. Schizophr Res 81:41–45, 2006

Busatto GF. Pilowsky LS. Costa DC, et al: Correlation between reduced in vivo benzodiazepine receptor binding and severity of psychotic symptoms in schizophrenia. Am J Psychiatry 154:56–63, 1997

Chen R, Classen J, Gerloff C, et al: Depression of motor cortex excitability by low-frequency transcranial magnetic stimulation. Neurology 48:1398–1403, 1997

Chibbaro G, Daniele M, Alagona G, et al: Repetitive transcranial magnetic stimulation in schizophrenic patients reporting auditory hallucinations. Neurosci Lett 383(1–2):54–57, 2005

Cohen E, Bernardo M, Masana J, et al: Repetitive transcranial magnetic stimulation in the treatment of chronic negative schizophrenia: a pilot study (letter). J Neurol Neurosurg Psychiatry 67:129–130, 1999

Cordes D, Haughton VM, Arfanakis K, et al: Mapping functionally related regions of brain with functional connectivity MR imaging. AJNR Am J Neuroradiol 21:1636–1644, 2000

Curra A, Modugno N, Inghilleri M, et al: Transcranial magnetic stimulation techniques in clinical investigation. Neurology 59:1851–1819, 2002

d'Alfonso AA, Aleman A, Kessels RP, et al: Transcranial magnetic stimulation of left auditory cortex in patients with schizophrenia: effects on hallucinations and neurocognition. J Neuropsychiatry Clin Neurosci 14:77–79, 2002

Daskalakis ZJ, Christensen BK, Chen R, et al: Evidence for impaired cortical inhibition in schizophrenia using transcranial magnetic stimulation. Arch Gen Psychiatry 59:347–354, 2002

Davey NJ, Puri BK, Lewis HS, et al: Effects of antipsychotic medication on electromyographic responses to transcranial magnetic stimulation of the motor cortex in schizophrenia. J Neurol Neurosurg Psychiatry 63:468–473, 1997

Dierks T, Linden DE, Jandl M, et al: Activation of Heschl's gyrus during auditory hallucinations. Neuron 22:615–621, 1999

Elwood RW: The California Verbal Learning Test: psychometric characteristics and clinical application. Neuropsychol Rev 5:173–201, 1995

Feinsod M, Kreinin B, Chistyakov A, et al: Preliminary evidence for a beneficial effect of low-frequency, repetitive transcranial magnetic stimulation in patients with major depression and schizophrenia. Depress Anxiety 7:65–68, 1998

Fiez JA, Raichle ME, Balota DA, et al: PET activation of posterior temporal regions during auditory word presentation and verb generation. Cereb Cortex 6:1–10, 1996

Fitzgerald PB, Brown TL, Daskalakis ZJ, et al: A study of transcallosal inhibition in schizophrenia using transcranial magnetic stimulation. Schizophr Res 56:199–209, 2002a

Fitzgerald PB, Brown TL, Daskalakis ZJ, et al: A transcranial magnetic stimulation study of inhibitory deficits in the motor cortex in patients with schizophrenia. Psychiatry Res 114:11–22, 2002b

Fitzgerald PB, Benitez J, Daskalakis ZJ, et al: A double-blind sham-controlled trial of repetitive transcranial magnetic stimulation in the treatment of refractory auditory hallucinations. J Clin Psychopharmacol 25:358–2005

Geller V, Grisaru N, Abarbanel JM, et al: Slow magnetic stimulation of prefrontal cortex in depression and schizophrenia. Prog Neuropsychopharmacol Biol Psychiatry 21:105–110, 1997

Gold JM, Carpenter C, Randolph C, et al: Auditory working memory and Wisconsin Card Sorting Test performance in schizophrenia. Arch Gen Psychiatry 54:159–165, 1997

Hampson M, Peterson BS, Skudlarski P, et al: Detection of functional connectivity using temporal correlations in MR images. Hum Brain Mapp 15:247–262, 2002

Hoffman RE, Boutros NN, Berman RM, et al: Transcranial magnetic stimulation of left temporoparietal cortex in three patients reporting hallucinated "voices." Biol Psychiatry 46:130–132, 1999

Hoffman RE, Boutros NN, Hu S, et al: Transcranial magnetic stimulation and auditory hallucinations in schizophrenia. Lancet 355:1073–1075, 2000

Hoffman RE, Hawkins KA, Gueorguieva R, et al: Transcranial magnetic stimulation of left temporoparietal cortex and medication-resistant auditory hallucinations. Arch Gen Psychiatry 60:49–56, 2003

Hoffman RE, Gueorguieva R, Hawkins KA, et al: Temporoparietal transcranial magnetic stimulation for auditory hallucinations: safety, efficacy and predictors in a fifty patient sample. Biol Psychiatry 58:97–104, 2005

Homan RW, Herman J, Purdy P: Cerebral location of the international 10–20 system electrode placement. Electroencephalogr Clin Neurophsyiol 66:376–382, 1987

Keefe RS, Arnold MC, Bayen UJ, et al: Source monitoring deficits in patients with schizophrenia: a multinomial modeling analysis. Psychol Med 29:903–914, 1999

Klein E, Kolsky Y, Puyerovsky M, et al: Right prefrontal slow repetitive transcranial magnetic stimulation in schizophrenia: a double-blind sham-controlled pilot study. Biol Psychiatry 46:1451–1454, 1999a

Klein E, Kreinin I, Chistyakov A, et al: Therapeutic efficacy of right prefrontal slow repetitive transcranial magnetic stimulation in major depression: a double-blind controlled study. Arch Gen Psychiatry 56:315–320, 1999b

Kraemer HC, Wilson GT, Fairburn CG, et al: Mediators and moderators of treatment effects in randomized clinical trials. Arch Gen Psychiatry 59:877–883, 2002

Lee S-H, Kim W, Chung Y-C, et al: A double-blind study showing that two weeks of daily repetitive TMS over the left or right temporoparietal cortex reduces symptoms in patients with schizophrenia who are having treatment-refractory auditory hallucinations. Neurosci Lett 376:177–181, 2005

Lennox BR, Park SB, Medley I, et al: The functional anatomy of auditory hallucinations in schizophrenia. Psychiatry Res 100:13–20, 2000

Lowe MJ, Mock BJ, Sorenson JA: Functional connectivity in single and multislice echo-planar imaging using resting-state fluctuations. Neuroimage 7:119–132, 1998

Lowe MJ, Lurito JT, Mathews VP, et al: Quantitative comparison of functional contrast from BOLD-weighted spin-echo and gradient-echo echoplanar imaging at 1.5 tesla and $H_2\ ^{15}O$ PET in the whole brain. J Cereb Blood Flow Metab 20:1331–1340, 2000

McIntosh AM, Semple D, Tasker K, et al: Transcranial magnetic stimulation for auditory hallucinations in schizophrenia. Psychiatry Res 127:9–17, 2004

Nahas Z, Lomarev M, Roberts DR, et al: Unilateral left prefrontal transcranial magnetic stimulation (TMS) produces intensity-dependent bilateral effects as measured by interleaved BOLD fMRI. Biol Psychiatry 50:712–720, 2001

Ojemann GA: Organization of short-term verbal memory of human cortex: evidence from electrical stimulation. Brain Lang 5:331–340, 1978

Ojemann GA: Cortical distribution of language. J Neurosci 11:2281–2287, 1991

Pascual-Leone A, Manoach DS, Birnbaum R, et al: Motor cortical excitability in schizophrenia. Biol Psychiatry 52:24–31, 2002

Post RM, Kimbrell TA, Frye M, et al: Implications of kindling and quenching for the possible frequency dependence of rTMS. CNS Spectr 2:54–60, 1997

Poulet E, Brunelin J, Bediou B, et al: Slow transcranial magnetic stimulation can rapidly reduce resistant auditory hallucinations in schizophrenia. Biol Psychiatry 57:188–191, 2005

Puri BK, Davey NJ, Ellaway PH, et al: An investigation of motor function in schizophrenia using transcranial magnetic stimulation of the motor cortex. Br J Psychiatry 169:690–695, 1996

Puri BK, Lekh SK, Nijran KS, et al: SPECT neuroimaging in schizophrenia with religious delusions. Int J Psychophysiol 40:143–148, 2001

Rollnik JD, Huber TJ, Mogk H, et al: High frequency repetitive transcranial magnetic stimulation (rTMS) of the dorsolateral prefrontal cortex in schizophrenic patients. Neuroreport 11:4013–4015, 2000

Schonfeldt-Lecuona C, Gron G, Walter H, et al: Stereotaxic rTMS for the treatment of auditory hallucinations in schizophrenia. Neuroreport 15:1669–1673, 2004

Schroder J, Buchsbaum MS, Siegel BV, et al: Cerebral metabolic activity correlates of subsyndromes in chronic schizophrenia. Schizophr Res 19:41–53, 1996

Shergill SS, Murray RM, McGuire PK: Auditory hallucinations: a review of psychological treatments. Schizophr Res 32:137–150, 1998

Shergill SS, Brammer MJ, Williams SCR, et al: Mapping auditory hallucinations in schizophrenia using functional magnetic resonance imaging. Arch Gen Psychiatry 57:1033–1038, 2000

Silbersweig DA, Stern E, Frith C, et al: A functional neuroanatomy of hallucinations in schizophrenia. Nature 378:176–179, 1995

Strafella AP, Paus T, Barrett J, et al: Repetitive transcranial magnetic stimulation of the human prefrontal cortex induces dopamine release in the caudate nucleus. J Neurosci 21:RC157, 2001

Swerdlow NR, Koob GF: Dopamine, schizophrenia, mania, depression: toward a unified hypothesis of cortico-striato-pallido-thalamic function. Behav Brain Sci 10:197–245, 1987

Volk DW, Pierri JN, Fritschy JM, et al: Reciprocal alterations in pre- and postsynaptic inhibitory markers at chandelier cell inputs to pyramidal neurons in schizophrenia. Cereb Cortex 12:1063–1070, 2002

Wassermann EM, Kimbrell TA, George MS, et al: Local and distant changes in cerebral glucose metabolism during repetitive transcranial magnetic stimulation (abstract). Neurology 48:A107–A108, 1997

Weinberger DR: Implications of normal brain development for the pathogenesis of schizophrenia. Arch Gen Psychiatry 44:660–669, 1987

Weinberger DR, Berman KF: Prefrontal function in schizophrenia: confounds and controversies. Philos Trans R Soc Lond B Biol Sci 351:1495–503, 1996

Wolkin A, Sanfilipo M, Wolf AP, et al: Negative symptoms and hypofrontality in chronic schizophrenia. Arch Gen Psychiatry 49:959–965, 1992

Xiong J, Parsons LM, Gao JH, et al: Interregional connectivity to primary motor cortex revealed using MRI resting state images. Hum Brain Mapp 8:151–156, 1999

Yu H-C, Liao K-K, Chang T-J, et al: Transcranial magnetic stimulation in schizophrenia (letter). Am J Psychiatry 159:494–495, 2002

9

TRANSCRANIAL MAGNETIC STIMULATION AND BRAIN IMAGING

Mark S. George, M.D.
Daryl E. Bohning, Ph.D.
Xingbao Li, M.D.
Ziad Nahas, M.D., M.S.C.R.
Stewart Denslow, Ph.D.
David Ramsey, M.S.
Christine Molnar, Ph.D.
Kevin A. Johnson, B.E.
Jejo Koola, B.S.
Paulien De Vries, M.S.

One of the more exciting areas of transcranial magnetic stimulation (TMS) involves combining TMS with brain imaging. Integrating imaging and TMS allows one to better place the TMS coil (see also Chapter 2 in this volume, "Methods of Administering Transcranial Magnetic Stimulation"), to understand more fully the effects of TMS on the brain, and to improve understanding of how the brain works by perturbing the brain and understanding different networks. In this chapter, we provide an overview of this rapidly advancing field.

USING IMAGING TO GUIDE COIL PLACEMENT IN TMS

Magnetic Resonance Imaging

One of the major problems confronting TMS research, especially when stimulating outside of primary motor or visual pathways, is trying to determine exactly where one is stimulating in the brain (George 2003; George et al. 1995, 1996, 1997). In many TMS studies the placement of the TMS coil was determined by referencing the stimulation a certain distance from a functionally determined spot, such as the motor area for thumb, by choosing an anatomical landmark (e.g., distance from the lateral canthus of the eye), or by using a variant of the electroencephalographic electrode placement system (Kahkonen et al. 2005). These techniques serve to standardize TMS placement, but it is well known that different individuals have widely varying brain size and morphology. In addition to differences in brain structure, there is even greater variation of functional location of behaviors across individuals, especially for behaviors other than simple movement or vision. Thus, in general, except for motor and visual studies (in which external monitoring of TMS effects may be possible), researchers have struggled to invent better methods for positioning the TMS coil.

Several different systems for positioning a TMS coil, based on a subject's structural magnetic resonance imaging (MRI) scan, are currently available. A widely used system, Brainsight, was developed at McGill University in Montreal, Quebec, and is illustrated in Figure 2–2 in Chapter 2 of this volume (Paus et al. 1997b; Peters et al. 1996). There are other systems for performing this same function either in a clinical laboratory (Neggers et al. 2004; Smith et al. 2005) or inside the MRI scanner (Bohning et al. 2003b). Initially one might think that the ideal way to determine where to place the TMS coil would be to invisibly peel away the scalp and skull and directly position the TMS coil on specific gyri. In fact, most neurosurgery departments now routinely employ MRI-guided presurgical mapping systems. These systems allow one to perform a brain MRI scan on a patient, with markers in key areas, and then place the MRI scan in a computer workstation. Next, with the subject sitting in a chair with a headholder, one can move an attached stereotactic wand to a position on the skull that is directly over a brain region. Alternatively, one can position the wand on the skull, and the system will electronically display the brain regions under the wand. This method can reliably determine where stimulation will occur. However, it is unclear at present how necessary this degree of coil positioning is for many TMS research and clinical applications.

As mentioned earlier, gyral anatomy and morphology vary a great deal between individuals. Additionally, it is no easy task, even with the brain fully exposed, to agree on specific gyri across individuals. Finally, as noted, even when the problems with structural differences are resolved, the location of different functions within the brain also varies. Even if one stimulates the same anatomical spot across individuals, there is no guarantee that one is stimulating the same functional location or equivalent.

Probabilistic Method

Some systems overlay information from large datasets onto an individual MRI scan. Then, a probabilistic coil placement adjusts for differences in skull size and shape but only loosely guarantees that the TMS coil is positioned over the part of an individual's brain involved in performance of a task. Some systems using this approach are relatively simple and straightforward to perform in a clinical setting and eliminate the need for a brain MRI scan (Evans et al. 1993; Herwig et al. 2003; Mazziotta et al. 1995).

Within-Individual Functional Mapping

Finally, the most sophisticated method of determining coil placement involves having the person perform a task within the scanner, determining his or her specific functional location, and finally placing the TMS coil on the scalp location designed to stimulate this region. However, it is no trivial task to determine, within an individual, the precise location involved in complex tasks. For example, Johnson and colleagues (2004) at the Medical University of South Carolina (MUSC) used a high-field MRI scanner (3.0 tesla [T]) to directly test the repeatability of functional MRI (fMRI) maps for potential TMS positioning. They scanned 25 right-handed healthy men twice while the subjects performed a working memory task. The authors found significant parietal activation in only 74% (37 of 50) of the fMRI scanning sessions. Only 56% (14 of 25) of the subjects had significant parietal activation on both days. Three subjects had hemispheric switches of their main activation region. Of the 11 subjects with target activation on the same side for both days, the average change in spot distance between days was 16.4 ± 10.0 mm, with random directional shift. With this amount of variance, scientists should exercise caution in using individual maps of cognitive brain function for TMS targeting.

With higher-field-strength MRI scanners and multichannel acquisition coils, there has been rapid progress recently in using fMRI to determine an individual's functional anatomy (e.g., Kozel et al. 2005), and the next few years should see improvements in this area for research studies. Whether the clinical applications of TMS would require individual MRI-guided application is still an unanswered question.

As mentioned in Chapter 5 ("Transcranial Magnetic Stimulation in Major Depression") in this volume, one of the key unanswered questions to be addressed over the next decade is whether there are some regions of the prefrontal cortex that might prove more effective in TMS as a treatment for depression. For example, one would assume that stimulation over a gyrus would be more clinically effective than placement over a sulcus. Additionally important is whether stimulation over one particular Brodmann region or aspect of the prefrontal cortex (e.g., medial, lateral, anterior) is more effective than another.

The current probabilistic approach to coil placement for depression treatment was developed and adopted initially in 1995 (George et al. 1995, 1996). Herwig and colleagues (2001, 2003), in Munich, elegantly described the limitations of this approach (Figure 9–1). In Figure 9–1, the individual Talairach coordinates before and after standard positioning of the coil are visualized in an individual surface-rendered brain MRI (white matter segmentation) that was transformed into Talairach space (viewed over the left frontal cortex). The small black dots indicate the optimal sites for abductor pollicis brevis muscle stimulation over the motor cortex (i.e., the region around the lateral edge of the hand knob). The larger dots indicate the rostral coil positions over the different Brodmann areas: red BA 6, blue BA 6/8 and 8, yellow BA 8/9 and 9. In some individuals, particularly those with large skulls, or individuals in whom the motor strip is posterior, the 5-centimeter rule results in stimulation of premotor cortex and not prefrontal cortex. It is likely that more sophisticated and flexible approaches to coil positioning and individual adjustment will be needed to optimize TMS as a treatment for depression and other neuropsychiatric illnesses.

Testing and Validation of TMS Coil Positioning Methods

An important background neuroscience question in attempting to validate various TMS placement methods is *whether TMS is stimulating the same brain regions that are normally involved in carrying out a task.* Numerous retrospective studies have compared the skull locations where TMS found an effect with the known structural neuroanatomy or with changes observed on a functional image. Several initial studies demonstrated that the TMS-determined motor area for thumb was close to the area revealed by positron emission tomography (PET) or fMRI scanning to be responsible for thumb movement (Roberts et al. 1997; Wassermann et al. 1996). These studies were reassuring in that the optimal TMS scalp location that caused thumb movement was located over the same cortex that was also implicated by more conventional functional imaging.

The actual story may be a bit more complicated, however. For example, Denslow and colleagues (2005a) at MUSC assessed the variation in location and

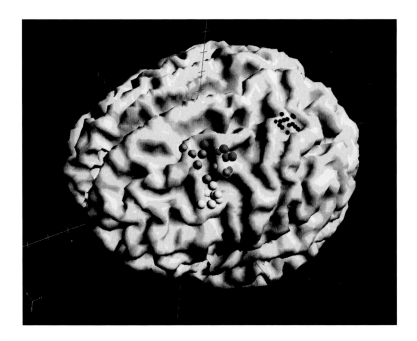

Figure 9–1. Range of prefrontal regions stimulated in different individuals using the current probabilistic placement method for transcranial magnetic stimulation (TMS).

Black dots represent the motor abductor pollicis brevis location, and the red, blue, and yellow dots represent the range of prefrontal locations. An important research issue for the field is to determine if TMS at different Brodmann locations, or prefrontal regions, affects antidepressant response.

Source. Reprinted from Herwig U, Padberg F, Unger J, et al.: "Transcranial Magnetic Stimulation in Therapy Studies: Examination of the Reliability of 'Standard' Coil Positioning by Neuronavigation," *Biological Psychiatry* 50:58–61, 2001, copyright 2001, with permission from the Society of Biological Psychiatry.

intensity of blood oxygen level–dependent (BOLD) contrast associated with movements induced by TMS or volition. The investigators scanned 11 healthy adults three times each at 1.5 T. They applied 1-Hz TMS, interleaved with fMRI, over motor cortex and alternated volition with TMS during the scans. The intrasubject standard deviations in BOLD locations ranged from 3 to 6 millimeters, allowing localization to subregions of the motor strip. Interestingly, coil placement relative to BOLD location varied more than did BOLD location ($SD_x = 9.5$ mm, $SD_y = 8.7$ mm, $SD_z = 9.0$ mm), with a consistent anterior displacement of the coil compared with where one would have predicted ($d_y = 21.8$ mm, $P < 0.025$; d_y = difference in y direction). There were no significant differences between TMS and volition BOLD locations or intensities. The high repeatability of location of TMS-induced BOLD activation suggests that TMS–fMRI stimulation could be used as a precise tool in investigation of cortical mechanisms.

The similarity between volition and TMS in the Denslow et al. (2005a) study suggests that TMS may act through "natural" brain movement circuits. Locations of the center of the TMS coil and its projection to the cortex, calculated from settings on the TMS holder, are shown in Figure 9–2. Although the locations were generally over the crown of the precentral gyrus, they clearly tended to be anterior to the location of the majority of Brodmann area 4 on the posterior bank of the central sulcus. These findings demonstrate that TMS stimulation, at 1 Hz and 110% of motor threshold (MT) for 21 seconds inducing twitch of the contralateral thumb, results in BOLD activation that varies little in anatomical location or intensity over repeated scans. The level of variance in location observed in this study sets a benchmark for what level of precision can be expected in the determination of anatomical sites of BOLD activity resulting from TMS.

The variations in location and intensity between TMS-induced and volitionally induced BOLD activations were similar (Denslow et al. 2005a). Also similar (but no statistically significant differences were found) were the absolute intensities, center-of-gravity locations, and time courses of the TMS-induced and volitionally induced BOLD responses. Further, whereas differences in BOLD response from different intensities of auditory stimulation were readily detectable, differences between TMS and volition activation intensities were not significantly different. The mean location of BOLD activation in the motor strip was approximately 10 ± 4 mm interior to the cortical surface, or about 5 mm below the locations found by others. These results also differ from the results of Epstein and colleagues (1990), who concluded that the point of stimulation occurs at a depth of about 6 mm. Epstein et al. did not measure a BOLD location but instead estimated stimulus site on the basis of electric field strength patterns from different coils. These differing results may imply that the point of initial triggering by the TMS-generated field is different than the point of maximum BOLD response. This situation might occur if the form of the BOLD response region was at least partially dependent on the particular arborization of the microvasculature and draining veins, which are the source of the BOLD signal (Logothetis et al. 2001; Menon et al. 1995; Weiskopf et al. 2003). It is also reasonable to suggest that TMS may initially trigger only axonal spiking depolarization rather than synaptic activity. Axonal spiking requires only small amounts of energy and thus may not produce a BOLD contrast increase. The signal from an initial spiking event might then activate more energy-intensive, synaptic activity in either an area of motor cortex somewhat displaced from the initial location of depolarization or an entirely separate cortical, subcortical, or spinal location. In the case of the spinal location, two groups have suggested that the mechanism producing motor region BOLD is the action of afferents returning signal from the affected muscle (Baudewig et al. 2001; Bestmann et al. 2003a, 2003b, 2004; Siebner et al. 1997–1999). The data from Denslow et al. (2005a) do not rule out this possibility.

In their precise study, Denslow and colleagues (2005a) also found a much larger variability in the placement of the TMS coil from scan to scan than in the location of the center of BOLD activation. A good deal of caution must be exercised when one is interpreting results on the basis of precise positioning of the TMS coil for stimulation of particular anatomy, especially when there is no outward physical sign such as a muscle twitch to be used as a guide for placement. A source of the observed wide range in TMS locations may be the great variability in the extent and locations of the shallowest portions of the motor cortex. The exponential fall-off in the field strength of the TMS coil from its face makes any TMS stimulation highly sensitive to the depth of the cortex from the scalp.

USING IMAGING TO UNDERSTAND THE BRAIN EFFECTS OF TMS

In addition to its role in validating positioning technique in TMS, brain imaging has been used to help researchers understand the effects of TMS. An example of the importance of using structural scanning to inform the field of TMS is illustrated by a series of studies from Kozel and colleagues. They initially acquired structural MRI scans in depressed subjects undergoing a depression treatment trial and measured the distance from the TMS coil (indicated by a marker or fiducial on the scan) to the closest edge of prefrontal cortex (George et al. 2000). This distance did not correlate with TMS antidepressant response. However, it did correlate with advancing age (the older the subject, the more space between scalp and cortex) (Kozel et al. 2000). However, in that trial and others (Figiel et al. 1998), TMS was not effective in treating older depressed subjects. In that trial, which used stimulation at 100% of MT, no subject with a distance greater than 1.6 mm (or an age greater than 50 years) responded. These MRI distance measurements suggested that the reason for TMS nonresponse in older depressed subjects might be that a higher intensity of stimulation is needed to reach cortex that is further away from the coil. The correlation of poor antidepressant response with greater prefrontal atrophy has been confirmed in another clinical study (Mosimann et al. 2002) and then elaborated in a single-photon emission computed tomography (SPECT) imaging study (Nahas et al. 2001b). In related work, approximately 60% of the between-subject variation in MT was found to be due to differences in the scalp-cortex distance (Kozel et al. 2000; McConnell et al. 2001). As one would expect, greater distance correlates with a higher MT.

Another method for determining where TMS is acting in the brain was developed by Bohning and colleagues. They discovered that one could use a modified TMS coil and a conventional MRI scanner to make a picture of the magnetic field

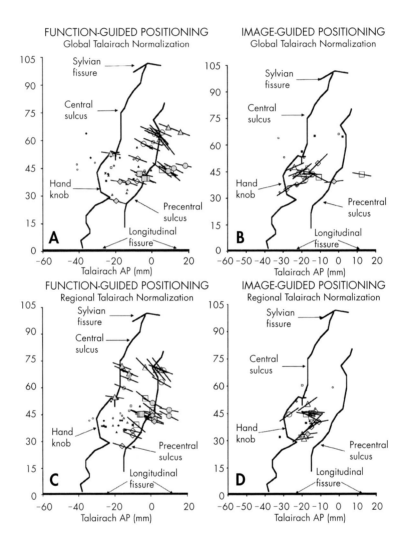

Figure 9–2. Locations of the center of the transcranial magnetic stimulation (TMS) coil and its projection to the cortex, calculated from settings on the TMS holder.

A: Function-guided results after global Talairach normalization, that is, using the AC point and maximum extents. Large symbols are TMS coil positions; lines through large symbols indicate direction of induced electric field; small symbols are COGs of BOLD activations. Different symbols are used for each subject's results. Sulcal paths are taken from the Talairach atlas. **B:** Image-guided results after global Talairach normalization, that is, using the AC point and maximum extents. Large symbols are TMS coil positions; lines through large symbols indicate direction of induced electric field; small symbols are COGs of BOLD activations. Different symbols are used for each subject's results. Sulcal paths are taken from the Talairach atlas. **C:** Function-guided results after regional Talairach normalization, that is, using landmarks along the central sulcus plus maximum extents. Large symbols are TMS coil positions; lines through large symbols indicate direction of induced electric field; small symbols are COGs of BOLD activations. Different symbols are used for each subject's results. Sulcal paths are taken from the Talairach atlas. Coil positions clustered over central and precentral sulci. **D:** Image-guided results after regional Talairach normalization, that is, using landmarks along the central sulcus plus maximum extents. Large symbols are TMS coil positions; lines through large symbols indicate direction of induced electric field; small symbols are COGs of BOLD activations. Different symbols are used for each subject's results. Sulcal paths are taken from the Talairach atlas. Coil positions clustered over the crown of the gyrus at the hand knob.

Note that in terms of repositioning the coil, magnetic resonance imaging (MRI) placement (right, images B and D) is much more accurate than placing the coil after hunting for the appropriate location (left images, A and C).

Source. Denslow S, Bohning DE, Bohning PA, et al.: "An Increased Precision Comparison of TMS-Induced Motor Cortex BOLD fMRI Response for Image-Guided Versus Function-Guided Coil Placement." *Cognitive Behavioral Neurology* 18:119–127, 2005. Copyright 2005 Lippincott Williams & Wilkins. Used with permission.

produced by a TMS coil. This image, called an *MRI phase map,* accurately displays the TMS magnetic field (Bohning et al. 1997). Current theories hold, however, that it is the induced electrical field that carries much of the neurobiological effect of TMS, and thus imaging the magnetic field is only partially the answer to knowing where TMS is acting in the brain (Wagner et al. 2004a, 2004b). However, new advances in MRI scanning might allow MRI also to image the TMS-induced electrical field—a development that would be enormously helpful in determining the neurobiological effects of TMS (Baumer et al. 2003; Le Bihan et al. 2001; Roth et al. 1994).

USING IMAGING TO ADDRESS THE SAFETY OF TMS

Nahas and colleagues (2000) performed MRI scans on depressed patients before and after a TMS treatment trial. They failed to find any radiographic evidence of TMS-induced changes, and careful measurement of prefrontal volume failed to find a difference before and after treatment. Diffusion tensor MRI allows one to examine the directional flow of water within the brain (Le Bihan et al. 2001). Diffusion tensor imaging (DTI) is therefore extremely sensitive to subtle brain trauma and is used in the acute management and detection of stroke (Koroshetz et al. 1997; Lutsep et al. 1997; Zivan et al. 1997). To investigate whether TMS changes diffusion, Li and colleagues (Duning et al. 2004) initially performed DTI scans on 14 depressed patients before and immediately after prefrontal TMS (1 Hz, 100% of MT, 147 pulses). They then used region-of-interest analysis guided by phase maps to compare DTI measurements in the prefrontal cortex before and after TMS. They failed to find any significant changes. However, Mottaghy and colleagues (2003) examined DTI before and after 1-Hz TMS (90% of MT, 12 minutes) over motor cortex and found a "temporary small restriction in diffusion" within the targeted left M1. Further studies are needed and are ongoing to resolve these two differing studies, which have important implications for TMS safety.

USING OTHER IMAGING TECHNIQUES TO STUDY TMS

TMS Studies Outside the Scanner

Fluorodeoxyglucose-PET

The first combination of TMS and functional neuroimaging in real time was performed with fluorodeoxyglucose (FDG)–PET in a patient before and after repetitive TMS (rTMS) treatment for refractory depression (George et al. 1995). Conclusions that can be drawn from this single case study are limited. However, the report clearly demonstrated the potential of combining TMS with functional imaging to begin to address clinical issues.

Many formal TMS studies with FDG-PET have been conducted. For example, a study of 1-Hz stimulation over the motor cortex for thumb showed decreased glucose uptake at the site of stimulation and in the contralateral motor cortex (Wassermann et al. 1997). Stimulation was performed at 1 Hz because FDG takes 20 minutes to settle into neurons and thus FDG-PET yields a composite picture of brain activity over 20 minutes. Stimulation at or around MT intensity at speeds faster than once per second carries the risk of a seizure. This paradoxical decrease in localized brain activity at the mirror or contralateral site during TMS has been confirmed by electrophysiology (Chae et al. 2004). A similar study by this same group of slow (1 Hz) rTMS over prefrontal cortex also found that TMS, compared with a baseline or sham condition, was associated with global reductions in blood flow, as well as localized reductions in activity in the left dorsolateral prefrontal cortex (the TMS site) and connected regions such as the caudate, orbitofrontal cortex bilaterally, and cerebellum (Kimbrell et al. 2002) (Figure 9–3). This work implies that 1-Hz prefrontal stimulation in healthy adults has profound brain effects both locally and remotely, perhaps explaining some of the more interesting clinical and research findings in mood regulation, obsessive-compulsive disorder, and working memory (Kimbrell et al. 2002).

The FDG-PET method has several limitations that detract somewhat from its utility in this area. The calculation of the models for determining the subtraction of one scan from the other is complex. The scanning technique also requires an arterial line for rapid sampling. Finally, as noted earlier, the final image is a summed picture of 20 minutes of brain activity. It is likely that TMS is having multiple different effects during that time: increased activity immediately upon stimulation, decreases during the rest time between TMS pulses, and dynamic changes across the 20 minutes as well. An important advantage of the FDG-PET method is that it yields information about absolute brain metabolism that is not possible to obtain with many other measures. Also, there is no concern about the TMS coil in the scanner causing artifact, because the TMS coil never enters the PET suite and is used only during tracer uptake away from the PET camera. After some disagreement in the literature (Paus 1999, 2001; Paus and Wolforth 1998; Paus et al. 1997a, 1997b, 1998, 1999), it appears that a TMS shield is not needed within the PET camera (Lancaster et al. 2004; Lee et al. 2003).

Perfusion SPECT

Another imaging tool that allows for tracer injection away from the camera is perfusion SPECT (George et al. 1991). In 8 healthy adults, George and colleagues (1999) used perfusion SPECT, which is taken up in 30–40 seconds, to image cerebral blood flow during fast (20-Hz) rTMS delivered to the left dorsolateral prefrontal cortex. Compared with a control scan with sham TMS, the authors reported relative decreases under the coil site and in the anterior cingulate and orbitofrontal cortex. TMS produced relative increases in blood flow in the brain stem and cerebellum.

Perfusion SPECT can only yield information about brain changes relative to other brain regions, not absolute brain activity. It is also unclear the exact amount of time that the image represents. This same group used SPECT to examine TMS-related changes in depressed subjects undergoing a treatment trial and found TMS-induced changes in limbic activity, especially in subjects who responded to TMS (Teneback et al. 1999).

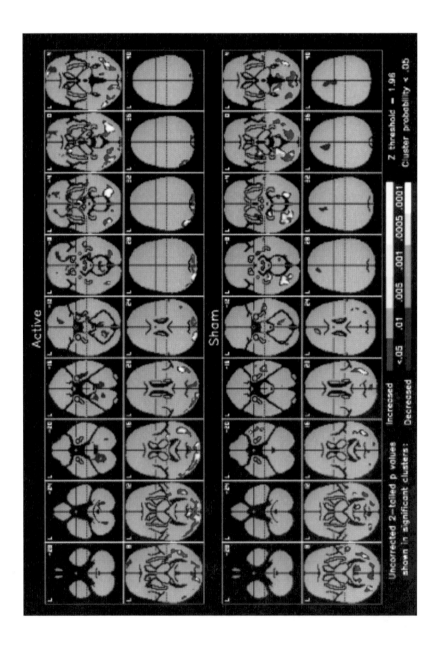

Figure 9–3. Global and localized reductions in blood flow with slow (1 Hz) repetitive transcranial magnetic stimulation (rTMS) over prefrontal cortex in 7 healthy control subjects.

Group images of the brain regions that significantly changed from before to after 1-Hz rTMS over the left prefrontal cortex for 20 minutes. The different axial slices start from the bottom of the brain (upper left) and progress with higher slices in the brain. Note that there are significant changes in the prefrontal cortex caused by TMS that are not seen with the sham condition.

Source. Adapted from Kimbrell et al. 2002.

Studies Within the Scanner

Oxygen-15 PET

Oxygen-15 (^{15}O)–labeled PET has a shorter time frame (approximately 1 minute for tracer uptake) than ^{18}FDG-PET (20–30 minutes). Paus and colleagues (1997a) were the first to publish a study combining ^{15}O-PET and TMS and found that intermittent fast (10-Hz) rTMS over the frontal eye fields for 1 minute caused dose-dependent increases in blood flow at the stimulation site and in visual cortex. That is, when Paus et al. increased the number of 10-Hz trains within the minute, blood flow increased. Surprisingly, when the investigators used the same rTMS parameters in the same subjects but shifted the coil to motor cortex, they found a dose-dependent reduction in cerebral blood flow (Paus et al. 1997b). In contrast, Fox and colleagues (1997) found that slow (1-Hz) rTMS over the motor cortex caused increased cerebral blood flow, although this effect was found in only four subjects. These paradoxical findings may imply that results seen at motor cortex will not necessarily be found in other brain regions. Alternatively, there may be large individual variation in TMS effects on blood flow either because of differences in cortical excitability, direct TMS effects on blood vessel smooth muscle, or differences in gyral anatomy. Again, these PET images are averages of 1 minute of activity during which the researcher has been intermittently stimulating and pausing, so the net picture is a combination of increases during TMS and changes during rest.

In a very interesting study with potential far-reaching implications for using TMS in clinical treatment, Speer and colleagues (2003) used ^{15}O-PET to scan depressed patients before and after 10 days of prefrontal TMS treatment. The cohort had some patients who received 1 Hz daily and the remainder who received 20 Hz. The authors found that 20-Hz rTMS applied over the left prefrontal cortex was associated only with increases in regional cerebral blood flow. Significant increases in regional cerebral blood flow across the group of all 10 patients were located in the prefrontal cortex (L>R), the cingulate gyrus (L>R), and the left amygdala, as well as bilateral insula, basal ganglia, uncus, hippocampus, parahippocampus, thalamus, and cerebellum. In contrast, 1-Hz rTMS was associated only with decreases in regional cerebral blood flow. Significant decreases in flow were noted in small areas of the right prefrontal cortex, left medial temporal cortex, left basal ganglia, and left amygdala. The changes in mood following the two rTMS frequencies were inversely related ($r=-0.78$, $P<0.005$, $n=10$) such that individuals who improved with one frequency worsened with the other. These data indicate that daily 20-Hz rTMS over the left prefrontal cortex at 100% of MT for 2 weeks induces persistent increases in regional cerebral blood flow in bilateral frontal, limbic, and paralimbic regions implicated in depression, whereas 1-Hz rTMS produces more circumscribed decreases (including in the left amygdala).

These data demonstrate frequency-dependent, opposite effects of high- and low-frequency rTMS on local and distant regional brain activity that may have important ramifications for clinical use of rTMS.

In another landmark study, Strafella and colleagues (2003) used ligand PET and showed that TMS over motor cortex caused dopamine release in the ipsilateral caudate. This study demonstrated the ability of focal electrical stimulation to cause site-specific neurochemical changes in distant regions of the brain.

Electroencephalography

Ilmoniemi and colleagues (1997) were the first to combine high-resolution electroencephalography (EEG) with TMS and reported regional changes in spectral content that shifted over very brief episodes of time and corresponded with known regional connections with primary motor cortex. High-resolution EEG clearly has the shortest and most precise temporal window of all of the imaging techniques (in the millisecond range), although the spatial resolution is poor. Recording EEG immediately after TMS is not simple, because TMS pulse produces a large artifact. Several additional groups have now been able to pursue this line of work (Boutros et al. 2000, 2001). The key hardware components include slew-rate limited preamplifiers to prevent saturation of the EEG system due to TMS (Thut et al. 2005).

BOLD fMRI

A promising but technically challenging imaging modality for TMS is combining TMS and fMRI. Bohning and colleagues (1998) first demonstrated the capability of interleaving TMS and blood flow imaging—BOLD fMRI—with good spatial and temporal resolution. This technique was initially thought impossible by many, because of concerns about introducing a focal TMS magnetic field (1–2 T) inside a clinical MRI scanner. Bohning et al. found that this technique, with the right precautions, is both feasible and safe. At least two research groups now have devised systems for interleaving TMS with functional MRI, which is also feasible at higher MRI scanner field strengths (2.0 and 3.0 T) (Baudewig et al. 2001; Bestmann et al. 2003a, 2003b, 2004; Bohning et al. 1998, 1999, 2000a, 2000b, 2003a, 2003b, 2003c; Siebner et al. 2003).

Figure 9–4 shows a group map for depressed subjects while they are being stimulated over the left prefrontal cortex, with areas of TMS-induced activation superimposed in color. Note that as the TMS machine is alternately triggered at 1 Hz for 7 seconds and then turned off, regional brain activity changes both underneath the coil and in deeper limbic regions.

Work to date has shown that interleaved TMS/fMRI is sensitive enough to detect subtle differences in brain blood flow response that result from changes in TMS intensity (Bohning et al. 1999; Nahas et al. 2001a). Additionally, direct

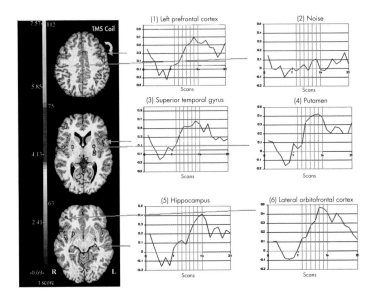

Figure 9–4. Statistical parametric map for 14 depressed patients receiving transcranial magnetic stimulation (TMS) applied over the left prefrontal cortex.

TMS (1 Hz) over the left prefrontal cortex at 100% of motor threshold produced significant increases relative to pre-rest in 14 depressed patients. A statistical parametric map shows voxels that occur within significant clusters ($t \geq 3.85$, $P_{uncorrected} < 0.001$; extend threshold $P_{corrected} < 0.05$), which are color coded according to their raw t value. L=left; R=right. Hemodynamic response curves: (**1**) left prefrontal cortex, (**2**) noise area, (**3**) left superior temporal gyrus, (**4**) left putamen, (**5**) left hippocampus, and (**6**) right lateral orbital cortex. Cluster analysis used t threshold = 3.85, cluster $P < 0.05$, $n = 14$.

Source.   Adapted from Li X, Nahas Z, Kozel FA, et al.: "Acute Left Prefrontal Transcranial Magnetic Stimulation in Depressed Patients Is Associated With Immediately Increased Activity in Prefrontal Cortical As Well As Subcortical Regions." *Biological Psychiatry* 55:882–890, 2004.

comparison of blood flow in motor cortex caused by TMS or by volition shows a similarity between TMS and normal movement. For example, the peak area of blood flow change is the same for TMS and normal movement (within 2 mm) (Bohning et al. 2000a). Also, stimulating at around 1 Hz and just at motor threshold activates roughly the same amount of brain tissue, and to the same degree. Thus, although many have the perception that TMS is causing supraphysiological changes in the brain, these fMRI studies imply that TMS at these parameters is acting remarkably like normal physiology (Denslow et al. 2004, 2005a, 2005b).

Ultimately, TMS combined with fMRI may allow for more exact positioning of the TMS coil, resulting in information obtained about the magnetic field as well as about alterations in physiology and biochemistry. The lines between imaging and pharmacology are blurring. For example, Li and colleagues (2004) at MUSC first used TMS combined with fMRI to investigate the brain effects of a central nervous system (CNS)–active compound. In the double-blind study, 10 healthy volunteers took either one dose of lamotrigine (325 mg) or placebo. Three hours later, they were scanned in a 1.5-T MRI scanner while also receiving intermittent TMS. The results showed that lamotrigine diffusely inhibited cortical activation induced by TMS applied over the motor cortex. In contrast, when TMS was applied over the prefrontal cortex, it increased TMS-induced activation of limbic regions, notably the orbitofrontal cortex and hippocampus. This study established a new method (TMS combined with fMRI) to understand the brain effect of CNS-active compounds.

Dynamic Causal Modeling and Combining TMS With Tractography

Combining TMS and imaging may help advance the field of functional imaging in addition to helping to sort out the mechanisms of TMS action. A major problem in the field of functional imaging or brain mapping to date has been the difficulty in causally linking changes seen on a brain image with a behavior in question. On any brain-mapping scan, is an activated brain region causing the behavior or inhibiting it, or has the study been poorly designed and is the activation not related to the behavior? The twin recent advances of being able to measure with certainty the exact magnetic field at a brain site and measure the brain metabolic changes associated with TMS allow the entire field of functional imaging to move one step further in establishing causal connections in brain-behavior relationships. Thus, one can now directly stimulate a region and know with certainty, by means of TMS/fMRI, that one is in the exact spot, and then use functional imaging to observe whether there are metabolic changes in the region that occur with changes in behavior. This development promises to move the entire functional imaging field forward.

The MUSC group recently demonstrated how one could use dynamic causal modeling (DCM) to analyze neural networks. Ten healthy subjects received TMS over their motor cortex in the TMS/fMRI setup. Four activated regions (primary motor area, supplementary motor area, thalamus, and cerebellum) were then analyzed using dynamic causal modeling (DCM). The initial results showed initial activation of the regions underneath the TMS coil that caused activation in the supplementary motor area, thalamus, and cerebellum (Li et al. 2005). This type of work can show the causal path of network activation.

Thus, by combining TMS and imaging, the field of functional imaging can now begin to directly address causal issues in the field of brain-behavior relationships. However, the distribution of functions within the brain is quite complex, and there may be only a few behaviors and even fewer regions for which there is a direct one-to-one necessary relationship. Our brain structure and function developed incrementally through evolution, and there are multiple redundant circuits for many behaviors (Maclean 1954, 1986, 1990, 1993). Thus, although combined TMS and imaging will allow the field to ask the questions of direct necessary causation, it is likely that many behaviors are modulated by multiple regions in circuits, and that stimulation of one node in the circuit will cause complex changes both in behavior and brain activity in other areas of the circuit. Nevertheless, combined TMS and imaging will likely help further understanding of the activity in distributed circuits as well, although perhaps not with the same causal rigor.

CONCLUSION

By combining TMS with imaging, one can both aid in understanding how TMS is affecting the brain and perhaps explain how the brain mediates behavior. This field is advancing rapidly. All the necessary tools are in place now for sophisticated functional imaging studies in which TMS is used to confirm whether a particular region is responsible for a behavior under study. MRI, with its proven ability to guide where to place the TMS coil, offers promise for determining the magnetic field at any given spot and then imaging changes in brain blood flow with stimulation. It is at least possible that in the near future a modified MRI scanner might be able to both image brain structure and function *and* stimulate the brain, perhaps even reaching deep structures with a combination of TMS coils in a deep array (Hallett 2000; Roth et al. 2005). This MRI/TMS machine would have powerful research applications and might even transform TMS therapeutics, allowing one to tailor the stimulation within an individual to regions of hypo- or hyperactivity. Before that dream can be realized, much work needs to be done with all aspects of TMS and imaging—an area that offers much promise.

REFERENCES

Baudewig J, Siebner HR, Bestmann S, et al: Functional MRI of cortical activations induced by transcranial magnetic stimulation (TMS). Neuroreport 12:3543–3548, 2001

Baumer T, Rothwell JC, Munchau A: Functional connectivity of the human premotor and motor cortex explored with TMS. Suppl Clin Neurophysiol 56:160–169, 2003

Bestmann S, Baudewig J, Siebner HR, et al: Is functional magnetic resonance imaging capable of mapping transcranial magnetic cortex stimulation? Suppl Clin Neurophysiol 56:55–62, 2003a

Bestmann S, Baudewig J, Siebner HR, et al: Subthreshold high-frequency TMS of human primary motor cortex modulates interconnected frontal motor areas as detected by interleaved fMRI-TMS. Neuroimage 20:1685–1696, 2003b

Bestmann S, Baudewig J, Siebner HR, et al: Functional MRI of the immediate impact of transcranial magnetic stimulation on cortical and subcortical motor circuits. Eur J Neurosci 19:1950–1962, 2004

Bohning DE, Pecheny AP, Epstein CM, et al: Mapping transcranial magnetic stimulation (TMS) fields in vivo with MRI. Neuroreport 8:2535–2538, 1997

Bohning DE, Shastri A, Nahas Z, et al: Echoplanar BOLD fMRI of brain activation induced by concurrent transcranial magnetic stimulation. Invest Radiol 33:336–340, 1998

Bohning DE, Shastri A, McConnell KA, et al: A combined TMS/fMRI study of intensity-dependent TMS over motor cortex. Biol Psychiatry 45:385–394, 1999

Bohning DE, Shastri A, McGavin L, et al: Motor cortex brain activity induced by 1-Hz transcranial magnetic stimulation is similar in location and level to that for volitional movement. Invest Radiol 35(11):676–683, 2000a

Bohning DE, Shastri A, Wassermann EM, et al: BOLD-fMRI response to single-pulse transcranial magnetic stimulation (TMS). J Magn Reson Imaging 11:569–574, 2000b

Bohning DE, Denslow S, Bohning PA, et al: Interleaving fMRI and rTMS. Suppl Clin Neurophysiol 56:42–54, 2003a

Bohning DE, Denslow S, Bohning PA, et al: A TMS coil positioning/holding system for MR image-guided TMS interleaved with fMRI. Clin Neurophysiol 114:2210–2219, 2003b

Bohning DE, Shastri A, Lomarev MP, et al: BOLD-fMRI response vs transcranial magnetic stimulation (TMS) pulse-train length: testing for linearity. J Magn Reson Imaging 17:279–290, 2003c

Boutros NN, Berman RM, Hoffman R, et al: Electroencephalogram and repetitive transcranial magnetic stimulation. Depress Anxiety 12:166–169, 2000

Boutros NN, Miano AP, Hoffman RE, et al: EEG monitoring in depressed patients undergoing repetitive transcranial magnetic stimulation. J Neuropsychiatry Clin Neurosci 13:197–205, 2001

Chae JH, Nahas Z, Wassermann E, et al: A pilot safety study of repetitive transcranial magnetic stimulation (rTMS) in Tourette's syndrome. Cogn Behav Neurol 17:109–117, 2004

Denslow S, Lomarev M, Bohning DE, et al: A high resolution assessment of the repeatability of relative location and intensity of transcranial magnetic stimulation-induced and volitionally induced blood oxygen level-dependent response in the motor cortex. Cogn Behav Neurol 17:163–173, 2004

Denslow S, Bohning DE, Bohning PA, et al: Increased precision comparison of TMS-induced motor cortex BOLD fMRI response for image-guided versus function-guided coil placement. Cogn Behav Neurol 18:119–127, 2005a

Denslow S, Lomarev M, George MS, et al: Cortical and subcortical brain effects of transcranial magnetic stimulation (TMS)–induced movement: an interleaved TMS/functional magnetic resonance imaging study. Biol Psychiatry 57:752–760, 2005b

Duning T, Rogalewski A, Steinstraeter O, et al: Repetitive TMS temporarily alters brain diffusion (comment; erratum appears in Neurology 62:2146, 2004). Neurology 62:2144; author reply, 2144–2145, 2004

Epstein CM, Schwartzenberg DG, Davey KR, et al: Localizing the site of magnetic brain stimulation in humans. Neurology 40:666–670, 1990

Evans AC, Collins DL, Mills SR, et al: 3-D Statistical neuroanatomical models from 305 MRI volumes, in Proceedings of the IEEE Nuclear Science Symposium and Medical Imaging Conference, 1993, San Francisco, CA, 31 October–6 November, 1993. Edited by Klaisner LA. Piscataway, NJ, IEEE Service Center, 1993, pp 1813–1817

Figiel GS, Epstein C, McDonald WM, et al: The use of rapid-rate transcranial magnetic stimulation (rTMS) in refractory depressed patients. J Neuropsychiatry Clin Neurosci 10:20–25, 1998

Fox P, Ingham R, George MS, et al: Imaging human intracerebral connectivity by PET during TMS. Neuroreport 8:2787–2791, 1997

George MS: Tickling the brain: the emerging new science of electrical brain stimulation. Sci Am 289:66–73, 2003

George MS, Ring HA, Costa DC, et al: Neuroactivation and Neuroimaging With SPECT. London, Springer-Verlag, 1991

George MS, Wassermann EM, Williams WA, et al: Daily repetitive transcranial magnetic stimulation (rTMS) improves mood in depression. Neuroreport 6:1853–1856, 1995

George MS, Wassermann EM, Williams WA, et al: Changes in mood and hormone levels after rapid-rate transcranial magnetic stimulation (rTMS) of the prefrontal cortex. J Neuropsychiatry Clin Neurosci 8:172–180, 1996

George MS, Wassermann EM, Williams WE, et al: Mood improvements following daily left prefrontal repetitive transcranial magnetic stimulation in patients with depression: a placebo-controlled crossover trial. Am J Psychiatry 154:1752–1756, 1997

George MS, Stallings LE, Speer AM, et al: Prefrontal repetitive transcranial magnetic stimulation (rTMS) changes relative perfusion locally and remotely. Hum Psychopharmacol 14:161–170, 1999

George MS, Nahas Z, Molloy M, et al: A controlled trial of daily left prefrontal cortex TMS for treating depression. Biol Psychiatry 48:962–970, 2000

Hallett M: Transcranial magnetic stimulation and the human brain. Nature 406(6792):147–150, 2000

Herwig U, Padberg F, Unger J, et al: Transcranial magnetic stimulation in therapy studies: examination of the reliability of "standard" coil positioning by neuronavigation. Bio Psychiatry 50:58–61, 2001

Herwig U, Satrapi P, Schonfeldt-Lecuona C: Using the international 10–20 EEG system for positioning of transcranial magnetic stimulation. Brain Topogr 16:95–99, 2003

Ilmoniemi RJ, Virtanen J, Ruohonen J, et al: Neuronal response to magnetic stimulation reveal cortical reactivity and connectivity. Neuroreport 8:3537–3540, 1997

Johnson KA, Mu Q, Yamanaka K, et al: Repeatability of within-individual blood oxygen level–dependent functional magnetic resonance imaging maps of a working memory task for transcranial magnetic stimulation targeting. Neuroscience Imaging 1:95–111, 2004

Kahkonen S, Komssi S, Wilenius J, et al: Prefrontal transcranial magnetic stimulation produces intensity-dependent EEG responses in humans. Neuroimage 24:955–960, 2005

Kimbrell TA, Dunn RT, George MS, et al: Left prefrontal-repetitive transcranial magnetic stimulation (rTMS) and regional cerebral glucose metabolism in normal volunteers. Psychiatry Res 115:101–113, 2002

Koroshetz WJ, Gonzalez G: Diffusion-weighted MRI: an ECG for "brain attack"? Ann Neurol 41:565–566, 1997

Kozel FA, Nahas Z, deBrux C, et al: How coil-cortex distance relates to age, motor threshold, and antidepressant response to repetitive transcranial magnetic stimulation. J Neuropsychiatry Clin Neurosci 12:376–384, 2000

Kozel FA, Johnson KA, Mu Q, et al: Detecting deception using functional magnetic resonance imaging. Biol Psychiatry 58:605–613, 2005

Lancaster JL, Narayana S, Wenzel D, et al: Evaluation of an image-guided, robotically positioned transcranial magnetic stimulation system. Human Brain Mapp 22:329–340, 2004

Le Bihan D, Mangin JF, Poupon C, et al: Diffusion tensor imaging: concepts and applications. J Magn Reson Imaging 13:534–546, 2001

Lee JS, Narayana S, Lancaster J, et al: Positron emission tomography during transcranial magnetic stimulation does not require micro-metal shielding. Neuroimage 19:1812–1819, 2003

Li X, Teneback CC, Nahas Z, et al: Interleaved transcranial magnetic stimulation/functional MRI confirms that lamotrigine inhibits cortical excitability in healthy young men. Neuropsychopharmacology 29:1395–1407, 2004

Li CS, Kosten TR, Sinha R: Sex differences in brain activation during stress imagery in abstinent cocaine users: a functional magnetic resonance imaging study. Biol Psychiatry 57:487–494, 2005

Logothetis NK, Pauls J, Augath M, et al: Neurophysiological investigation of the basis of the fMRI signal. Nature 412:150–157, 2001

Lutsep HL, Albers GW, deCrespigny A, et al: Clinical utility of diffusion-weighted magnetic resonance imaging in the assessment of ischemic stroke. Ann Neurol 41:574–580, 1997

Maclean PD: The limbic system and its hippocampal formation; studies in the animals and their possible application to man. J Neurosurg 11:29–44, 1954

Maclean PD: Culminating developments in the evolution of the limbic system: the thalamocingulate division, in The Limbic System: Functional Organization and Clinical Disorders. Edited by Doane BK, Livingston KE. New York, Raven, 1986, pp 172–189

Maclean PD: The Triune Brain in Evolution: Role in Paleocerebral Functions. New York, Plenum, 1990

Maclean PD: Introduction: perspectives on cingulate cortex in the limbic system, in Neurobiology of Cingulate Cortex and Limbic Thalamus: A Comprehensive Handbook. Edited by Vogt BA, Gabriel M. Boston, MA, Birkhauser, 1993, pp 1–19

Mazziotta JC, Toga AW, Evans A, et al: A probabilistic atlas of the human brain: theory and rationale for its development. Neuroimage 2:89–101, 1995

McConnell KA, Nahas Z, Shastri A, et al: The transcranial magnetic stimulation motor threshold depends on the distance from coil to underlying cortex: a replication in healthy adults comparing two methods of assessing the distance to cortex. Biol Psychiatry 49:454–459, 2001

Menon RS, Ogawa S, Hu X, et al: BOLD based functional MRI at 4 Tesla includes a capillary bed contribution: echoplanar imaging correlates with previous optical imaging using intrinsic signals. Magn Reson Med 33:453–459, 1995

Mosimann UP, Marre SC, Werlen S, et al: Antidepressant effects of repetitive transcranial magnetic stimulation in the elderly: correlation between effect size and coil-cortex distance. Arch Gen Psychiatry 59:560–561, 2002

Mottaghy FM, Gangitano M, Horkan C, et al: Repetitive TMS temporarily alters brain diffusion (see comment). Neurology 60:1539–1541, 2003

Nahas Z, DeBrux C, Chandler V, et al: Lack of significant changes on magnetic resonance scans before and after 2 weeks of daily left prefrontal repetitive transcranial magnetic stimulation for depression. J ECT 16:380–390, 2000

Nahas Z, Lomarev M, Roberts DR, et al: Unilateral left prefrontal transcranial magnetic stimulation (TMS) produces intensity-dependent bilateral effects as measured by interleaved BOLD fMRI. Biol Psychiatry 50:712–720, 2001a

Nahas Z, Teneback HC, Kozel A, et al: Brain effects of TMS delivered over prefrontal cortex in depressed adults: role of stimulation frequency and coil-cortex distance. J Neuropsychiatry Clin Neurosci 13:459–470, 2001b

Neggers SF, Langerak TR, Schutter DJ, et al: A stereotactic method for image-guided transcranial magnetic stimulation validated with fMRI and motor-evoked potentials. Neuroimage 21:1805–1817, 2004

Paus T: Imaging the brain before, during, and after transcranial magnetic stimulation. Neuropsychologia 37:219–224, 1999

Paus T: Integration of transcranial magnetic stimulation and brain imaging (abstract). Biol Psychiatry 49:6S-#21, 2001

Paus T, Wolforth M: Transcranial magnetic stimulation during PET: reaching and verifying the target site. Hum Brain Mapp 6:399–402, 1998

Paus T, Jech R, Thompson CJ, et al: Dose-dependent reduction of cerebral blood flow during rapid-rate transcranial magnetic stimulation of the human sensorimotor cortex. J Neurophysiol 79:1102–1107, 1997a

Paus T, Jech R, Thompson CJ, et al: Transcranial magnetic stimulation during positron emission tomography: a new method for studying connectivity of the human cerebral cortex. J Neurosci 17:3178–3184, 1997b

Paus T, Jech R, Thompson CJ, et al: Dose-dependent reduction of cerebral blood flow during rapid-rate transcranial magnetic stimulation of the human sensorimotor cortex. J Neurophysiol 79:1102–1107, 1998

Peters T, Davey B, Munger P, et al: Three-dimensional multi-modal image guidance for neurosurgery. IEEE Trans Med Imaging 15:121–128, 1996

Roberts DR, Vincent DJ, Speer AM, et al: Multi-modality mapping of motor cortex: comparing echoplanar BOLD fMRI and transcranial magnetic stimulation. J Neural Transm 104:833–843, 1997

Roth BJ, Momen S, Turner R: Algorithm for the design of magnetic stimulation coils. Med Biol Eng Comput 32:214–216, 1994

Roth Y, Zangen A, Voller B, et al: Transcranial magnetic stimulation of deep brain regions: evidence for efficacy of the H-coil. Clin Neurophysiol 116:775–779, 2005

Siebner HR, Lee L, Bestmann S: Interleaving TMS with functional MRI: now that it is technically feasible how should it be used? (comment). Clin Neurophysiol 114:1997–1999, 2003

Smith DT, Jackson SR, Rorden C: Transcranial magnetic stimulation of the left human frontal eye fields eliminates the cost of invalid endogenous cues. Neuropsychologia 43:1288–1296, 2005

Speer AM, Willis MW, Herscovitch P, et al: Intensity-dependent regional cerebral blood flow during 1-Hz repetitive transcranial magnetic stimulation (rTMS) in healthy volunteers studied with $H_2^{15}O$ positron emission tomography, II. effects of prefrontal cortex rTMS. Biol Psychiatry 54:826–832, 2003

Strafella AP, Paus T, Fraraccio M, et al: Striatal dopamine release induced by repetitive transcranial magnetic stimulation of the human motor cortex. Brain 126:2609–2615, 2003

Teneback CC, Nahas Z, Speer AM, et al: Changes in prefrontal cortex and paralimbic activity in depression following two weeks of daily left prefrontal TMS. J Neuropsychiatry Clin Neurosci 11:426–435, 1999

Thut G, Ives JR, Kampmann F, et al: A new device and protocol for combining TMS and online recordings of EEG and evoked potentials. J Neurosci Meth 141:207–217, 2005

Wagner TA, Gangitano M, Romero R, et al: Intracranial measurement of current densities induced by transcranial magnetic stimulation in the human brain. Neurosci Lett 354:91–94, 2004a

Wagner TA, Zahn M, Grodzinsky AJ, et al: Three-dimensional head model simulation of transcranial magnetic stimulation. IEEE Trans Biomed Eng 51:1586–1598, 2004b

Wassermann EM, Wang B, Zeffiro TA, et al: Locating the motor cortex on the MRI with transcranial magnetic stimulation and PET. Neuroimage 3:1–9, 1996

Wassermann EM, Kimbrell TA, George MS, et al: Local and distant changes in cerebral glucose metabolism during repetitive transcranial magnetic stimulation (rTMS) (abstract). Neurology 48:A107-P102.049, 1997

Weiskopf N, Veit R, Erb M, et al: Physiological self-regulation of regional brain activity using real-time functional magnetic resonance imaging (fMRI): methodology and exemplary data. Neuroimage 19:577–586, 2003

Zivan JA: Diffusion-weighted MRI for diagnosis and treatment of ischemic stroke. Ann Neurol 41:567–568, 1997

10

REPETITIVE TRANSCRANIAL MAGNETIC STIMULATION AND RELATED SOMATIC THERAPIES

Prospects for the Future

Robert M. Post, M.D.
Andrew M. Speer, M.D.

REPETITIVE TMS AND THE SEARCH FOR OPTIMAL PARAMETERS

The most robust literature on repetitive transcranial magnetic stimulation (rTMS) of the brain in the treatment of neuropsychiatric syndromes consists of studies of its potential as a therapy for depression. Although the observed incidence and magnitude of antidepressant effects of rTMS differ substantially across studies, there are several areas of convergence and emerging consensus. Most meta-analyses of rTMS in depression have found positive antidepressant effects and modest effect sizes ranging from 0.53 to 0.81 (Burt et al. 2002; Holtzheimer et al. 2001; Kozel and George 2002; McNamara et al. 2001), with the exception of Martin and colleagues (2003), in which the effect size was 0.35.

A major focus of this type of work in the future will necessarily continue to be on optimizing parameters for improving individual and overall clinical efficacy and for developing paradigms to increase the persistence of therapeutic effect (Schule et al. 2003) and establish prophylactic regimens. It is also likely that many of the same parametric issues studied for treatment of depression will be revisited as attempts are initiated to apply rTMS for therapeutic purposes in other neuro-psychiatric illnesses.

Lateralized Effects

Table 10–1 selectively summarizes several studies that suggest a lateralized effect of rTMS as a function of frequency. Documentation of lateralized effects of rTMS would be of great interest because the evidence of laterality based on positron emission tomography (PET) in the depressive syndromes themselves is not well delineated (Ketter et al. 1996, 1997, 1999).

As noted in Table 10–1, high-frequency rTMS (10–20 Hz) appears to be capable of inducing moderate to strong antidepressant effects in some patients when administered over the left prefrontal cortex, as initially explored by Mark George in our laboratory and then by many others (George et al. 1995, 1997a, 1997b; Pascual-Leone et al. 1996b; Kirkcaldie et al. 1997). These same parameters, however, do not appear to be effective when applied over the right frontal cortex or occiput (Pascual-Leone et al. 1996a). Conversely, 20-Hz rTMS over the right prefrontal cortex appears to be associated with antimanic effects, whereas the same stimulation on the left side is ineffective in mania (Grisaru et al. 1998).

Frequency Effects

Lower-frequency rTMS may also be associated with lateralized antidepressant effects opposite to those found using higher frequencies. That is, 1-Hz TMS applied over the right prefrontal cortex appears to be associated with antidepressant effects (Kirkcaldie et al. 1997; Klein et al. 1999), whereas the same parameters over the left usually are ineffective (but see Nahas et al. 2003).

Together, these data suggest that the relative ratio of increasing neural excitability on the left with higher frequencies and decreasing it on the right with lower frequencies may alter the ratio in favor of antidepressant effects, perhaps in the subgroup of patients with the classic unipolar pattern of hypofrontality (Dunn et al. 2002; George et al. 1993; Ketter et al. 1993, 1996, 1997; Kimbrell et al. 1999). Consistent with this view is the efficacy of combined left high-frequency and right low-frequency stimulation in the studies of Garcia-Toro and colleagues (2006).

Thus, it would appear that different frequencies of stimulation have different physiological and perhaps clinical effects as they interact with the laterality of stimulation. The prediction that low-frequency rTMS would decrease blood flow and metabolism, whereas higher frequencies would increase them, is derived from an extensive physiological literature on long-term depression (LTD) versus long-term potentiation (LTP) and kindling, as discussed elsewhere (Post et al. 1997; Weiss

Table 10–1. Affective responses to repetitive transcranial magnetic stimulation (rTMS) as a function of interaction between frequency and hemisphere laterality

rTMS Frequency	Frontal cortex rTMS stimulation	
	Left	Right
High (20 Hz)	+20 Hz vs. sham (George et al. 1997b) 20 Hz in multiple studies[a] +20 Hz with a baseline hypometabolism predicts response (Kimbrell et al. 1999) −20 Hz not effective for mania	+20 Hz antimanic effect (Grisaru et al. 1998; Kaptsan et al. 2003)
Medium (5–10 Hz)	+10 Hz antidepressant (Pascual-Leone et al. 1996a, 1996b) +10 Hz is as effective as ECT (Grunhaus et al. 2000) +5 Hz antidepressant (Nahas et al. 2003)	−10 Hz not effective
Low (1 Hz)	−1 Hz not effective +1 Hz with baseline hyperactivity predicts response (Kimbrell et al. 2002a)	+1 Hz antidepressant (Feinsod et al. 1998) +1 Hz antidepressant vs. sham (Fitzgerald et al. 2003; Kauffman et al. 2004; Klein et al. 1999)

Note. ECT=electroconvulsive therapy; +=positive study; −=negative or nonsignificant study.
[a]See several meta-analyses noted in introduction to this chapter.

et al. 1997, 1998b). PET data in depressed patients from our laboratory are consistent with the predictions that high-frequency rTMS would increase neural activity, whereas low frequency rTMS would inhibit it, as described below (see subsection "Frequency Effects on Blood Flow and Metabolism" below).

Opposite Effects of High- and Low-Frequency rTMS on Mood

Individual patients stimulated over the same left prefrontal area of the brain respond differently to high- and low-frequency rTMS, with their depressive symptoms improving at high or low frequency and deteriorating at the opposite
frequency (Figure 10–1). This dichotomous response within patients was initially
observed by Kimbrell and colleagues (1999) in a randomized comparison of 1-Hz
and 20-Hz rTMS versus sham stimulation at 80% of motor threshold (MT). In
that study, the direction of change in depression measured on the Hamilton Depression Rating Scale (Ham-D) following 2 weeks of 1-Hz stimulation was inversely correlated with the direction of change in Ham-D in that same patient
following 2 weeks of 20-Hz rTMS ($r=-0.797$, $P<0.004$, $n=10$). These findings
of differential mood response in individual patients as a function of frequency have
been replicated by Speer and colleagues (2000), using the same frequencies (1 Hz
vs. 20 Hz) but at a higher intensity (i.e., 100% of MT) ($r=-0.592$, $P<0.02$,
$n=15$).

Frequency Effects on Blood Flow and Metabolism

In individual cases, high-frequency rTMS has been shown to increase metabolism
in many areas of the brain in patients with bipolar disorder (George et al. 1995),
whereas low-frequency (1-Hz) stimulation of the right frontal cortex appeared to
decrease cerebral metabolism in two patients with posttraumatic stress disorder
(PTSD) and comorbid depression (McCann et al. 1998).

   These preliminary case observations have been extended by Kimbrell and associates (2002a) in a study indicating that even acute treatment with 1-Hz rTMS
over the left frontal cortex in one group of normal volunteers compared with sham
stimulation in another group is associated with decreases in bifrontal and caudate
metabolism, as well as significant decreases in the contralateral amygdala.

   Although there are discrepancies in the literature about the resultant effects of
acute rTMS on blood flow and metabolism as assessed by functional magnetic resonance imaging (fMRI) or PET (Fox et al. 1997; Kimbrell et al. 2002a; Paus et al.
1997, 1998; Speer et al. 2003a, 2003b; Li et al. 2004), depending on a variety of
parametric and methodological factors, there appears to be greater agreement on
the effects of more long-term stimulation (George et al. 1995; Kimbrell et al.
1999; McCann et al. 1998; Speer et al. 2000; A.M. Speer, B.E. Benson, T.A.
Kimbrell, et al., unpublished data, 2006; Shajahan et al. 2002; Teneback et al.
1999). The data are generally consistent with the hypothesis that low frequencies
(1 Hz) attenuate, whereas higher frequencies (5–20 Hz) increase blood flow and
metabolism, not only locally at the site of rTMS but also, in some instances, in a
widespread downstream fashion as well.

   In our first systematic rTMS study, Speer and associates (2000), using PET
and measuring ^{15}O blood flow, observed that 20-Hz rTMS at 100% of MT for

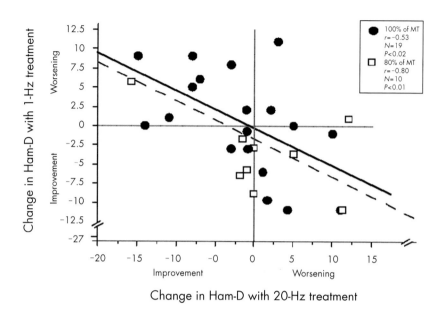

Figure 10–1. Inverse relationship between degree of antidepressant response achieved with 1-Hz versus 20-Hz repetitive transcranial magnetic stimulation (rTMS).

Studies by Kimbrell et al. (1999) of 1-Hz vs. 20-Hz rTMS at 80% of motor threshold and by Speer et al. (2000) of 1-Hz vs. 20-Hz rTMS at 100% of motor threshold show an inverse relationship between the degree of antidepressant response achieved in the same patient (as measured by the Hamilton Depression Rating Scale) at 1-Hz rTMS (vertical axis) compared with 20-Hz rTMS (horizontal axis).

2 weeks in patients with depression was associated 72 hours later with increases in blood flow bilaterally in widespread and transynaptically connected areas of the brain, whereas 1-Hz rTMS at 100% of MT induced more circumscribed decreases in blood flow, as predicted (Figure 10–2). These opposite effects on neural activity persisted for at least 3 days following a series of 10 treatments.

These findings have been replicated and extended in a larger group of patients studied at 100% of MT (A.M. Speer et al., unpublished data, 2006) and also replicated in a new randomized, parallel-group study using 1 Hz vs. 20 Hz vs. sham rTMS over left prefrontal cortex at 110% of MT for 3 weeks (A.M. Speer et al., unpublished data, 2006). One-hertz decreased blood flow locally in a widespread and more intense fashion than seen in the first study (Speer et al. 2000; Figure 10–2), and 20 Hz increased blood flow dramatically, whereas sham stimulation for 3 weeks produced no effect. There were no potentially confounding prior effects

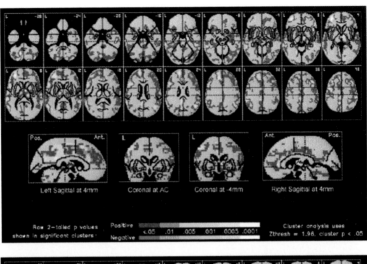

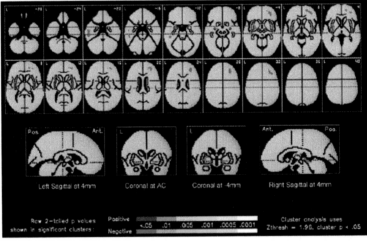

Figure 10–2. Association of transcranial magnetic stimulation (rTMS) with regional cerebral blood flow (rCBF) in patients with depression.

Top: Significant increases were found in absolute rCBF 72 hours after 2 weeks of 20-Hz repetitive rTMS over the left prefrontal cortex at 100% of motor threshold relative to the pretreatment baseline in the group of 10 depressed patients. A statistical parametric map shows voxels that occur within significant clusters and is color coded according to their raw *P* value. Increases in rCBF are displayed with a red–orange–yellow color scale; there were no areas of decreases in rCBF displayed with a dark blue–light blue color scale. Nonsignificant values are displayed as gray on the positron emission tomography template. The number in the top right corner of each horizontal section (*top two rows*) indicates its position in millimeters with respect to the anterior commissure (AC)–posterior commissure plane. Twenty-hertz rTMS resulted in widespread increases in rCBF in the following regions: prefrontal cortex (L>R), cingulate gyrus (L>R), bilateral insula, basal ganglia, uncus, hippocampus, parahippocampus, thalamus, cerebellum, and left amygdala. Note the distal effects in bilateral cortical and subcortical structures following stimulation over the left prefrontal cortex. Coronal sections (*middle, bottom row*) are displayed at the AC and 4 mm behind it to maximize visualization of the amygdala. Increases in the left amygdala, but not the right amygdala, are best viewed in horizontal sections at 20, 16, and 12 mm, however. Sagittal sections are 4 mm to the left and right of midline to illustrate the greater increases in the left cingulate gyrus relative to the right. L="left" side of image. **Bottom:** Significant decreases in absolute rCBF 72 hours after 2 weeks of 1-Hz repetitive rTMS over the left prefrontal cortex at 100% of motor threshold relative to the pretreatment baseline in the same group of 10 depressed patients. Horizontal, sagittal, and coronal images are illustrated as in the top part of the figure. Focal decreases in rCBF were present in the right prefrontal cortex (horizontal sections –4 to +32 mm), left medial temporal cortex (–20 to –12 mm), left basal ganglia (–14 to +8 mm), and left amygdala (–12 to –8 mm). Note the opposite effect of rTMS frequency on rCBF in the left amygdala (horizontal section= –12 mm) in the top part of the figure.

of the opposite frequency as in the first study because patients were not crossed over to the other frequency. This series of three studies provides strong documentation of the predicted opposing effects on neural activity of high vs. low frequency rTMS (Post et al. 1997).

Interestingly, the illustrated increases in blood flow after 20-Hz stimulation at 100% of MT (Figure 10–2) were only slightly more prominent on the left side of the prefrontal cortex, where rTMS was applied, than on the right, and they were present over the entire extent of the cingulate gyrus on the left side (Speer et al. 2000). This latter effect is particularly noteworthy in relation to studies indicating that in patients with unipolar depression, the degree of cingulate hypometabolism was inversely correlated with Ham-D scores (i.e., those patients with the most marked decrements in cingulate metabolism were most severely depressed) (Kimbrell et al. 2002b). These cingulate correlations with severity of depression were greatest on the left side and were present over the full extent of the cingulate gyrus. If this reduced cingulate activity is part of the etiopathophysiology of depression, reversal of it with high-frequency rTMS should be therapeutic and correlated with degree of improvement, a proposition that can now be directly tested.

Patterns of Brain Imaging Alterations and rTMS Stimulation Parameters

Targeting Regional Pathological Changes

Mayberg and colleagues (1997) have also reported differential degrees of pharmacological response depending on whether the pregenual cingulate cortex is hypoactive or hyperactive. The ability to robustly modulate cingulate activity with rTMS noted above raises the possibility that high frequencies could be used in hypoactive nonresponders. The data of Mayberg et al. also converge with the well-replicated observations of Wu and colleagues (Wu and Bunney 1990; Wu et al. 1992) and Ebert and associates (Ebert and Berger 1998; Ebert et al. 1991) that baseline hyperactivity in various limbic and paralimbic areas of the brain (particularly in the amygdala and anterior cingulate) is associated with positive antidepressant effects of one night's sleep deprivation.

Thus, frequency and location of stimulation, and a variety of other parameters (Table 10–2), remain to be systematically explored in patients with different patterns of neural activity revealed with functional brain imaging. Will some patients also require rTMS stimulation over the temporal lobes to better modulate activity dysfunction in this area and in the underlying deep limbic structures thought to modulate affective and affiliative behavior (Figure 10–3)? One could also ask whether cerebellar rTMS would induce some of the therapeutic effects originally observed by Heath and colleagues (1980), who used electrical stimulation with implanted electrodes over the cerebellum in patients with intractable behavioral disorders and epilepsy.

Differentiating Primary Pathological From Secondary Compensation Abnormalities

As different depression subtypes and cerebral topographies become better defined (Ketter et al. 2001), different frequencies and locations of rTMS may then be required. Whether one should aim for normalization of the baseline pattern of flow or metabolism, or attempt to drive a given brain region even further from normal, depends on whether the initial changes reflect the primary pathology of depression or its secondary adaptations (Post and Weiss 1992, 1996).

Hypotheses about whether altered activity in a given brain area reflects the primary pathology to be ameliorated or secondary attempts at compensations to

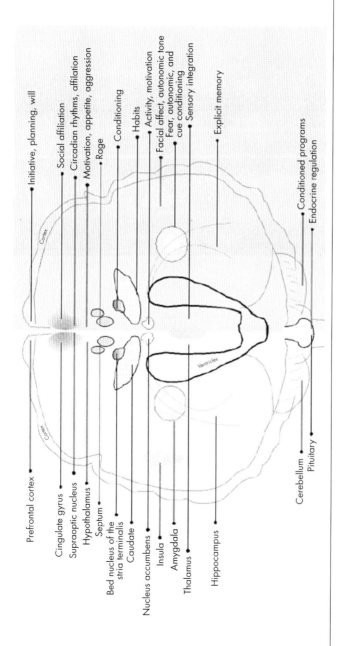

Figure 10–3. Neuroanatomy of emotion and affiliation.

Areas of brain (*left labels*) are linked in a highly preliminary way with some of the emotional and affiliative functions (*right labels*) they modulate. Further and more precise definition of the neuroanatomy of the emotional homunculus and its neuroplasticity (similar to that revealed for the distorted representations of the body surface for sensory function in the parietal cortex) should help in the delineation of the physioanatomy of the major psychiatric illnesses.

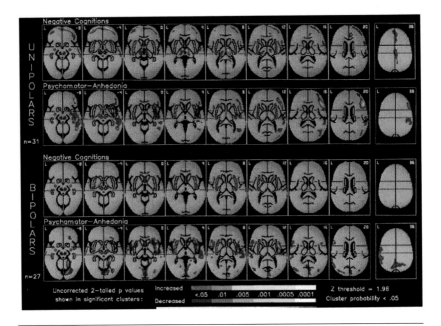

Figure 10–4. Frontal hypometabolism proportional to the degree of negative cognition in patients with unipolar depression.

Correlative topographies of the negative cognitions and psychomotor-anhedonia components with absolute regional cerebral metabolism in patients with unipolar and bipolar depression at illustrative slices from 8 mm below to 36 mm above the anterior commissure (AC)–posterior commissure (PC) plane. Cool colors indicate negative correlations and warm colors indicate positive correlations. Multiple comparisons were controlled for by cluster analysis.

be further enhanced (i.e., the abnormalities exacerbated) can be directly tested by using rTMS. This would be particularly pertinent to the finding of Dunn and colleagues (2002) of frontal hypometabolism in proportion to the degree of negative cognition (guilt or rumination) in patients with unipolar depression (Figure 10–4). Yet, right insula hypometabolism was correlated with the degree of anhedonia and psychomotor retardation in both unipolar and bipolar depressed patients, and the optimal ways of changing activity in this brain region could likewise now readily be explored.

Intermediate Stimulation Frequencies: 10-Hz rTMS Versus Electroconvulsive Therapy

Five relatively small studies have compared the efficacy of rTMS (at 10 Hz and 90%–110% of MT delivered to left prefrontal cortex) with that of electroconvul-

Table 10–2. Parameters to explore for optimizing antidepressant effects of repetitive transcranial magnetic stimulation

- Intensity (current range: 80%–120% of motor threshold; will an expansion of this range be necessary?)
- Location (left vs. right; frontal [dorsal vs. basal; medial vs. lateral] vs. temporal, parietal, cerebellar)
- Frequency (current range: 1–25 Hz; ultra-low to higher frequencies may be required)
- Pulse width
- Intertrain interval
- Coil type (focal vs. diffuse; figure-eight vs. circular; other designs for greater penetrance)
- Duration (length of session; number of stimulations)
- Number of sessions
- Interval between sessions
- Time of day (circadian rhythms)
- Dependence of parameters on prior brain activity
- Experience-dependent factors
- Augmentation with drugs and other modalities

sive therapy (ECT) and found similar results in patients with nonpsychotic depression (Grunhaus et al. 2000, 2003; Janicak et al. 2002; Pridmore et al. 2000; Schulze-Rauschenbach et al. 2005). These observations raise the possibility that midrange rTMS (10 Hz) will prove to be more effective for depression than either very high (20 Hz) or low (1 Hz) rTMS. This midrange frequency would be practically as well as theoretically valuable and might suggest that 20-Hz or 1-Hz rTMS is too strong, over- and under-driving neural activity, respectively, and potentially leading to compensating opposing adaptations and loss of therapeutic effect. The intermediate range (10 Hz) is close to the normal alpha frequency and is at the midpoint between low frequency–producing hippocampal LTD and higher (>10 Hz) frequency–producing LTP (Malenka 1995; Post et al. 1997). Driving neural systems at a frequency less far from their normal patterning with 10-Hz rTMS could theoretically be more effective than the more marked changes (Figure 10–2) induced by very low or high frequencies. These more profound changes could lead to more concerted attempts at engaging compensatory mechanisms, eventually either blunting or reversing the initial direction of rTMS effects, as we have preliminarily observed in some follow-up PET scans in patients who have or have not lost the positive effects of continued rTMS (A.M. Speer et al., unpublished data, 2006).

OTHER POTENTIAL STRATEGIES FOR OPTIMIZING rTMS

Given the unique ability of rTMS to be administered to the awake patient during normal conversation and recall, a variety of possibilities for therapeutics and interactions with other modalities emerge (Figure 10–5).

The literature about experience-dependent neuroplasticity is very extensive, indicating that synaptic strength is modified only under conditions of neuronal firing and activation (Li et al. 1998; Linden 1994; Malenka 1995; Xu et al. 1997). This pattern of neuronal firing and activation also appears to be a fundamental tenet of the Hebbian synapse, which is thought to be the major principle underlying learning and memory. Those synapses that fire coincidentally with each other are selectively modulated for either increases or decreases in synaptic efficacy. The neural mechanisms underlying this phenomenon are just beginning to be elucidated and are thought to include activity-dependent expression of neurotrophic factors (Korte et al. 1996; Marty et al. 1997; Smith et al. 1995) and other elements that are involved in the long-term modulation of synaptic efficacy.

Activity-Dependent Synaptic Modulation

Given this perspective one can begin to envision the process of selective tuning and modulation of neural pathways related to specific behaviors and memories. In contrast to ECT, which applies a large amount of electrical stimulation to the whole brain to induce a generalized major motor seizure, rTMS offers the potential for much more discrete enhancement or inhibition of areas of the brain and of synapses selectively brought online by appropriate memory and other neuropsychological retrieval strategies (Paus et al. 2001; Post et al. 1997). When a given memory engram is thus activated, theoretically, one can imagine its enhancement or inhibition not only with appropriate psychological cuing and extinction processes, respectively, but also with further intervention and modulation by the appropriate frequencies of rTMS.

For example, pairing a pungent smell with a seizure aura may abort the development of a generalized seizure (Efron 1956) and, hypothetically, recalling traumatic memories in the context of physiological interference based on attention to alternate visual stimuli (Carlson et al. 1998; Shapiro 1996; Wilson et al. 1997) might be a mechanism of desensitization. One could take these types of intervention to the next level with rTMS by enhancing counter-regulatory circuits, and even more specifically, by attempting to apply LTD-like depotentiation strategies targeting the specific synapses that have already been putatively potentiated by a trauma. Thus, the application of low-frequency (1-Hz) stimulation in the context of traumatic recall would be postulated to be more effective than 1-Hz rTMS in the resting state. Interestingly, Cohen

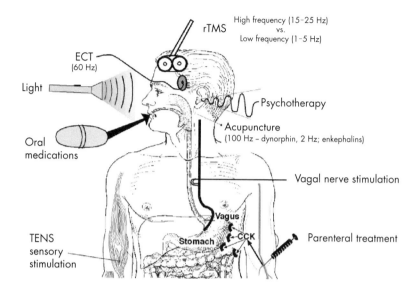

Figure 10–5. Possible therapeutic modalities that could be combined with repetitive transcranial magnetic stimulation (rTMS).

CCK = cholecystokinin; ECT = electroconvulsive therapy; TENS = transcutaneous electrical nerve stimulation.

and colleagues (2004) found that 10-Hz rTMS, but not 1-Hz or sham rTMS, over right prefrontal cortex was associated with positive effects in PTSD, although in this study there was no apparent attempt to manipulate traumatic recall or bring online alternative processes to be enhanced.

rTMS in the Context of Directed Psychotherapy

By researchers pursuing these types of new directions for TMS application, a new level of neurophysiologically facilitated psychotherapy could eventually be created. One could envision not only the future development of specific psychotherapies directed toward specific neuropsychiatric syndromes (as is the case with cognitive-behavioral therapy of depression and anxiety disorders) but also the further specific reconfiguration of these paradigms to maximize their interaction with physiological brain stimulation (rTMS). Attempting to increase the activity of frontal cortical systems to better modulate overactive subcortical ones in bipolar illness and schizophrenia would be one example.

rTMS in Poststroke Depression and Disorders Secondary to Primary CNS Illnesses

Jorge and colleagues (2004) reported on the efficacy of 10-Hz rTMS at 110% of MT, with 20 trains of 5-second duration for 10 sessions, in patients with antidepressant-refractory poststroke depression. Given the remarkable preclinical data on the utility of stimulants in motor rehabilitation in poststroke depression, rTMS could also be studied for its effects on neurological recovery, especially when the hypertensive effects of stimulants may be contraindicated. The ability of rTMS to release dopamine in the striatum acutely (Strafella et al. 2001, 2003) and modulate neural activity in the striatum on a longer-lasting basis (Speer et al. 2000) provides further convergent rationales for such a study.

rTMS in Substance Abuse

The ability of rTMS to affect the striatum also raises other possibilities. Habit memory is thought to involve striatal rather than the medial temporal structures (the amygdala and hippocampus) that are linked to representational memory (Mishkin and Appenzeller 1987). Automatic or unconscious processes that underlie some syndromes such as substance abuse craving and cue-related relapse also may be approached in this fashion with rTMS. Perhaps one could facilitate deconditioning in the habit/memory system of the links between drug cues and substance craving. Alternatively, because such new learning requires active N-methyl-D-aspartate (NMDA) receptor–related processes in the cortex, rTMS could be used to enhance this process similar to the use of glutamate co-agonists to potentiate active desensitization (Walker and Davis 2004).

Enhancement of Neural Plasticity in Neural Implants and Spinal Cord Repair

Another potential use for rTMS could be to facilitate appropriate survival and reconnection of neural implants in a variety of psychiatric disorders. Implants of neonatal striatal (Kordower et al. 1998a, 1998b) and adrenal medulla tissue (Date 1996) are now being used to treat Parkinson's disease with some success regarding both cell survival and differentiation of the cells into dopaminergic neurons with extension of their axons in the appropriate direction toward striatal conductivity (Kordower et al. 1997, 1998a, 1998b; Lindvall 1997). One can envision a time when implant incorporation is facilitated by appropriate stimulation with rTMS so that some of the patterns of activity-dependent wiring of the CNS involving neurotrophic factors that were evident in initial phases of CNS development could be reactivated in relation to this new level of synapse formation (Yurek et al. 1996; Zhou et al. 1997). Neuronal activity is crucial for the matching and maintenance of neural connections during development, and rTMS may, in a similar fashion, be able to further enhance this process in adults.

Such a process could also be considered in attempting to bridge and repair spinal cord trauma associated with paraplegia and quadriplegia. Considerable progress has been made in the area of preparing the structural and neurosurgical basis for axonal regrowth (Bregman et al. 1997; Falci et al. 1997; Olson et al. 1998; Schwab and Bartholdi 1996; Tuszynski et al. 1998), but the appropriate experimental conditions have not been adequately delineated such that the regrowth is adequately functional. One could imagine the possibility that rTMS-driven neural activity from above could be matched with appropriate stimulated motor patterning from below such that activity-dependent neuroplasticity is used for axonal guidance on a physiological basis in addition to its structural facilitation with appropriate neurosurgical repair.

Interaction of rTMS With Low-Level Magnetic Fields

Recent work by McLean and associates (Holcomb et al. 2000; McLean et al. 2003a; Segal et al. 2001) has indicated the potential clinical relevance of low-level magnetic fields (LLMFs) in the prevention of pain and epileptic discharges. These investigators found that specially constructed quadri-polar alternating magnetic fields, which produce a constant LLMF with an inverted volcano-shaped hole in the center of the field, are able to block the painful sensations and accompanying electrophysiological discharges of the C-afferent pain fibers following subcutaneous injection of capsaicin. This normally excruciating pain with capsaicin is ameliorated to the point where it is tolerable, with ratings decreasing from the maximum pain score of 10 seen with a sham magnet to about 3 or 4 with the active magnet. In addition to these ameliorating effects on capsaicin-induced pain, the application of these magnets in a variety of natural and endogenously induced pain syndromes is associated with a therapeutic effect in a very high percentage of patients.

McLean and colleagues also found that application of these unique magnets is capable of preventing epileptiform discharges in brain slice preparations in vitro (McLean et al. 1995) and in strains of rats in vivo (McLean et al. 2003b). This LLMF is effective in some seizure models on its own and markedly potentiates the anticonvulsant effects of phenytoin when doses of this drug are in themselves not effective (McLean et al. 2003b).

McLean and associates have now gone on to use a constant LLMF from a specially constructed electromagnet and found similar degrees of efficacy against seizures. Thus, whereas effects on mood have not been directly tested with this type of constant LLMF, it is noteworthy that other anticonvulsant modalities such as valproate, carbamazepine, and lamotrigine do exert positive therapeutic effects in patients with bipolar illness. It is possible that whatever is engendering the transcranial anticonvulsant effects of these LLMFs could eventually have implications for the treatment of other neuropsychiatric syndromes beyond those of the seizure disorders.

Given these promising clinical and preclinical data and their potential application to not only clinical paroxysmal pain and ictal syndromes but also neuropsychiatric dysregulation in a variety of other illnesses such as panic and depression, one could imagine applying LLMFs to achieve one level of constant background physiological alteration, while simultaneously administering rTMS for superimposed frequency-modulated effects. In this fashion one might be able to achieve a much larger signal-to-noise ratio, or enhancement or inhibition of specifically targeted pathways while others are blocked by such an LLMF. In the paroxysmal pain syndromes, application of the magnet exerting a constant LLMF for a relatively short period of time (days to weeks) is often sufficient to allow the attenuation of even chronic pain syndromes, after which the application of the magnet is no longer required (Holcomb et al. 2000).

Transcranial Direct Current Stimulation

Paulus (2003) has described another and perhaps closely related mechanism for delivering low levels of constant direct current that is achieved with the applications of an active and inactive electrode rather than a magnet (i.e., transcranial direct current stimulation [DCS]). Paulus and his associates found across a series of studies that low-density anodal stimulation tends to be excitatory, whereas cathodal stimulation is inhibitory, with aftereffects lasting at least 3 minutes. Thus, direction of current flow appears to be important. Interestingly, carbamazepine eliminated the anodal-induced transcranial DCS aftereffects on rTMS-induced motor evoked potentials while leaving cathodal effects unchanged. Moreover, NMDA antagonists abolished the transcranial DCS–induced aftereffects, suggesting potential linkage to LTP, which also requires activation of NMDA glutamate receptors.

Depending on the parameters and lengths of the transcranial DCS, increases and decreases in excitability can be achieved for about 1 hour, and preliminary data suggest that these changes could have differential effects on different neuropsychological tasks, with anodal stimulation better for initial learning tasks and cathodal stimulation improving skill in overlearned tasks (Nitsche et al. 2003c). A study by Kincses and colleagues (2004) indicated that implicit learning in a probabilistic classification paradigm could be improved by weak anodal transcranial DCS over the prefrontal cortex, suggesting that increases in excitability in this area could have effects on learning and memory similar to the changes observed over motor cortex. Matsunaga and colleagues (2004) also reported effects of transcranial DCS over the sensory motor cortex on somatosensory evoked potentials in man. Nitsche and colleagues (2003a) further documented selective effects of carbamazepine and flunarizine on eliminating excitability enhancement induced by anodal stimulation during and after transcranial DCS.

Nitsche and colleagues (2003b) have outlined safety parameters for transcranial DCS, indicating that current densities that they used were 1,000 times lower than those thought to be associated with brain injury. They also reported on the safety of their parameters of transcranial DCS in that they did not cause heating under the electrodes, did not elevate serum neuron-specific enolase levels (which are a marker of neuronal damage), and did not result in abnormal findings on patients' MRI scans or electroencephalograms (EEGs). They further suggested the importance of placing the nonstimulating or remote electrode in a position to avoid current flow through the brain stem, which could, at least theoretically, affect respiratory or cardiac function.

Echo-Planar Magnetic Resonance Spectroscopic Imaging

The most recent novel approach to brain stimulation treatment for patients with bipolar disorder was discovered by accident by colleagues at McLean Hospital. As first reported at the December 2003 American College of Neuropsychopharmacology (ACNP) meeting, these investigators were using echo-planar magnetic resonance spectroscopic imaging (EP-MRSI) during a study to determine how the brain chemistry of bipolar patients differs from that of people without the illness, when several depressed patients with bipolar disorder emerged from the scanner happier than when they went in. Some patients were even laughing when they came out. The researchers conducting the original study told Dr. B. Cohen, Chief Psychiatrist at McLean Hospital, and Dr. P. Renshaw, Director of the Brain Imaging Center at McLean Hospital, of their observations. With Dr. M. Rohan, an imaging specialist, they decided to conduct a study using active EP-MRSI versus sham EP-MRSI.

In the study of Rohan and colleagues (2004), 30 patients with bipolar illness received active EP-MRSI; 10 patients with bipolar disorder received sham EP-MRSI; and 14 healthy subjects (without bipolar disorder) also received active EP-MRSI. The patients with bipolar disorder had received a diagnosis of either bipolar I or bipolar II and were between the ages of 18 and 65. None of the participants in the study were aware that the EP-MRSI evaluation was being investigated for mood effects, and they could not tell the difference between sham and active EP-MRSI. The active treatment consisted of four EP-MRSI sequences lasting a total of 20.5 minutes. Each sequence produced a series of 512 alternating pulses 0.256 milliseconds long, repeated every 2 seconds for 4 minutes.

In 23 of the 30 patients with bipolar disorder, mild to marked mood improvement was seen, particularly in all 11 of the patients who were not taking medication at the time. Improvement in patients with sham EP-MRSI was seen in only 3 of 10 patients. Four of the 14 control subjects without bipolar illness, who received active EP-MRSI, also felt better. The eventual clinical significance of this magnitude of improvement, and whether it can be converted into a time frame yielding lasting effects, remain to be ascertained.

Despite these ambiguities, there is keen interest in this potential new technique because it uses ultra LLMFs (100–1,000 times weaker than rTMS fields). The electrical field (0.7 V/m) is some 500 times lower than that generated in the rTMS paradigm (1–500 V/m). The sequence used by Rohan and colleagues yielded a frequency stimulation of 1 kHz, or about 1,000 times higher frequency than the 1–20 Hz that is typically generated with rTMS. Rohan and colleagues believe it is this ultra-high frequency, and not the ultra LLMF (which is also unidirectional in character like that in transcranial DCS), that yields the acute therapeutic effects of the EP-MRSI sequence, but this remains to be directly demonstrated. Some neurons fire this fast (at 1 kHz) naturally, and it is thought these ultra-high-frequency, unidirectional low-level fields might somehow retrain dysfunctional neural pathways to fire in a more organized fashion. Whether the rapid frequencies or the LLMF of transcranial DCS magnetics is the key ingredient to the positive effects on mood can now be systematically assessed.

Potentiation of rTMS Effects

It is just such longer-term adaptations that one is seeking in the therapeutics of a variety of psychiatric syndromes with rTMS. However, to date, the effects of rTMS have not been consistently clinically robust, reliable, or lasting enough to meet the specifications of the anticipated clinical therapeutic intervention. A variety of parametric issues remain to be explored with rTMS itself, particularly location, frequency, duration, wave and train characteristics, and number of repetitions (Table 10–2), It is also possible that the clinical effects might eventually be enhanced with concomitant use of psychopharmacological agents (Schule et al. 2003) that provide a background of appropriate pharmacological neuromodulations.

For example, as noted previously, McLean and associates (2003b) found that application of LLMFs together with an anticonvulsant such as phenytoin provides complete protection against convulsions in epilepsy-prone rodents, whereas either procedure alone is only partially effective. With the potentially longer-lasting attributes of LLMFs and pharmacotherapy in concert with rTMS, one could imagine the possibility of a new level of clinical therapeutics that has not as yet been possible in a number of the most prominent psychiatric illnesses, such as panic disorder and affective illness. In both these disorders, remissions are typically often achieved with pharmacological intervention, but long-term prophylactic treatment is generally required in order to maintain such a remission.

In other words, the underlying neurobiological vulnerability, based on genetic or environmental/experiential impact on gene expression, remains relatively unchanged. As long as the drug treatment is present, the threshold for symptomatic expression is not exceeded because of the appropriate therapeutic targeting with, for example, serotonin-selective antidepressants or anticonvulsants to block overexcitation or enhance inhibition through glutamate and GABA (γ-aminobutyric acid)–ergic circuits, respectively. Perhaps with appropriate combination treatments involving rTMS and other modalities, longer-lasting and ameliorative, if not curative, effects could eventually be achieved.

PRIMING, PRECONDITIONING, AND METAPLASTICITY EFFECTS

Pretreatment with electrical stimulation can have inhibitory or excitatory effects on subsequent electrical stimulation depending on the interval between the two stimulations as revealed in the paired-pulse potentiation paradigm; shorter interstimulus intervals are associated with inhibition of, and longer ones increased excitation of, the second stimulus. Metaplasticity effects have also been noted in which an initial high-frequency (100-Hz) burst in hippocampal slices leads to greater degrees of LTD-like phenomena.

In the amygdala, the effects of such priming stimulation on metaplasticity can be even more dramatic. Li and associates (1998) showed that 1-Hz stimulation of basolateral amygdala neurons in the amygdala slice preparation for 15 minutes was usually associated with gradual onset of LTP. However, if a pretreatment 100-Hz stimulation was induced, the opposite effects of 15 minutes of 1-Hz stimulation were produced. Instead of the long-lasting increases in excitation (LTP) produced by 1-Hz stimulation in naive slices, Li et al. found that LTD was induced in neurons pretreated by high-frequency stimulation. These investigators also showed that this metaplastic change (from LTP to LTD) was inhibited by antagonists of type 2 metabotropic glutamate receptors, implicating these, and not NMDA receptors, as having a role in this type of metaplasticity.

Priming, if not metaplastic changes, can be induced in humans as well. Iyer and colleagues (2003) showed that subthreshold rTMS (6 Hz) could prime the motor cortex to produce increased amounts of cortical depression following suprathreshold 1-Hz stimulation. These investigators noted that 6 Hz primes both 1-Hz rTMS-induced depression and LTD.

Likewise, Siebner and colleagues (2004) reported preconditioning of 1-Hz rTMS with transcranial DCS. They found "facilitatory preconditioning" with anodal transcranial DCS causes a subsequent period of reduced corticospinal excitability following 1-Hz rTMS. Conversely, inhibitory preconditioning with cathodal transcranial DCS resulted in increasing corticospinal excitability for at least 20 minutes following 1-Hz rTMS. These data indicate that changing the initial state of motor cortex excitability by a period of DC polarization could exert metaplastic effects on the effects of 1-Hz rTMS. It is noteworthy that these effects were dependent on the direction of the DC current and were specific to the left primary motor cortex being stimulated. These authors suggested that the preconditioning effects of transcranial DCS suggested the existence of homeostatic mechanisms in human motor cortex that stabilize corticospinal excitability within a physiologically useful range.

We would add that in addition to these possible differential therapeutic effects induced, one should consider the possibility that naturalistic previous preconditioning effects induced by normal and pathological neural processes, such as those engaged in PTSD, could themselves be associated with metaplastic changes and that these should be taken into account in the assessment of the appropriate therapeutic modalities of rTMS. For example, one might see enhanced excitatory effects of 1-Hz stimulation similar to that shown by Li and colleagues (1998) in naive unstimulated neurons in the amygdala slice preparation, but to the extent that PTSD-related events induce trains of prior high frequency stimulation, one might then predict that 1-Hz stimulation reaching the amygdala in patients with PTSD could, as in the amygdala slide preparation, induce LTD instead of LTP.

Parenthetically, a more recent clinical study, noted previously, reported potential therapeutic effects of higher-frequency rTMS over the right prefrontal cortex in patients with PTSD and no effect of 1 Hz (Cohen et al. 2004). These findings could be related to the primary areas of the brain being facilitated or inhibited by such stimulation. It is possible that increased prefrontal cortical excitability is necessary for new learning, including extinction learning (Davis et al. 2003). Thus, enhancement of cortical excitability in prefrontal areas could be involved not only in suppression of limbic hyperexcitability that has been reported in some PTSD paradigms, but also in facilitating new learning and desensitization mechanisms. Such interactions of 1) the potential effects of pathological primary effects by prior experience; 2) brain area affected; 3) region of the brain targeted for rTMS and other stimulation paradigms; and 4) parameters of stimulation chosen could all markedly affect psychological and therapeutic effects.

Long-Term Amelioration and Primary Prevention

It has typically been thought that brain implants or more direct gene therapy techniques that use viral and other vectors to deliver appropriate alterations in DNA would be required for longer-lasting therapeutic interventions in the neuropsychiatric disorders so that deficient systems in a given syndrome could begin expressing the appropriate chemical normally. An example of such a system that might respond to genetic amelioration is the epilepsy-prone rodent model, in which a deficit in cholecystokinin (CCK) production has been shown (Zhang et al. 1992, 1997). When a viral or other vector containing the message for CCK gene transcription is administered, increased amounts of CCK protein are expressed in the hippocampus of these animals, and for the duration of time of increased CCK expression, the rodents show a decreased susceptibility to seizures.

Thus, to the extent that long-term gene therapy can be appropriately delivered (a significant feat), one could envision the more basic amelioration of underlying pathophysiological processes conveying long-term vulnerability to a given syndrome. However, because this may be difficult, dangerous, or prohibitively expensive with viral and other vectors, one might alternatively envision attempts to alter basic processes of pathophysiological vulnerability in different syndromes using a combination of endogenous and exogenous mechanisms.

What we are suggesting is that perhaps using pharmacotherapy with rTMS that proceeds acutely, intensively, or chronically enough and with suitable patterning and frequency modulation, a system that is pathologically deficient in a given neurotransmitter or peptide may be induced to sufficiently increase production of the relevant compounds such that long-lasting amelioration of the related syndrome is possible. A long-lasting depression of specific hippocampal and amygdala synapses has been achievable with appropriate in vitro low-frequency stimulation-producing LTD (Li et al. 1998; Malenka 1995), so it is possible that similar LTD-like effects could be achieved in the future by rTMS, if some of the augmentation strategies discussed previously (or others) prove effective. Moderately lasting suppression of auditory persistent hallucinations achieved by rTMS has already been reported in patients with schizophrenia who were not responsive to antipsychotic medications (D'Alfonso et al. 2002; Hoffman et al. 2003).

It is also possible, with the application of appropriate parameters of rTMS stimulation, that some degenerative processes of the CNS could be altered or prevented from the outset. That is, in a patient with susceptibility to progression in Parkinson's disease, Huntington's disease, or Alzheimer's disease, application of appropriate neural stimulation may be able to induce gene expression of neurotrophic and other survival factors that counter the ongoing processes of excitotoxic and apoptotic cell death.

We know this to be more than a theoretical possibility because Huntington's disease–doomed cells in the striatum function quite adequately for a significant proportion of an individual's adult life. It is only when the pathophysiology of the abnormal huntingtin protein reaches some critical threshold, perhaps interacting with aging and other aspects of neurodevelopment, that the process of cell death begins to be triggered at a rate that brings the onset of illness-related dementia (The Huntington's Disease Collaborative Research Group 1993).

What we are suggesting is that the patterns of neuronal activity and biochemistry that trigger this process of apoptotic or excitotoxic cell death could be delayed or ameliorated. It is possible that counter-regulatory processes could become involved, enabling and enhancing neural systems that would ordinarily provide neurotrophic and other protective factors that prevent the onset of such cell death. Lithium and a host of other neurotrophic and protective agents (Chen et al. 1999; Chuang et al. 1992, 2002; Mason et al. 1999; Nonaka and Chuang 1998, Nonaka et al. 1998a, 1998b) may ultimately be used for this purpose in conjunction with appropriately patterned rTMS to achieve the more region-specific anticipated primary preventive strategies.

Quenching of Kindled Excitability

We have preliminarily observed long-term increases in amygdala afterdischarge and seizure thresholds in kindled animals following quenching with low-level direct current delivered intracerebrally in the amygdala (Weiss et al. 1998a, 2001). The effects of low-level direct current are intensity- and duration-dependent. The mechanisms of the effect and whether it can be achieved without inducing a focal lesion remain to be further explored. The quenching effect has been associated with local increases in the induction of mRNA for glial fibrillary acidic protein and possibly upregulation of benzodiazepine receptor binding. Intracerebral low-level direct current, in addition to that achieved extracranially by LLMF, transcranial DCS, or EP-MRSI, thus reveals another mode of potential brain stimulation that could be explored in the search for more enduring effects.

There is a long history of studies, both controlled and uncontrolled, predominantly in the Russian literature, suggesting that low levels of current may be capable of alleviating a number of neuropsychiatric conditions (Ayrapetov et al. 1985; Erishev et al. 1988; Gariti et al. 1992; Grinenko et al. 1988; Klawansky et al. 1995; Krupitsky et al. 1991; Stinus et al. 1990). One could envision much more specific targeting of the appropriate neural substrates (Figures 10–3, 10–4, and 10–5) with combinations of low-level direct current and frequency-dependent neural firing driven by rTMS, perhaps even in conjunction with pharmacological augmentation as well.

Online Brain Mapping and Treatment Assessment

Early in his work in our laboratory, Dr. George envisioned patients in one setting having fMRI assessments and therapeutic rTMS interventions based on, and targeted to, the observed abnormalities. In this way, rTMS-induced adaptive changes could be monitored online with periodic assessments with fMRI. Such a prospect would appear to be technically feasible in the near future.

CONCLUSION

Although one would be justified in greeting with amusement, if not ridicule and derision, some of the speculations in this chapter about the future uses of rTMS, one need only look at the exponential explosion in neuroscience knowledge in the latter part of the twentieth century to envision the possibility of dramatic therapeutic interventions in the near future. In the early 1970s, one of us (R.M.P.) was impressed with how rapidly the Buck Rogers–type space walk of his childhood was transformed from pure science fiction to reality (and a relatively routine one at that) at the height of the U.S. and Russian space exploration ventures and competition. This generated speculations about what aspects of neuroscience might have equally unexpected advances that would result in a conversion of CNS science fiction to readily available therapeutic modalities. Many of these speculations written in an unpublished manuscript in the early 1970s and predicted for the far distant future have already come to fruition, including brain implants for Parkinson's disease, gene therapy, and manipulation of the CNS with the application of focal magnetic fields.

Given such a rapid transition from science fiction fantasy to clinical reality in recent years, one might reconsider and reevaluate such seemingly far-fetched possibilities as those presented in this chapter, and many other even more outrageous ones, as potentially attainable within a young person's lifetime. We thus look forward to the application of existing technologies, the rapid development of new and currently unimagined ones, and their rapid application to the clinical therapeutics of neuropsychiatric illnesses.

We can envision a set of rTMS therapeutics that are more targeted and have greater efficacy-to-side-effects ratios and, ultimately, perhaps the shift from exclusively interventional strategies to those of secondary and even primary prevention. Within the known universe, the brain appears to be one of the more unimaginably complex creations, capable of enormous changes and plasticity with development and maturation. The brain's inherent neuroplasticity—suited for both engendering its own development and acquiring knowledge based on learning and memory—would appear almost infinitely malleable and adaptive. If polio can be immunized against and prevented by inoculations evoking appropriate adaptive defenses, why is it not possible to envision appropriate physiological, pharmacological, and neuropsychological approaches to cerebral-targeted prevention strategies for individuals who are at high risk for certain neuropsychiatric illnesses, such that sufficient adaptive mechanisms are evoked and the syndrome is never even expressed?

It appears that we are presently in possession of many of the essential tools for such adventures, and we need only the critical studies and expansion of an empirical database and experience to achieve the development of rTMS and related strategies for therapeutic purposes and clinical practice. Thus, we surmise that such exciting possibilities are nearer at hand than one might imagine.

REFERENCES

Ayrapetov LN, Zaychik AM, Trukchmanov MS, et al: Change of the brain and cerebrospinal fluid endorphin levels after transcranial electro analgesia. Physiol J USSR 51:56–64, 1985

Bregman BS, Diener PS, McAtee M, et al: Intervention strategies to enhance anatomical plasticity and recovery of function after spinal cord injury. Adv Neurol 72:257–275, 1997

Burt T, Lisanby SH, Sackeim HA: Neuropsychiatric applications of transcranial magnetic stimulation: a meta analysis. Int J Neuropsychopharmacol 5:73–103, 2002

Carlson JG, Chemtob CM, Rusnak K, et al: Eye movement desensitization and reprocessing (EDMR) treatment for combat-related posttraumatic stress disorder. J Trauma Stress 11:3–24, 1998

Chen G, Zeng WZ, Yuan PX, et al: The mood-stabilizing agents lithium and valproate robustly increase the levels of the neuroprotective protein bcl-2 in the CNS. J Neurochem 72:879–882, 1999

Chuang DM, Gao XM, Paul SM: N-methyl-D-aspartate exposure blocks glutamate toxicity in cultured cerebellar granule cells. Mol Pharmacol 42:210–216, 1992

Chuang DM, Chen RW, Chalecka-Franaszek E, et al: Neuroprotective effects of lithium in cultured cells and animal models of diseases. Bipolar Disord 4:129–136, 2002

Cohen H, Kaplan Z, Kotler M, et al: Repetitive transcranial magnetic stimulation of the right dorsolateral prefrontal cortex in posttraumatic stress disorder: a double-blind, placebo-controlled study. Am J Psychiatry 161:515–524, 2004

D'Alfonso AA, Aleman A, Kessels RP, et al: Transcranial magnetic stimulation of left auditory cortex in patients with schizophrenia: effects on hallucinations and neurocognition. J Neuropsychiatry Clin Neurosci 14:77–79, 2002

Date I: Parkinson's disease, trophic factors, and adrenal medullary chromaffin cell grafting: basic and clinical studies. Brain Res Bull 40:1–19, 1996

Davis M, Walker DL, Myers KM: Role of the amygdala in fear extinction measured with potentiated startle. Ann NY Acad Sci 985:218–232, 2003

Dunn RT, Kimbrell TA, Ketter TA, et al: Principal components of the Beck Depression Inventory and regional cerebral metabolism in unipolar and bipolar depression. Biol Psychiatry 51:387–399, 2002

Ebert D, Berger M: Neurobiological similarities in antidepressant sleep deprivation and psychostimulant use: a psychostimulant theory of antidepressant sleep deprivation. Psychopharmacology (Berl) 140:1–10, 1998

Ebert D, Feistel H, Barocka A: Effects of sleep deprivation on the limbic system and the frontal lobes in affective disorders: a study with Tc-99m-HMPAO SPECT. Psychiatry Res 40:247–251, 1991

Efron R: The effect of olfactory stimuli in arresting uncinate fits. Brain 79:267–281, 1956

Erishev OF, Balashova TM, Ribakova TG: Affective disorders in recovery-alcoholics, in The Problems of Clinical Therapy and Pathogenesis of Alcoholism. Edited by Kovalev V. Moscow, Moscow Research Institute of Psychiatry, 1988, pp 49–53

Falci S, Holtz A, Akesson E, et al: Obliteration of a posttraumatic spinal cord cyst with solid human embryonic spinal cord grafts: first clinical attempt. J Neurotrauma 14:875–884, 1997

Feinsod M, Kreinin B, Chistyakov A, et al: Preliminary evidence for a beneficial effect of low-frequency, repetitive transcranial magnetic stimulation in patients with major depression and schizophrenia. Depress Anxiety 7:65–68, 1998

Fitzgerald PB, Brown TL, Marston NA, et al: Transcranial magnetic stimulation in the treatment of depression: a double-blind, placebo-controlled trial. Arch Gen Psychiatry 60:1002–1008, 2003

Fox P, Ingham R, George MS, et al: Imaging human intracerebral connectivity by PET during TMS. Neuroreport 8:2787–2791, 1997

Garcia-Toro M, Salva J, Daumal J, et al: High (20-Hz) and low (1-Hz) frequency transcranial magnetic stimulation as adjuvant treatment in medication-resistant depression. Psychiatry Res 146:53–57, 2006

Gariti P, Auriacombe M, Incmikoski R, et al: A randomized double-blind study of neuroelectric therapy in opiate and cocaine detoxification. J Subst Abuse 4:299–308, 1992

George MS, Ketter TA, Post RM: SPECT and PET imaging in mood disorders. J Clin Psychiatry 54 (suppl):6–13, 1993

George MS, Wassermann EM, Williams WA, et al: Daily repetitive transcranial magnetic stimulation (rTMS) improves mood in depression. Neuroreport 6:1853–1856, 1995

George MS, Speer AM, Wassermann EM, et al: Repetitive TMS as a probe of mood in health and disease. CNS Spectrums 2:39–44, 1997a

George MS, Wassermann EM, Kimbrell TA, et al: Mood improvement following daily left prefrontal repetitive transcranial magnetic stimulation in patients with depression: a placebo-controlled crossover trial. Am J Psychiatry 154:1752–1756, 1997b

Grinenko AJ, Krupitskiy EM, Lebedev VP, et al: Metabolism of biogenic amines during the treatment of alcohol withdrawal syndrome by transcranial electric treatment. Biogenic Amines 5:427–436, 1988

Grisaru N, Chudakov B, Yaroslavsky Y, et al: Transcranial magnetic stimulation in mania: a controlled study. Am J Psychiatry 155:1608–1610, 1998

Grunhaus L, Dannon PN, Schreiber S, et al: Repetitive transcranial magnetic stimulation is as effective as electroconvulsive therapy in the treatment of nondelusional major depressive disorder: an open study. Biol Psychiatry 47:314–324, 2000

Grunhaus L, Schreiber S, Dolberg OT, et al: A randomized controlled comparison of electroconvulsive therapy and repetitive transcranial magnetic stimulation in severe and resistant nonpsychotic major depression. Biol Psychiatry 53:324–331, 2003

Heath RG, Llewellyn RC, Rouchell AM: The cerebellar pacemaker for intractable behavioral disorders and epilepsy: follow-up report. Biol Psychiatry 15:243–256, 1980

Hoffman RE, Hawkins KA, Gueorguieva R, et al: Transcranial magnetic stimulation of left temporoparietal cortex and medication-resistant auditory hallucinations. Arch Gen Psychiatry 60:49–56, 2003

Holcomb RR, Worthington WB, McCullough BA, et al: Static magnetic field therapy for pain in the abdomen and genitals. Pediatr Neurol 23:261–264, 2000

Holtzheimer PE III, Russo J, Avery DH: A meta-analysis of repetitive transcranial magnetic stimulation in the treatment of depression. Psychopharmacol Bull 35:149–169, 2001

The Huntington's Disease Collaborative Research Group: A novel gene containing a tri-nucleotide repeat that is expanded and unstable on Huntington's disease chromosomes. Cell 72:971–983, 1993

Iyer MB, Schleper N, Wassermann EM: Priming stimulation enhances the depressant effect of low-frequency repetitive transcranial magnetic stimulation. J Neurosci 23:10867–10872, 2003

Janicak PG, Dowd SM, Martis B, et al: Repetitive transcranial magnetic stimulation versus electroconvulsive therapy for major depression: preliminary results of a randomized trial. Biol Psychiatry 51:659–667, 2002

Jorge RE, Robinson RG, Tateno A, et al: Repetitive transcranial magnetic stimulation as treatment of poststroke depression: a preliminary study. Biol Psychiatry 55:398–405, 2004

Kaptsan A, Yaroslavsky Y, Applebaum J, et al: Right prefrontal TMS versus sham treatment of mania: a controlled study. Bipolar Disord 5:36–39, 2003

Kauffman CD, Cheema MA, Miller BE: Slow right prefrontal transcranial magnetic stimulation as a treatment for medication-resistant depression: a double-blind, placebo-controlled study. Depress Anxiety 19:59–62, 2004

Ketter TA, Andreason PJ, George MS, et al: Reduced resting frontal lobe CBF in mood disorders (NR298), in 1993 New Research and Abstracts, American Psychiatric Association 146th Annual Meeting, San Francisco, CA, May 22–27, 1993. Washington, DC, American Psychiatric Association, 1993

Ketter TA, George MS, Kimbrell TA, et al: Functional brain imaging, limbic function, and affective disorders. The Neuroscientist 2:55–65, 1996

Ketter TA, George MS, Kimbrell TA, et al: Functional brain imaging in mood and anxiety disorders: current review of mood and anxiety disorders. 1:95–112, 1997

Ketter TA, Kimbrell TA, George MS, et al: Baseline cerebral hypermetabolism associated with carbamazepine response, and hypometabolism with nimodipine response in mood disorders. Biol Psychiatry 46:1364–1374, 1999

Ketter TA, Kimbrell TA, George MS, et al: Effects of mood and subtype on cerebral glucose metabolism in treatment-resistant bipolar disorder. Biol Psychiatry 49:97–109, 2001

Kimbrell TA, Little JT, Dunn RT, et al: Frequency dependence of antidepressant response to left prefrontal repetitive transcranial magnetic stimulation (rTMS) as a function of baseline cerebral glucose metabolism. Biol Psychiatry 46:1603–1613, 1999

Kimbrell TA, Dunn RT, George MS, et al: Left prefrontal-repetitive transcranial magnetic stimulation (rTMS) and regional cerebral glucose metabolism in normal volunteers. Psychiatry Res 115:101–113, 2002a

Kimbrell TA, Ketter TA, George MS, et al: Regional cerebral glucose utilization in patients with a range of severities of unipolar depression. Biol Psychiatry 51:237–252, 2002b

Kincses TZ, Antal A, Nitsche MA, et al: Facilitation of probabilistic classification learning by transcranial direct current stimulation of the prefrontal cortex in the human. Neuropsychologia 42:113–117, 2004

Kirkcaldie MT, Pridmore SA, Pascual-Leone A: Transcranial magnetic stimulation as therapy for depression and other disorders. Aust NZ J Psychiatry 31:264–272, 1997

Klawansky S, Yeung A, Berkey C, et al: Meta-analysis of randomized controlled trials of cranial electrostimulation: efficacy in treating selected psychological and physiological conditions. J Nerv Ment Dis 183:478–484, 1995

Klein E, Kreinin I, Chistyakov A, et al: Therapeutic efficacy of right prefrontal slow repetitive transcranial magnetic stimulation in major depression: a double-blind controlled study. Arch Gen Psychiatry 56:315–320, 1999

Kordower JH, Goetz CG, Freeman TB, et al: Dopaminergic transplants in patients with Parkinson's disease: neuroanatomical correlates of clinical recovery. Exp Neurol 144:41–46, 1997

Kordower JH, Freeman TB, Chen EY, et al: Fetal nigral grafts survive and mediate clinical benefit in a patient with Parkinson's disease. Mov Disord 13:383–393, 1998a

Kordower JH, Freeman TB, Olanow CW: Neuropathology of fetal nigral grafts in patients with Parkinson's disease. Mov Disord 13 (suppl 1):88–95, 1998b

Korte M, Staiger V, Griesbeck O, et al: The involvement of brain-derived neurotrophic factor in hippocampal long-term potentiation revealed by gene targeting experiments. J Physiol Paris 90:157–164, 1996

Kozel FA, George MS: Meta-analysis of left prefrontal repetitive transcranial magnetic stimulation (rTMS) to treat depression. J Psychiatr Pract 8:270–275, 2002

Krupitsky EM, Burakov AM, Karandashova GF, et al: The administration of transcranial electric treatment for affective disturbances therapy in alcoholic patients. Drug Alcohol Depend 27:1–6, 1991

Li H, Weiss SR, Chuang DM, et al: Bidirectional synaptic plasticity in the rat basolateral amygdala: characterization of an activity-dependent switch sensitive to the presynaptic metabotropic glutamate receptor antagonist 2S-alpha-ethylglutamic acid. J Neurosci 18:1662–1670, 1998

Li X, Nahas Z, Kozel FA, et al: Acute left prefrontal transcranial magnetic stimulation in depressed patients is associated with immediately increased activity in prefrontal cortical as well as subcortical regions. Biol Psychiatry 55:882–890, 2004

Linden DJ: Long-term synaptic depression in the mammalian brain. Neuron 12:457–472, 1994

Lindvall O: Neural transplantation: a hope for patients with Parkinson's disease. Neuroreport 8:iii–ix, 1997

Malenka RC: LTP and LTD: dynamic and interactive processes of synaptic plasticity. The Neuroscientist 1:35–42, 1995

Martin JL, Barbanoj MJ, Schlaepfer TE, et al: Repetitive transcranial magnetic stimulation for the treatment of depression: systematic review and meta-analysis. Br J Psychiatry 182:480–491, 2003

Marty S, Berzaghi MP, Berninger B: Neurotrophins and activity-dependent plasticity of cortical interneurons. Trends Neurosci 20:198–202, 1997

Mason RP, Leeds PR, Jacob RF, et al: Inhibition of excessive neuronal apoptosis by the calcium antagonist amlodipine and antioxidants in cerebellar granule cells. J Neurochem 72:1448–1456, 1999

Matsunaga K, Nitsche MA, Tsuji S, et al: Effect of transcranial DC sensorimotor cortex stimulation on somatosensory evoked potentials in humans. Clin Neurophysiol 115:456–460, 2004

Mayberg HS, Brannan SK, Mahurin RK, et al: Cingulate function in depression: a potential predictor of treatment response. Neuroreport 8:1057–1061, 1997

McCann UD, Kimbrell TA, Morgan CM, et al: Repetitive transcranial magnetic stimulation for posttraumatic stress disorder. Arch Gen Psychiatry 55:276–279, 1998

McLean MJ, Holcomb RR, Wamil AW, et al: Blockade of sensory neuron action potentials by a static magnetic field in the 10 mT range. Bioelectromagnetics 16:20–32, 1995

McLean MJ, Engstrom S, Holcomb RR: Magnetotherapy: Potential Therapeutic Benefits and Adverse Effects. New York, TFG Press, 2003a

McLean MJ, Engstrom S, Holcomb RR, et al: A static magnetic field modulates severity of audiogenic seizures and anticonvulsant effects of phenytoin in DBA/2 mice. Epilepsy Res 55:105–116, 2003b

McNamara B, Ray JL, Arthurs OJ, et al: Transcranial magnetic stimulation for depression and other psychiatric disorders. Psychol Med 31:1141–1146, 2001

Mishkin M, Appenzeller T. The anatomy of memory. Sci Am 256:80–89, 1987

Nahas Z, Kozel FA, Li X, et al: Left prefrontal transcranial magnetic stimulation (TMS) treatment of depression in bipolar affective disorder: a pilot study of acute safety and efficacy. Bipolar Disord 5:40–47, 2003

Nitsche MA, Fricke K, Henschke U, et al: Pharmacological modulation of cortical excitability shifts induced by transcranial direct current stimulation in humans. J Physiol 553:293–301, 2003a

Nitsche MA, Liebetanz D, Lang N, et al: Safety criteria for transcranial direct current stimulation (tDCS) in humans. Clin Neurophysiol 114:2220–2222, 2003b

Nitsche MA, Schauenburg A, Lang N, et al: Facilitation of implicit motor learning by weak transcranial direct current stimulation of the primary motor cortex in the human. J Cogn Neurosci 15:619–626, 2003c

Nonaka S, Chuang DM: Neuroprotective effects of chronic lithium on focal cerebral ischemia in rats. Neuroreport 9:2081–2084, 1998

Nonaka S, Hough CJ, Chuang DM: Chronic lithium treatment robustly protects neurons in the central nervous system against excitotoxicity by inhibiting N-methyl-D-aspartate receptor–mediated calcium influx. Proc Natl Acad Sci USA 95:2642–2647, 1998a

Nonaka S, Katsube N, Chuang DM: Lithium protects rat cerebellar granule cells against apoptosis induced by anticonvulsants, phenytoin and carbamazepine. J Pharmacol Exp Ther 286:539–547, 1998b

Olson L, Cheng H, Zetterstrom RH, et al: On CNS repair and protection strategies: novel approaches with implications for spinal cord injury and Parkinson's disease. Brain Res Brain Res Rev 26:302–305, 1998

Pascual-Leone A, Catala MD, Pascual-Leone Pascual A: Lateralized effect of rapid-rate transcranial magnetic stimulation of the prefrontal cortex on mood. Neurology 46:499–502, 1996a

Pascual-Leone A, Rubio B, Pallardo F, et al: Rapid-rate transcranial magnetic stimulation of left dorsolateral prefrontal cortex in drug-resistant depression. Lancet 348:233–237, 1996b

Paulus W: Transcranial direct current stimulation (tDCS). Suppl Clin Neurophysiol 56:349–354, 2003

Paus T, Jech R, Thompson CJ, et al: Transcranial magnetic stimulation during positron emission tomography: a new method for studying connectivity of the human cerebral cortex. J Neurosci 17:3178–3184, 1997

Paus T, Jech R, Thompson CJ, et al: Dose-dependent reduction of cerebral blood flow during rapid-rate transcranial magnetic stimulation of the human sensorimotor cortex. J Neurophysiol 79:1102–1107, 1998

Paus T, Castro-Alamancos MA, Petrides M: Cortico-cortical connectivity of the human mid-dorsolateral frontal cortex and its modulation by repetitive transcranial magnetic stimulation. Eur J Neurosci 14:1405–1411, 2001

Post RM, Weiss SR: Ziskind-Somerfeld Research Award 1992. Endogenous biochemical abnormalities in affective illness: therapeutic versus pathogenic. Biol Psychiatry 32:469–484, 1992

Post RM, Weiss SRB: A speculative model of affective illness cyclicity based on patterns of drug tolerance observed in amygdala-kindled seizures. Mol Neurobiol 13:33–60, 1996

Post RM, Kimbrell T, Frye M, et al: Implications of kindling and quenching for the possible frequency dependence of rTMS. CNS Spectr 2:54–60, 1997

Pridmore S, Bruno R, Turnier-Shea Y, et al: Comparison of unlimited numbers of rapid transcranial magnetic stimulation (rTMS) and ECT treatment sessions in major depressive episode. Int J Neuropsychopharmacol 3:129–134, 2000

Rohan M, Parow A, Stoll AL, et al: Low-field magnetic stimulation in bipolar depression using an MRI-based stimulator. Am J Psychiatry 161:93–98, 2004

Schule C, Zwanzger P, Baghai T, et al: Effects of antidepressant pharmacotherapy after repetitive transcranial magnetic stimulation in major depression: an open follow-up study. J Psychiatr Res 37:145–153, 2003

Schulze-Rauschenbach SC, Harms U, Schlaepfer TE, et al: Distinctive neurocognitive effects of repetitive transcranial magnetic stimulation and electroconvulsive therapy in major depression. Br J Psychiatry 186:410–416, 2005

Schwab ME, Bartholdi D: Degeneration and regeneration of axons in the lesioned spinal cord. Physiol Rev 76:319–370, 1996

Segal NA, Toda Y, Huston J, et al: Two configurations of static magnetic fields for treating rheumatoid arthritis of the knee: a double-blind clinical trial. Arch Phys Med Rehabil 82:1453–1460, 2001

Shajahan PM, Glabus MF, Steele JD, et al: Left dorsolateral repetitive transcranial magnetic stimulation affects cortical excitability and functional connectivity, but does not impair cognition in major depression. Prog Neuropsychopharmacol Biol Psychiatry 26:945–954, 2002

Shapiro F: Eye movement desensitization and reprocessing (EMDR): evaluation of controlled PTSD research. J Behav Ther Exp Psychiatry 27:209–218, 1996

Siebner HR, Lang N, Rizzo V, et al: Preconditioning of low-frequency repetitive transcranial magnetic stimulation with transcranial direct current stimulation: evidence for homeostatic plasticity in the human motor cortex. J Neurosci 24:3379–3385, 2004

Smith MA, Makino S, Kvetnansky R, et al: Stress and glucocorticoids affect the expression of brain-derived neurotrophic factor and neurotrophin-3 mRNAs in the hippocampus. J Neurosci 15:1768–1777, 1995

Speer AM, Kimbrell TA, Wassermann EM, et al: Opposite effects of high and low frequency rTMS on regional brain activity in depressed patients. Biol Psychiatry 48:1133–1141, 2000

Speer AM, Willis MW, Herscovitch P, et al: Intensity-dependent regional cerebral blood flow during 1-Hz repetitive transcranial magnetic stimulation (rTMS) in healthy volunteers studied with $H_2^{15}O$ positron emission tomography, I: effects of primary motor cortex rTMS. Biol Psychiatry 54:818–825, 2003a

Speer AM, Willis MW, Herscovitch P, et al: Intensity-dependent regional cerebral blood flow (rCBF) during 1-Hz repetitive transcranial magnetic stimulation in healthy volunteers studied with $H_2^{15}O$ positron emission tomography, II: effects of prefrontal cortex rTMS. Biol Psychiatry 54:826–832, 2003b

Stinus L, Auriacombe M, Tignol J, et al: Transcranial electrical stimulation with high frequency intermittent current (Limoge's) potentiates opiate-induced analgesia: blind studies. Pain 42:351–363, 1990

Strafella AP, Paus T, Barrett J, et al: Repetitive transcranial magnetic stimulation of the human prefrontal cortex induces dopamine release in the caudate nucleus. J Neurosci 21:1–4, 2001

Strafella AP, Paus T, Fraraccio M, et al: Striatal dopamine release induced by repetitive transcranial magnetic stimulation of the human motor cortex. Brain 126:2609–2615, 2003

Teneback CC, Nahas Z, Speer AM, et al: Changes in prefrontal cortex and paralimbic activity in depression following two weeks of daily left prefrontal TMS. J Neuropsychiatry Clin Neurosci 11:426–435, 1999

Tuszynski MH, Weidner N, McCormack M, et al: Grafts of genetically modified Schwann cells to the spinal cord: survival, axon growth, and myelination. Cell Transplant 7:187–196, 1998

Walker DL, Davis M: Are fear memories made and maintained by the same NMDA receptor–dependent mechanisms? Neuron 41:680–682, 2004

Weiss SRB, Li X-L, Heynen T, et al: Kindling and quenching: conceptual links to rTMS. CNS Spectr 2:32–35;-65–68, 1997

Weiss SR, Eidsath A, Li XL, et al: Quenching revisited: low level direct current inhibits amygdala-kindled seizures. Exp Neurol 154:185–192, 1998a

Weiss SRB, Li X-L, Noguera EC, et al: Quenching: persistent alterations in seizure and afterdischarge threshold following low-frequency stimulation, in Kindling 5. Edited by Corcoran M, Moshe S. New York, Plenum, 1998b, pp 101–119

Weiss SRB, Eidsath A, Heynen T, et al: Role of low level direct current in quenching amygdala-kindled seizure development and expression, in Epilepsy Surgery. Edited by Luders HO, Comair Y. Philadelphia, PA, Lippincott-Raven, 2001, pp 829–836

Wilson SA, Becker LA, Tinker RH: Fifteen-month follow-up of eye movement desensitization and reprocessing (EMDR) treatment for posttraumatic stress disorder and psychological trauma. J Consult Clin Psychol 65:1047–1056, 1997

Wu JC, Bunney WE: The biological basis of an antidepressant response to sleep deprivation and relapse: review and hypothesis. Am J Psychiatry 147:14–21, 1990

Wu JC, Gillin JC, Buchsbaum MS, et al: Effect of sleep deprivation on brain metabolism of depressed patients. Am J Psychiatry 149:538–543, 1992

Xu L, Anwyl R, Rowan MJ: Behavioural stress facilitates the induction of long-term depression in the hippocampus. Nature 387:497–500, 1997

Yurek DM, Lu W, Hipkens S, et al: BDNF enhances the functional reinnervation of the striatum by grafted fetal dopamine neurons. Exp Neurol 137:105–118, 1996

Zhang LX, Wu M, Han JS: Suppression of audiogenic epileptic seizures by intracerebral injection of a CCK gene vector. Neuroreport 3:700–702, 1992

Zhang LX, Li XL, Smith MA, et al: Lipofectin-facilitated transfer of cholecystokinin gene corrects behavioral abnormalities of rats with audiogenic seizures. Neuroscience 77:15–22, 1997

Zhou J, Bradford HF, Stern GM: Influence of BDNF on the expression of the dopaminergic phenotype of tissue used for brain transplants. Brain Res Dev Brain Res 100:43–51, 1997

EPILOGUE FOR THE CLINICIAN

Mark S. George, M.D.
R. H. Belmaker, M.D.

The previous chapters have outlined the history of modern transcranial magnetic stimulation (TMS), reviewed its physics and safety, discussed the methods used, and then synthesized what is known about TMS in the context of several neuropsychiatric conditions. The field is rapidly evolving, and there is much optimism that this relatively non-invasive technique will continue to evolve as a research tool. TMS is really the first new treatment in psychiatry with an entirely new mechanism or mechanisms to come along in quite a while and, with the exception of vagus nerve stimulation (George et al. 2000, 2005; Rush et al. 2000, 2005a, 2005b), the first to go from discovery to treatment approval in 20 years. This raises reasonable hope for the future that there are many new treatments for patients that are waiting to be discovered. The example of TMS should justify further investment by the public in psychiatric research. However, what is the clinical psychiatrist, neurologist, or psychologist to make of this new technique? What are the take-home messages from the earlier chapters? How and when should clinicians use TMS in their practice?

TMS AS PART OF A NEW BRANCH OF NEUROPSYCHIATRIC MEDICINE

At the time of this writing, one TMS company has completed a large multisite clinical trial of TMS in depression and has submitted the results to the U.S. Food and Drug Administration (FDA) for potential approval of the treatment. Thus, it is likely that clinicians soon will have a new treatment tool, unlike virtually anything they are familiar with. There are some similarities between TMS and electroconvulsive therapy (ECT) (George and Wassermann 1994). However, the non-invasive nature of TMS, combined with its ability to interact with only specific parts of the brain, makes it something entirely new under the sun.

Although psychiatry has long had somatic nonpharmacological treatments such as cold wet body wraps, TMS and other brain stimulation techniques do not fit with any prior healing traditions. TMS is not like allopathy, homeopathy, osteopathy, or surgery. There are many names being used to describe this new field (e.g. neuromodulation, brain stimulation), and there is also a dizzying array of new techniques (some of which are outlined in Table 11–1). TMS is unique within this class for several reasons. First, it is remarkably safe, with few unwanted side effects even at high doses (Anderson et al. 2006). The decision tree concerning when and in whom to use it is thus quite different from that of the more invasive brain stimulation techniques such as deep brain stimulation (DBS) and vagus nerve stimulation (VNS). TMS is also largely focal and thus differs from ECT, in which the entire brain is involved in a generalized seizure. TMS also directly interacts with neurons, in contrast to techniques that act secondarily through other connections into the brain (e.g., TENS, acupuncture). Finally, TMS has many brain effects even when it does not cause a seizure—a feature that differentiates it from ECT, magnetic seizure therapy (MST), and focal electrical alternating current seizure therapy (FEAST).

USE OF TMS IN TREATMENT OF DEPRESSION

Most of the studies using TMS in depression have studied depressed patients with some degree of treatment resistance. Unfortunately, until very recently the degree of treatment resistance of the patients in these studies was not well documented. The labeling of the FDA approval will likely reflect the enrollment in the multisite clinical trial and suggest that TMS be used in unipolar patients with treatment-resistant depression who are not taking medication and who are actively depressed. Because the pivotal trial excluded patients with psychotic depression, these will not be part of the labeling. But TMS to date has proven remarkably safe and non-invasive.

Figure 11–1 illustrates a potential method for determining when to use TMS. By now, multiple studies have shown that TMS is effective when used adjunctively with other antidepressants (Avery et al. 2006; Kirkcaldie et al. 1997; Pridmore 2000). We have no evidence that concomitant medications hinder the antidepressant response. Thus, it would seem reasonable to use TMS in patients who are taking medications (except those that increase the risk of seizures, such as theophylline

Table 11–1. Brain stimulation techniques

Technique	Full name	Convulsive?	Site	MDE evidence
ECT	Electroconvulsive therapy	C	Cortical	RCT
rTMS	Repetitive transcranial magnetic stimulation		Cortical	RCT
MST	Magnetic seizure therapy	C	Cortical	Open series
DBS	Deep brain stimulation		Subcortical	Open series
tDCS	Transcranial direct current stimulation		Cortical	T
TENS	Transcutaneous electrical nerve stimulation		Peripheral nerves	
VNS	Vagus nerve stimulation		Cranial nerve	Open series
EPI-fMRI	Echoplanar imaging—functional MRI		Subcortical?	Open series
FEAT	Focal electrical alternating current therapy		Cortical	T
FEAST	Focal electrical alternating current seizure therapy	C	Cortical	T

Note. C=convulsive; MDE=major depressive episode; RCT=randomized, controlled trial; T=theoretical, no data yet.

or stimulants). Additionally, since TMS is safe and without side effects, it would seem reasonable to use TMS in patients who are less treatment resistant, or even patients who are not treatment resistant but rather are medication intolerant (cannot take medications because of side effects). Thus, the typical TMS patient would be actively depressed and probably would have tried and experienced failed trials with one or two antidepressant medications (either nonresponsive or intolerant), along with some form of talking therapy. Because of the side effects and risks of ECT, patients would likely try TMS prior to ECT, unless the patient was known to respond to ECT without marked cognitive side effects. TMS would certainly be used prior to trying the other brain stimulation therapies such as VNS or DBS.

Surprisingly little is known about maintenance TMS, although there are case reports showing that this is possibly effective in some patients (Li et al. 2002; O'Reardon et al. 2005).

ADMINISTRATION AND SETTING OF TMS

Because of the need to dose TMS relative to motor threshold, and the risk of seizures, TMS will need to be prescribed and supervised by trained physicians, most likely psychiatrists and neurologists. There is no need for an anesthesiologist, and thus the procedure can be done in any medical setting where precautions and equipment exist for staff to handle a seizure or other medical emergency. In many of the treatment trials, TMS has been administered by nurses or other trained medical personnel. It is likely that the TMS devices developed by the different manufacturers will become increasingly easier to use. In most TMS clinical trial work to date, subjects have simply rested in the chair during treatment sessions, doing nothing in particular other than staying awake.

A most important area for the near future is whether to have subjects perform certain tasks while they are receiving TMS. In general, in neuroscience a circuit is easier to modify if the neurons are actively engaged as a circuit (Bartsch and van Hemmen 2001; Stanton and Sejnowsky 1989). Thus, some practitioners will likely use 20- to 30-minute treatment sessions to perform supportive or cognitive-behavioral therapy. There is, however, no evidence as to whether this approach improves or worsens outcomes.

The Medical University of South Carolina (MUSC) group, working with Dr. Chip Epstein at Emory University, built a portable TMS device that might serve as a prototype for an at-home device. Thus, in the near future patients might receive an acute TMS course at a physician's office. If they respond, and a reasonable maintenance schedule is found, one can envision prescribing TMS at home. However, these at-home devices have yet to be manufactured on a large scale.

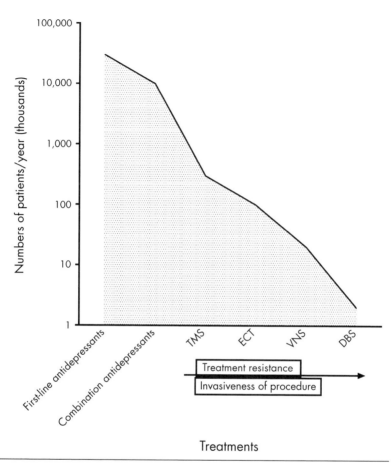

Figure 11–1. Proposed algorithm for using transcranial magnetic stimulation (TMS) in treatment-resistant depression.

It is unclear when clinicians should use TMS. On the *y* axis, the figure shows approximate numbers of patients treated per year for depression in the United States. On the *x* axis, it shows levels of treatment resistance in these patients and *proposed* points at which the different types of treatments, arranged by increasing degree of invasiveness, would be appropriate based on the level of treatment resistance. This graph places the use of TMS for depression in a general context in the near future, assuming TMS is approved by the U.S. Food and Drug Administration and that deep brain stimulation (DBS) is also approved and available. Because of the difficulties with daily commutes to a physician's office, it is not likely that TMS will be used as a first-line treatment. Estimates are that 1 in 10 American women are taking an oral antidepressant medication, with slightly lower rates in men. If oral medications do not work, or if the patient experiences intolerable side effects, one would potentially try TMS. Because of its non-invasiveness, one would use TMS before trying more invasive treatments such as electroconvulsive therapy (ECT), vagus nerve stimulation (VNS), or DBS.

OTHER DISORDERS IN WHICH TMS MIGHT PLAY A ROLE

Although TMS will be approved for the treatment of depression, it is probable that clinicians will rapidly begin using it for other disorders. The best evidence to date exists for its use in acute pain syndromes (Borckardt et al., in press), hallucinations in schizophrenia, and anxiety disorders, particularly OCD.

TRAINING AND CERTIFICATION FOR TMS

A continuing medical education course in TMS is offered each year at the annual meeting of the American Psychiatric Association (APA). The APA is also considering formal training requirements for TMS. With ECT, each hospital has to certify the hospital privilege, and thus each clinician must demonstrate competence to the local hospital board before performing ECT. Because TMS is not limited to hospitals, that safeguard does not exist for ensuring the competence of TMS operators. The International Society for Transcranial Stimulation (ISTS) lists training courses on its Web site (http://www.ists.unibe.ch).

PRIORITIES FOR RESEARCH ON TMS IN THE NEAR FUTURE

In general, the main TMS methods of delivery remain unexamined, following protocols in early studies that found antidepressant efficacy (George et al. 1995, 1997). Thus, it is unclear whether stimulation at different scalp locations, with different use parameters or dosing strategies or with different coils (Roth et al. 2002, 2005), will affect clinical outcomes. The TMS use parameters, derived largely from best-guess assumptions, are expensive and slow to work out in clinical trials. Thus, a key step for TMS clinical advancement would be to develop quick-change, laboratory-based measures that relate to ultimate antidepressant response. TMS has rapidly progressed from an interesting technique, outside of most paradigms, to an FDA-approved treatment for depression. It will likely not be restricted to use in depression for long.

REFERENCES

Anderson B, Mishory A, Nahas Z, et al: Tolerability and safety of high daily doses of repetitive transcranial magnetic stimulation in healthy young men. J ECT 22:49–53, 2006

Avery DH, Holtzheimer PE 3rd, Fawaz W, et al: A controlled study of repetitive transcranial magnetic stimulation in medication-resistant major depression. Biol Psychiatry 59:187–194, 2006

Bartsch AP, van Hemmen JL: Combined Hebbian development of geniculocortical and lateral connectivity in a model of primary visual cortex. Biol Cybern 84:41–55, 2001

Borckardt JJ, Weinstein M, Reeves ST, et al: Postoperative left prefrontal repetitive transcranial magnetic stimulation (rTMS) reduces patient-controlled analgesia use. Anesthesiology (in press)

George MS, Wassermann EM: Rapid-rate transcranial magnetic stimulation and ECT. Convuls Ther 10:251–254; discussion 255–258, 1994

George MS, Wassermann EM, Williams WA, et al: Daily repetitive transcranial magnetic stimulation (rTMS) improves mood in depression. Neuroreport 6:1853–1856, 1995

George MS, Wassermann EM, Kimbrell TA, et al: Mood improvement following daily left prefrontal repetitive transcranial magnetic stimulation in patients with depression: a placebo-controlled crossover trial. Am J Psychiatry 154:1752–1756, 1997

George MS, Sackeim HA, Rush AJ, et al: Vagus nerve stimulation: a new tool for brain research and therapy. Biol Psychiatry 47:287–295, 2000

George MS, Rush AJ, Marangell LB, et al: A one-year comparison of vagus nerve stimulation with treatment as usual for treatment-resistant depression. Biol Psychiatry 58:364–373, 2005

Kirkcaldie MT, Pridmore SA, Pascual-Leone A: Transcranial magnetic stimulation as therapy for depression and other disorders. Aust NZ J Psychiatry 31:264–272, 1997

Li X, Nahas Z, Anderson B, et al: Can left prefrontal rTMS be used as a maintenance treatment for bipolar depression? A series treated for one year. Presentation at the International Society for Transcranial Stimulation Annual Meeting, Philadelphia, PA, May 12–14, 2002

O'Reardon JP, Blumner KH, Peshek AD, et al: Long-term maintenance therapy for major depressive disorder with rTMS. J Clin Psychiatry 66:1524–1528, 2005

Pridmore S: Substitution of rapid transcranial magnetic stimulation treatments for electroconvulsive therapy treatments in a course of electroconvulsive therapy. Depress Anxiety 12:118–123, 2000

Roth Y, Zangen A, Hallett M: A coil design for transcranial magnetic stimulation of deep brain regions. J Clin Neurophysiol 19:361–370, 2002

Roth Y, Zangen A, Voller B, et al: Transcranial magnetic stimulation of deep brain regions: evidence for efficacy of the H-coil. Clin Neurophysiol 116:775–779, 2005

Rush AJ, George MS, Sackeim HA, et al: Vagus nerve stimulation (VNS) for treatment-resistant depressions: a multicenter study. Biol Psychiatry 47:276–286, 2000

Rush AJ, Marangell LB, Sackeim HA, et al: Vagus nerve stimulation for treatment-resistant depression: a randomized, controlled acute phase trial. Biol Psychiatry 58:347–354, 2005a

Rush AJ, Sackeim HA, Marangell LB, et al: Effects of 12 months of vagus nerve stimulation in treatment-resistant depression: a naturalistic study. Biol Psychiatry 58:355–363, 2005b

Stanton PK, Sejnowsky TJ: Associative long-term depression in the hippocampus induced by Hebbian covariance. Nature 339:215–218, 1989

INDEX

*Page numbers printed in **boldface** type refer to tables or figures.*

schizophrenia and assessment of, 180–186

Motor cortical inhibition. *See also* Cerebellar inhibition of the motor cortex
depression and, 124
schizophrenia and, 180–186

Motor evoked potential (MEP)
amplitude/intensity curve for, 64–65, 74
chronic fatigue syndrome and, 123–124
maps of, 65–66, 74
recording of, 43–44
schizophrenia and, 181

Motor evoked potential-electromyography (MEP-EMG), **46**

Motor threshold (MT). *See also* Resting motor threshold
algorithms for, 44
measurement of motor cortical excitability and, 63–64, 74
measurement of nervous system excitability and, 51
protocols and determination of, 43–45
schizophrenia and, 180–181
seizures and, 85

Movement disorders, and applications of TMS under development, 95–99

National Institute of Mental Health, 141

Needle stimulation, of spinal roots, 60

NEO Personality Inventory—Revised (NEO PI-R), 174–175

Nervous system excitability, TMS administration and measures of, 51–55

Neural implants, 238–239

Neural tissue, effects of TMS on, 29–30

Neuroanatomy. *See also* Brain; Neurophysiological studies
of emotion and affiliation, **233**
models of pathophysiology of obsessive-compulsive disorder and, 166–169

Neuroimaging, and pathophysiology of obsessive-compulsive disorder and, 167–169. *See also* Brain imaging

Neuroleptics, and TMS as add-on treatment for mania, 154, 157

Neurological examination, and seizures, 54

Neuromodulators
anticonvulsants and, 91
MEP intensity curve and, 64–65
short-interval intracortical inhibition and, 69

Neurophysiological studies. *See also* Neuroanatomy
epilepsy and, 89–91
importance of, 59
measures of motor cortical connectivity and, 60–62
measures of motor cortical excitability and, 63–72

Neuropsychiatric medicine, and TMS, 257–258

Neurosurgery, and neuroanatomy of obsessive-compulsive disorder, 167–169

NMDA antagonists, and intracortical facilitation, 70

NMDA receptor blockers, and short-interval intracortical inhibition, 69

Obsessive-compulsive disorder, 166–172, 175

Ohm's law, 16

Orbitofrontal cortex, and obsessive-compulsive disorder, 167

Oxygen-15 PET, 214–215

Pacemakers, 30

Pain and pain disorders
applications of TMS under development for, 99–104
low-level magnetic fields (LLMFs) and, 239, 240

Paired-pulse measurement, of nervous system excitability, 51, 52, 54